CLINICAL EFFECTS OF INTERACTION BETWEEN DRUGS

Clinical effects of interaction between drugs

Editors:

L. E. Cluff

Department of Medicine, University of Florida, Gainesville, Florida, U.S.A.

and

J. C. Petrie

Department of Therapeutics and Clinical Pharmacology, University of Aberdeen, Aberdeen, United Kingdom

Excerpta Medica, Amsterdam

1974 American Elsevier Publishing Company, Inc., New York

ISBN Excerpta Medica: 90 219 2045 X
ISBN American Elsevier: 0 444 15140 0
Library of Congress Catalogue Card Number: 73-90559

Publishers

Excerpta Medica, Amsterdam

Sole distributors for the U.S.A. and Canada

American Elsevier Publishing Company, Inc.
52 Vanderbilt Avenue, New York, N.Y. 10017

Printed in The Netherlands

Preface

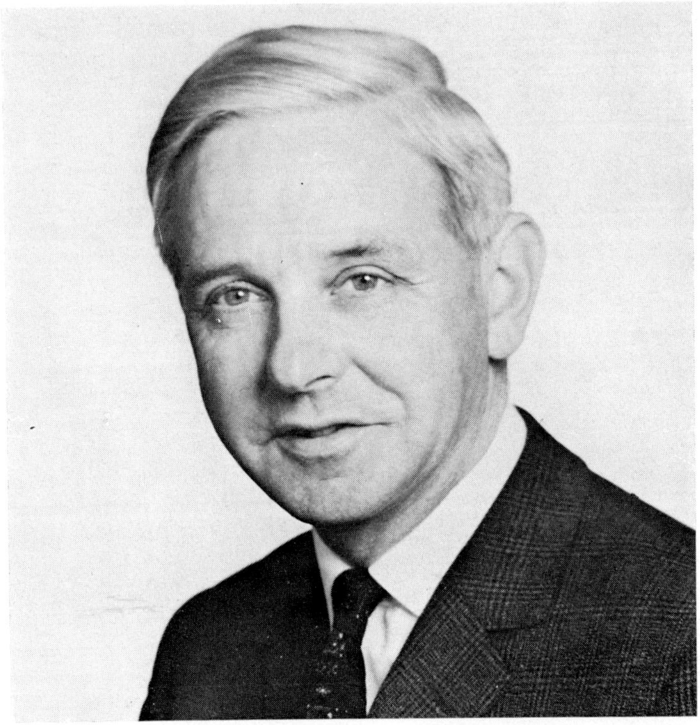

Alistair G. Macgregor (1919-1972)

B.Sc., M.D., F.R.C.P. (Ed., Glasg., Lond.)
Regius Professor of Materia Medica, University of Aberdeen, Scotland, U.K.

'A lifelong and tireless proponent of rational therapeutics and clinical pharmacology'

This monograph is dedicated to the memory of the late Professor A. G. Macgregor, who planned the outline and was delighted with the ready willingness of the authors to undertake the reviews. It is hoped that these contributions will increase the understanding of some aspects of the clinical effects of drug interaction and will encourage the further development of rational therapeutics of which he was such a forceful and inspiring advocate.

List of contributors

E. J. Ariëns – Department of Pharmacology, University of Nijmegen, Nijmegen, The Netherlands **ch. 5**

A. Bartelink – Department of Medicine, University Hospital, Groningen, The Netherlands **ch. 6**

L. E. Cluff – Department of Medicine, University of Florida, Gainesville, Florida 32610, U.S.A. **chs. 1, 3**

J. Crooks – Department of Pharmacology and Therapeutics, The University of Dundee, Dundee DD1 4HN, United Kingdom **ch. 13**

L. Dettli – Department of Internal Medicine, University of Basel, 4000 Basel, Switzerland **ch. 4**

C. T. Dollery – Royal Postgraduate Medical School, Hammersmith Hospital, London W12, United Kingdom **ch. 7**

D. Durno – Department of General Practice, University of Aberdeen, Foresterhill, Aberdeen AB9 2ZD, United Kingdom **ch. 12**

C. F. George – Faculty of Medicine, The University of Southampton, Southampton General Hospital, Southampton SO9 4XY, United Kingdom **ch. 7**

A. Herxheimer – Department of Pharmacology and Therapeutics, The London Hospital, Medical College, London E1 2AD, United Kingdom **ch. 14**

J. G. R. Howie – Department of General Practice, University of Aberdeen, Foresterhill, Aberdeen AB9 2ZD, United Kingdom **ch. 12**

H. W. Kosterlitz – Unit of Addictive Drugs, University of Aberdeen, Foresterhill, Aberdeen AB9 1AS, United Kingdom **ch. 11**

L. Lasagna – Department of Pharmacology and Toxicology, University of Rochester, Rochester, N.Y. 14642, U.S.A. **ch. 2**

M. D. Milne – Westminster Medical School, St. John's Gardens, London SW1 2AP, United Kingdom **ch. 10**

D. C. Moir – Department of Community Medicine, University of Aberdeen, Foresterhill, Aberdeen AB9 2ZD, United Kingdom **ch. 13**

M. L'E. Orme – Royal Postgraduate Medical School, Hammersmith Hospital, London W12, United Kingdom **ch. 7**

K. N. V. Palmer – Department of Medicine, University of Aberdeen, Foresterhill, Aberdeen AB9 2ZD, United Kingdom **ch. 8**

J. W. Paterson – Asthma Research Council, Department of Medicine, Brompton Hospital, London SW3, United Kingdom **ch. 8**

J. C. Petrie – Department of Therapeutics and Clinical Pharmacology, University of Aberdeen, Foresterhill, Aberdeen AB9 2ZD, United Kingdom **chs. 1, 12**

J. R. Philp – Department of Medicine, The Bowman-Gray School of Medicine, Winston-Salem, North Carolina 27103, U.S.A. **ch. 9**

A. M. Simonis – Department of Pharmacology, University of Nijmegen, Nijmegen, The Netherlands **ch. 5**

R. B. Stewart – College of Pharmacy, University of Florida, Gainesville, Florida 32610, U.S.A. **ch. 3**

Contents

CHAPTER 1

Introduction

JAMES C. PETRIE AND LEIGHTON E. CLUFF

Patients often take more than one drug, and may be given fifty or more different drugs while in hospital. Individuals also take a varying number of drugs as self-medication. Furthermore, some drug products contain several different pharmacologically active ingredients. Increasingly, more than one physician is responsible for the care of each patient and this may lead to the prescription of more drugs. All of these factors are responsible for potential drug interactions which may have beneficial or adverse effects. Unfortunately, physicians often do not have the information necessary to control or prevent adverse drug interactions, and may not be familiar with the beneficial effects which may occasionally be obtained by the administration of more than one drug.

This monograph emphasises the clinical aspects of drug interactions, but also includes presentations of the underlying pharmacological mechanisms which are important to the understanding of the clinical effects. It is hoped that this approach will prove useful to clinicians and pharmacologists, and will be valuable to the specialist and practitioner. Maintenance of this emphasis has been achieved by the authors, most of whom are active clinicians.

Many adverse, and perhaps some beneficial, drug interactions have not yet been identified. Methods for studying drug interactions are therefore discussed in some detail. The pharmacokinetic and pharmacodynamic mechanisms and concepts of drug interactions are emphasised, as an understanding of these mechanisms is essential in studies of drug interactions.

Organisation of information and presentation of data or concepts about different classes of drugs or certain aspects of drug interactions, inevitably results in repetition. No attempt has been made to avoid undue repetition as it occurs in different contexts and the comprehensiveness of each chapter has not been sacrificed for the sake of obligatory brevity.

The principles and problems of drug interactions are extensive and embrace all of medicine. Omissions in this monograph, therefore, are admitted freely. In particular, detailed discussions of interactions involving monoamine oxidase inhibitors, anaesthetic agents, and alcohol are not provided. It is hoped that the reader will understand these omissions and will appreciate the effort to emphasise concepts and principles rather than to cover comprehensively all aspects of drug interactions.

During the past several years the development and availability of drugs have reached astronomical proportions, and there has been a corresponding increase in the use of drugs. This has magnified the difficulty in the selection of those drugs appropriate in any particular instance, and makes it almost impossible to possess or memorise the requisite information to be able to discriminate between more than a few drugs in a rational way. Improved systems for handling information about drug prescribing and the use of drugs could provide the basis for avoiding drug interactions about which the physician and patient are unfamiliar. However the voluminous use of drugs would necessitate the application of computer systems for storage, retrieval, and analysis of such information. Until such systems are developed and established, the dispensing pharmacist could play an important role to improve drug utilisation and to prevent and avoid adverse drug interactions, as the pharmacist is a key link in the chain of drug availability, prescribing and drug dispensing. This role of the pharmacist would not diminish the responsibility of the physician but could augment the appropriateness and effectiveness of his prescribing practices. Patients also have a responsibility to use drugs discriminately and an improved understanding of drug interactions by physicians and pharmacists could assist patients in using drugs more safely.

CHAPTER 2

The clinical importance of drug interactions

LOUIS LASAGNA

1 The present situation

Today's clinician, unless he has somehow managed to avoid all contact with colleagues or the world literature, is likely to feel overwhelmed by the avalanche of reports dealing with drug interactions. Is this the appropriate or inevitable response? Or can the clinician achieve some perspective and a set of principles that will help him achieve both peace of mind and a rational approach to the problem?

Old-fashioned notions about drugs were often delightfully simple – a drug produced one or more effects, the occurrence of which was related to dosage and route of administration, but not much else. We now recognize this fallacy for the mirage that it is. A drug represents just one variable in the biological situation. It may be a prepotent variable, but there are almost always other variables, some of which may at times be of more importance than the drug itself.

It is commonplace to speak of drug interactions as if one were usually concerned only with drug–drug interactions. Since there are many important drug–non-drug interactions, we might do worse than to consider a few of these first.

Take, for instance, the variable of body size. We are immediately faced with a remarkable paradox: pharmacologists pay an enormous 'lip-service' to the notion of dosing per body surface area, but usually dose their animals on the basis of body weight, and clinicians usually prescribe doses (at least for adults) without concern for *either* body surface or body weight!

The arguments favoring the use of body surface are in part theoretical and in part empirical. Body surface is supposed to predict 'metabolic mass' better than does body weight, although certain of these past calculations have been based on both assumptions and observations of questionable validity (Krovetz, 1965). Pragmatically, equieffective doses in species varying tremendously in average size can often be made to look a great deal more similar when recalculated on the basis of 'body surface' (actually a mathematical transformation of body weight by one or another 'finagle' factor).

In man, the data sometimes look better when calculated on the basis of body surface, but at other times body weight appears more useful as a standard of calculation (Lasagna, 1956). Since drugs differ in their propensities for fat depots, and in being metabolized to either active or inactive metabolites, there are at least theoretical reasons for being suspicious of those who unremittingly advance body surface as *the* right basis for all situations.

Early in life, body weight and surface area are confounded with age, with the addition of a number of complicating variables, such as immaturity of metabolizing enzymes or renal function. In old age, the percentage of muscle mass tends to decrease and fat to increase, even with no change in total body weight, although there are huge interindividual differences in this regard.

Occasionally, an animal species will demonstrate a dramatic sex difference in response to a drug, but convincing human examples of this sort are rare, beyond the obvious sex-linked differences in the genitourinary and endocrine apparatus. Perhaps the most important interaction between sex and drugs in the human occurs from the unique ability of females to become pregnant, thus allowing for the unwitting exposure of two patients to a drug's effects instead of one.

Devotees of the 'plasma level school' believe that most (if not all) of our pharmacological cares would vanish if dosing were such as to achieve comparable plasma levels in all subjects and species. (It is really equal levels at the receptors, of course, that we want to achieve, but plasma level is at least an achievable approximation.) Theoretically and empirically one can adduce impressive arguments in favor of such an approach, but it has limitations as well. It requires, e.g., readily available methodology to allow the measurements to be made. It is most applicable, also, when both good and bad effects of a drug are related to either parent compound or one major metabolite. And, unfortunately, there are relatively few drugs for which solid evidence exists that plasma levels *do* correlate with the biological effect, and at least a few where it seems fairly clear that they do *not* (Lasagna, 1970).

In real life, it often turns out that specific individual variables such as genetic factors or the presence of disease are vastly more important then any general principles about age, weight, or sex. A thin, highly anxious old lady may require a sleeping draught that would overwhelm a complacent 200-pound young athlete. The acute schizophrenic tolerates doses of tranquilizer that he himself will not be able to withstand when he is over the acute phase of his disease. An individual who has acquired cellular or metabolic tolerance to heroin, alcohol, or barbiturates will be able to function at plasma concentrations of these agents that might be fatal to non-tolerant individuals. Kindred have been described in the medical literature who are genetically resistant or genetically hypersensitive to indirect-acting anticoagulants despite normal metabolism of these agents.

The list of disease–drug interactions is endless: allergies; the existence of a diseased myocardium; kidneys that cannot excrete drugs taken into the body, etc., etc. While most of these interactions are likely to make the patient's treatment more difficult or perilous, occasionally it works the other way – as in the patient with bacterial meningitis, whose inflamed meninges allow antibiotics to pass through barriers that ordinarily would bar such access.

One of the most important areas of interaction might be termed the socio-psychological sphere of therapeutics. While the placebo phenomenon has perhaps received the most publicity, other factors are of interest and deserving of attention. The attitudes of doctors as well as their patients toward drugs may affect the performance of the latter. Patient and doctor may differ not only in their expectations and goals but in their assessment of change. The inability of many patients to follow directions on prescriptions, has now been documented over and over again in patients suffering from almost all types of illness.

The other contributions in this volume will document fully the ways in which drugs may interact with each other, e.g. altering absorption, biotransformation, excretion, protein binding, action at receptor sites, etc. Here I wish merely to point out that these drug–drug interactions, like drug–non-drug interactions, may be either beneficial or harmful to the patient. We tend to think of such interactions as nuisances, by and large, yet who would want to practice medicine without such interactions as isoniazid–paramino-salicylic acid in tuberculosis, diuretic–antihypertensive drugs in hypertension, or nalorphine–morphine in narcotic poisoning?

So much for 'perspective'. Can we agree on some guidelines, a sort of breviary for the therapeutically perplexed? Let me try to put down such a list:

(1) The practicing clinician needs to have precise data on not only the existence of an interaction but its frequency of occurrence and the biological importance of the event. A man is not a mouse, and the hundreds of drug interactions observed in lower animals are not necessarily going to be seen in human beings, or at least not in such a way as to affect therapy significantly (Conney et al. 1972). With all the controversy, for instance, about chloral hydrate and its capacity to alter the effect of anticoagulant drugs,

there is a paucity of reported cases where the interaction was clinically significant.

Even where clinical significance exists potentially, we need *data*, and not glittering generalities. When premature infants readily get into trouble with chloramphenicol because their metabolic enzymes are inadequate, *that* is important information. If, on the contrary, an infant requires larger doses of a drug than would be expected on the basis of his body weight, we must know *that* as well. Specific, quantified interactions that allow effective management of patients are very useful; clichés about 'the young' and 'the old' are generally not (especially when the ravages of acquired disease are confused with chronological age).

(2) A corollary of (1) is that the clinician should know well those interactions that *are* well documented and quantified, *especially* for the drugs that he prescribes with some frequency.

(3) Keep in mind especially those possible drug interactions where the result is likely to be clinically important, e.g. hypertensive crisis, serious drops in blood pressure, haemorrhage, seizures, cardiac arrhythmias, hypoglycaemia.

(4) Whenever possible, a ranking of important interacting variables in a given clinical situation should be made, assigning importance to those factors that seem, on the basis of general experience and of specific knowledge about the given patient, likely to prove most important in determining therapeutic outcome.

(5) Do not neglect the information to be obtained from a history of the patient's past experiences with drugs. Trouble in the past often presages trouble in the future.

(6) It is unpardonable not to 'prevent the preventable'. A patient who has once had a dreadful allergic reaction to penicillin is not a good candidate for penicillin therapy.

(7) It makes good sense to avoid, whenever possible, drugs that have a high likelihood of undesirable interactions, e.g. monoamine oxidase inhibitors.

(8) Disease characteristics that are often associated with drug interactions should be kept prominently in mind, e.g. renal insufficiency.

(9) In general, the fewer drugs taken simultaneously, the better. (It goes without saying that no drug should be administered without good reason.)

(10) In general, the less frequently a drug has to be taken during the day, and the clearer the directions, the better.

(11) Drug treatment should not be continued any longer than necessary.

(12) When proper precautions are taken, the benefits of drug therapy far outweigh the risks of therapy.

(13) When the taking of drugs together is not contraindicated, or the

patient is actually *better* off for taking the drugs together, obviously (9) is not applicable.

(14) A fixed-ratio combination of tested efficacy and safety (e.g., oral contraceptives) is often to be preferred to idiosyncratic ratios decided upon by the physician without adequate clinical testing.

(15) Consider the possibility of a drug–drug or drug–non-drug interaction when the patient is not doing as well as expected.

(16) There are numerous possibilities for unhappy interactions to occur when drugs are added to the contents of a flask hooked up to an intravenous needle. Since such i.v. administration occurs almost always within hospital, mischief is most effectively prevented if the responsibility for such 'mixing' is placed squarely on the shoulders of a person likely to be au courant with the area, i.e., the hospital pharmacist.

2 The future

The short list of suggestions above is clearly not a completely satisfactory answer to the problem of drug interactions. What can we do to help the doctor in the years ahead? One possibility is to use computers as monitors, advisers, protectors of the patient and doctor. It is not ridiculous to imagine physicians sitting at a keyboard recording the pertinent anamnestic, physical, and laboratory characteristics of a patient, posing the therapeutic problems, and receiving back almost immediately a display of available remedies, recommended doses, warnings about interactions, probability estimates for benefit, toxicity, cost, etc. Science has outsmarted itself in the sense that there is too much drug information to be kept within any one doctor's head. The use of computers would avoid any pretense that the doctor does in fact possess all the required information.

Such usage of computers assumes that adequate 'software' would be devised. (The 'hardware' is already available.) It assumes that competent physicians, pharmacologists, toxicologists, pharmacists, etc., would cooperate in writing the programmes and would keep updating them as new information accrued. The task appears difficult but not impossible, and it may constitute the only way for the doctor of 1980 to keep abreast of 'the clinical importance of drug interactions'.

References

Conney, A. H., Chang, R., Levin, W. M., Garbut, A., Munro-Faure, A. D., Peck, A. W. and Bye, A. (1972): Effects of piperonyl butoxide on drug metabolism in rodents and man. *Arch. environ. Health*, **24**, 97.

Krovetz, L. J. (1965): The physiologic significance of body surface area. *J. Pediat.*, **67**, 841.
Lasagna, L. (1956): Drug effects as modified by aging. *J. chronic Dis.*, **3**, 567.
Lasagna, L. (1970): Correlation of clinical effects with blood levels of drugs. In: The Physiological Equivalence of Drug Dosage Forms (Symposium, Food and Drug Directorate, Ottawa, Canada, June 26, 27, 1969).

CHAPTER 3

Methods of study of drug interactions

RONALD B. STEWART AND LEIGHTON E. CLUFF

1 Historical background

Drug interaction is the phenomenon which results when the effect of one drug is modified by the prior or concurrent administration of another drug. The resultant effect may be an enhanced or diminished activity of the drugs and may be desirable or undesirable. The possibility that such interaction could occur has been repeatedly suggested in the medical literature. Loewe (1953) attempted to apply scientific principles to the study of interactions between drugs over two decades ago. However, he was never able to devise a satisfactory method for the simultaneous study of the effect of more than two drugs in combination.

Within the past several years increasing numbers of drug interaction reports have been appearing in the literature. These reports have been a cause for concern by the physician, pharmacist and the patient. As the level of awareness continues to increase methods must be developed to identify possible interactions, and determine their clinical significance.

The magnitude of the problem of drug interactions is at present unknown but is probably largely due to the number of agents used. A chemist working in the laboratory would never add twenty chemicals at random to a test tube without first making some preparation for possible explosive consequences. Yet, this number and even more drugs are often given almost randomly to people without a clear understanding of possible untoward consequences. This random drug administration has no doubt led to increasingly frequent and serious adverse effects as a result of chemical or pharmacological interactions. The ease of rationalizing expected therapeutic benefit from prescribing many drugs contrasts with the predictability of deleterious effects.

The problem of drug interaction is further compounded by the use of over-the-counter remedies. The practice of self-medication is deeply embedded in history, and frequently we have been described as a drug oriented society. This practice is further perpetuated today by the continuous advertising of non-prescription drugs.

The drug interaction problem is complicated to a greater extent since by definition the interaction may result in an absence or lack of effect. Compare this for example to the problem of adverse drug reactions where one looks for an undesirable or unintended response to a therapeutic agent. Studying drug interactions one must be aware, for instance, that failure of tetracycline therapy may have resulted from concurrent treatment of peptic ulcer disease with aluminium hydroxide or that a patient's hypertension which was previously well controlled by guanethidine is now out of control as a result of therapy with a new tricyclic antidepressant drug.

It took nearly 80 years of clinical experience to relate gastric haemorrhage with the administration of aspirin (Meyler, 1968). Similarly, thalidomide was heralded as an ideal tranquilizing agent for nearly three years before its teratogenic effects were fully appreciated (Taussig, 1962). These examples depict the difficulty of identifying relationships between a single drug and an undesirable side effect. The possibility that an adverse effect may be attributable to concurrent administration of two drugs becomes even more difficult.

The complexity of drug action in the human introduces variables which are difficult to control. The response to a drug by a patient may vary, based on factors such as dosage, absorption, volume of distribution, protein binding, etc. As more work is done to elucidate the mechanism of drug action one finds that a single drug may have a multiplicity of effects on the organism. In the course of any disease, improvement of the patient's condition may be independent of drug effects and may in fact result from a placebo effect.

Drug–drug interactions may occur in many different ways. When two or more drugs are administered to a patient the possibility exists that their effect will be additive (i.e. duplication of pharmacological actions will occur). If the combined effects of the drugs are greater than those of the active component alone the response is termed synergism. A possibility also exists that the drugs will have opposing pharmacological activity and antagonism will result. Actual mechanisms by which these effects are produced are numerous and include such phenomena as modification of absorption, distribution, transport across cell membranes, protein binding, receptor site sensitivity, metabolism and renal clearance. Interactions do not necessarily have to occur in vivo but can take place prior to administration as a result of direct chemical or physical interaction. One of the most common examples of an in vitro interaction is observed in the various intravenous admixtures given to hospitalized patients. These interactions may produce visible signs of incompatibility such as precipitates, turbidity, or colour changes. However inactivation of the drugs may occur with no overt indication.

Drug interactions may also occur as a result of predisposing factors in a susceptible host. An interaction may not result when a drug combination is administered to the 'average patient', however when that same combination of drugs is given to an elderly patient with renal and liver disease toxicity may result. Other host factors such as genetic predisposition, and the psyche may also influence the interaction.

It is difficult to control variables such as medication habits of patients and prescribing habits of physicians, yet it is in this setting where drug interactions are most liable to occur and should be identified. Investigation of drug interactions in natural settings, involving sick patients using a variety of prescription and non-prescription drugs is essential. The physician is not likely to administer together drugs known or suspected to interact adversely, and is less likely to administer several test drugs simultaneously to sick patients. It is with this background that the approaches used up to now and proposed in this chapter have been developed.

The complex clinical effects of interactions between drugs requires a multidirectional approach to their investigation. Drug interactions can be studied initially in patients, laboratory animals or in vitro models. Suspicions arising from clinical observations can lead to laboratory investigation or this process may occur in the reverse order.

Unfortunately one can never control all the variables in the clinical setting. Perhaps the best that can be accomplished at the present time is to develop approaches with an awareness and insight into the existing variables. Therefore, the purpose of this chapter will be to identify problem areas confronting drug interaction investigation, review methods that have been employed to study interactions and suggest future approaches to the problem.

2 Factors to be considered in the investigation of drug interactions

2.1 INTRODUCTION

An unintended or unexpected response to a drug exhibited by a patient is difficult to predict and may result from a multitude of factors. Investigation of drug interactions requires that careful consideration be given to three major determinants. These are: the peculiar properties of each drug; the physical and psychological status of the patient and, the total number of drugs to which the patient is exposed. Goodman (1964) has described numerous factors entering into the study of drug efficacy, and many of these factors are equally applicable to the study of drug interactions. Response to drug therapy is a complex phenomenon and is influenced by the drug taken, the patient receiving it and the physician prescribing it (Table I). Several of these factors will be discussed as examples although all bear careful consideration when studying drug interactions.

TABLE I

The problem of drug efficacy

A. Drug factors	
Doses employed	Tolerance
Multiple effects	Side-effects
Absorption	Toxicity
Distribution	Idiosyncrasy, hypersensitivity
Metabolic fate	Margin of safety
Excretion	Precautions
Duration of effect	Contraindications
Route, duration of administration	Pharmaceutical properties
Habituation	Chemical properties
Addiction liability	Drug interactions
B. Patient factors	
Sex, age	Contraindications, precautions
Body size and weight	Toxicity
Pregnancy	Margin of safety
Pharmacogenetic factors	Concomitant therapy
Biochemical status	Personality factors
Nutritional status	Attitude toward disease, drugs, doctors
Drug metabolism	Halo and milieu influences
Disease (vast multiplicity of factors)	Cost
Idiosyncrasy, hypersensitivity	
C. Physician factors	
Training	Attitude toward drug therapy
Diagnostic skill	Attitude toward patient
Therapeutic skill	Attitude toward disease
Experience with drugs	Halo and milieu influences
Concomitant therapy	
Factors affecting drug efficacy[a]	

[a] From Goodman (1964).

2.2 DRUG DETERMINANTS

A drug's physical and chemical properties are important to consider when studying it's potential to interact with other drugs. Whether a drug is absorbed depends on properties such as water solubility, partition coefficient, dissociation constant, molecular weight, etc. Binding properties of a drug to tissue and plasma proteins can influence factors such as it's distribution, rate of passage through membranes and the magnitude of pharmacological effect. Knowledge of these physical and chemical properties may enable one to suspect and predict potential interactions. For example, information concerning the pK_a of a drug will allow one to predict whether a concurrently administered agent such as sodium bicarbonate can alter the pH of the urine to a degree necessary to significantly affect elimination.

A thorough understanding of a drug's mechanism of action may enable the physician to suspect these types of interactions between drugs, but the number of different drugs available makes it almost inconceivable for a physician to possess this understanding completely.

Few drugs have precise and narrow ranges of action. Salicylates, for example, produce many different effects (Woodbury, 1971) including: (1) local irritant effects to mucosa; (2) changes in the EEG; (3) direct stimulation of respiration; (4) increased volume of bile; (5) reduced plasma-prothrombin levels; (6) increased urinary excretion of urates; (7) decreased aggregation of thrombocytes; (8) negative nitrogen balance in large doses; (9) alteration of acid–base balance; (10) uncoupling of oxidative phosphorylation with inhibitory action of many ATP-dependent reactions. Any drug having effects similar or opposite to these actions may interact with salicylates producing additive or antagonistic effects.

The effect of one drug may be altered leading to an adverse reaction not because of drug–drug interaction but because of drug–host–drug influences. Thiazide diuretics, for example, when used in conjunction with digitalis in the management of congestive heart failure may produce a hypokalaemia which can increase the toxic manifestation of cardiac glycosides. Similarly, paralysis of skeletal muscle may result from the same potassium-depleting mechanisms especially in patients receiving a neuromuscular blocking agent.

Many drugs are metabolized by hepatic microsomal enzymes which change the lipid-soluble active compound into a more polar metabolite. In this form the drug is more readily eliminated by renal clearance mechanisms. Many drugs have an ability to increase the amount of enzyme substance (enzyme induction) and thereby induce not only their own metabolism but also the metabolism of a variety of other drugs. A change in the rate of a drug's metabolism may produce clinically significant effects on the patient. Modifying the biological half-life of a drug by the administration of other drugs complicates therapy and can result in serious consequences to the patient such as those observed with barbiturates and Warfarin. When the investigator of drug interactions considers properties of a drug such as enzyme induction possible interactions can be predicted.

It is also essential that the investigator be cognizant of 'hidden ingredients' in trade name combination drug products. Drugs given for dissimilar therapeutic purposes may have common or similar pharmacological effects causing adverse reactions. Use of Combid ® for nausea, Histospan ® for a cold, Benadryl ® for leg cramps, Tofranil ® for depression, Donnatal ® and Kolantyl Wafers ® for dyspepsia in a middle aged woman produced additive anticholinergic activity. Routine use of all six of these seemingly unrelated drugs provides six different chemicals with anticholinergic activity and may result in significantly decreased intestinal motility and other adverse effects.

While most physicians recognize the variations that exist among drugs and patients, they may not consider that a more subtle difference exists between 'identical' drugs produced by different manufacturers. Inequivalence of drug products must be considered as a variable when investigating interactions between drugs.

Since drug brands vary from hospital to hospital and clinic to clinic so too, results of interaction studies may vary because of this difference in drug products. This suggests the possibility that epidemiological investigations identifying an interaction at one institution using brand A, may not be duplicated in another institution employing brand B.

Evidence for this has been well documented in recent years. There have been very few reports of controlled studies in which two or more commercial drug products, containing the same drug in the same type dosage form were compared in man. Although, approximately 3000 drugs were involved in the Drug Efficacy Study of the National Academy of Science only 12 drugs in two or more commercial drug products have been studied in man under controlled conditions to evaluate bioavailability (Wagner, 1971). For 7 of the 12 drugs studied (58%), large differences in the bioavailability of the drugs from different manufacturers' products were found. The 7 drugs included riboflavin, aspirin, *p*-aminosalicylic acid, chloramphenicol, diphenylhydantoin, tetracycline and oxytetracycline.

Glazko et al. (1968) studied the absorption characteristics of four different chloramphenicol preparations. Subjects were given a single 500 mg oral dose of chloramphenicol, and one product produced plasma levels which were nearly twice as great as a product by a different manufacturer. These observations emphasize the need for caution when assuming that absorption is the same for different products containing identical amounts of drug.

Variations in the biological availability of digoxin from four manufacturers was recently documented by Lindenbaum et al. (1971). In this cross-over study, identical doses of digoxin from different manufacturers were administered to patients. Significant differences in serum digoxin levels were achieved, with one product producing peak serum levels 7-fold greater than those obtained with another product. Significant variations were also observed between different lots of the same manufacturer's product.

Since the intensity of pharmacological response elicited by many drugs is probably directly related to the concentration or activity of the drug in the immediate vicinity of the receptor site in the body, it would follow that when interactions occur the intensity would also depend on the concentrations of the drug at that site. Although controlled absorption studies have only been performed on a few drugs the results indicate that significant differences do exist between different drug brands. In view of these findings it is likely that similar variations could be found among many other products and this factor should be considered when evaluating drug interaction results and reports.

2.3 HOST DETERMINANTS

Each time a physician prescribes a drug or drug combination he is in essence performing a new experiment. Every individual will have a peculiar set of characteristics which may alter the response to a given drug. Determinants such as age, sex, genetic make-up, environment, willingness to comply with the prescribed regimen and disease state all may have a bearing on drug response.

2.4 AGE AND SEX

Age is a most important determinant of drug response and therefore plays a significant role in the problem of drug interaction. A well-known example which illustrates the effect age may have on response to drugs is the 'grey syndrome'. Lowe (1968) described a study in which premature infants receiving prophylactic chloramphenicol died at a much higher rate than those receiving other antibiotics. The infants developed a peculiar grey cyanosis, hypothermia or irregular respiration, and expired. Eventually, it was found that blood levels were higher and the half-life of the drug was prolonged in these infants as compared to adults. Ewy et al. (1969) have shown that digoxin, a drug primarily eliminated by the kidney, has a longer half-life in older patients. It has been suggested (Fingl and Woodbury, 1971) that elderly patients may respond to drugs in an abnormal manner, often because of decreased ability to inactivate or excrete drugs or because of concurrent pathological changes.

Sex differences in response to drug therapy are less clearly defined. Sex differences in the rate of drug metabolism have not been observed in species other than the rat (Goldstein et al., 1968). Jick et al. (1968) have reported that there is a higher risk of bleeding in women over 60 years of age receiving heparin therapy.

2.5 HEREDITY

The genetic make-up of a patient may significantly influence drug interaction. Recent advances in pharmacogenetics have revealed the precise mechanism of several adverse drug effects previously not well understood. Normal variation of drug response in man is usually continuous and gives a unimodal frequency distribution curve for the drug action measured. These unimodal distribution curves are characteristic of multi-factorial inheritance. Several drugs, including succinylcholine and isoniazid, have shown a discontinuous variation depicted as bimodal, trimodal distribution. These multi modal distribution curves of drug response are usually the result of modifications in drug metabolism and may cause increased sensitivity to a drug.

Adverse drug reactions may also be characterized as following a bimodal distribution curve. For example, in a group of patients receiving ampicillin there will be a large patient distribution with a normal therapeutic response, exhibiting no sign of hypersensitivity and a smaller number experiencing rash and fever.

Variations in the metabolic conversion of isoniazid was reported by Hughes et al. (1954), which suggested that certain groups were genetically susceptible to developing peripheral neuropathy. It was subsequently determined that isoniazid and related drugs are inactivated by acetylation in the liver and considerable variation may exist from person to person in the ability to acetylate this drug. In fact, Evans et al. (1960) studied isoniazid metabolism in large populations and were able to show a bimodal distribution characterized as slow inactivators and rapid inactivators.

A different type of hereditary drug anomaly is resistance to the pharmacological action. This observation was made by O'Reilly et al. (1964) in an elderly man receiving Warfarin prophylactically after a myocardial infarction. Usual therapeutic doses were ineffective and therapeutic ranges of prothrombin times were achieved only when the patient was given a daily dose of 145 mg (i.e. 20 times the usual dose). Subsequent studies revealed the patient was not metabolizing the anticoagulant at an abnormally rapid rate since serum levels and distribution in the tissues were normal after normal doses. It was also found that there was a 20-fold sensitivity to the antidotal effects of vitamin K in the patients resistant to Warfarin. Further tests identified five other members of the family with a similar resistance to Warfarin. The patient's identical twin also had shown anticoagulant resistance after a myocardial infarction and the metabolic trait was believed to be inherited as an autosomal dominant. Lewis et al. (1967) in a later report have identified resistance to the anticoagulant effect of this drug based on rapid drug metabolism.

One can easily see from these reports how genetic factors may affect a study of drug interactions. An idiosyncratic reaction to a drug combination may be genetically based and one must be cautious not to identify such a response as a drug interaction. For example, suppose that a study is being conducted to document clinical evidence of the reported interaction of isoniazid and diphenylhydantoin (i.e. isoniazid inhibits the metabolism of diphenylhydantoin). If only a small number of patients are observed it is possible they would be rapid acetylators and no diphenylhydantoin intoxication would result. Many isolated drug interactions reported in the literature may have resulted from genetic factors and may not be duplicated by other investigators.

2.6 ENVIRONMENT

The interaction of the host with his environment may significantly alter the response to drugs. Environmental factors such as food, beverages, and exposure to insecticides are important to consider especially in a study of drug interactions conducted among ambulant patients. For these reasons it is advisable to maintain patients in a controlled environment and on a constant diet during drug interaction studies.

Food may interfere with drugs either by producing changes in absorption or elimination or by virtue of pharmacological properties of food. For instance, absorption of tetracycline is impaired by milk and milk products (Kunin and Finland, 1961). There is a growing interest in the use of natural food products and with this an increase in the consumption of vitamins. Frequently one observes patients who have taken large quantities of vitamins including A, C, and E. The use of large doses of vitamin C (up to 5 g daily) as a prophylactic measure for the common cold is not without hazard (Medical Letter, 1971) and may alter urinary pH sufficiently to influence the clinical response to some drugs by altering their rate of excretion. Foods rich in vitamin K are capable of altering the prothrombin time of the patient stabilized on anticoagulant drugs. Foods containing pharmacologically active substances may alter the response of a concomitantly administered drug. A classic example of this effect is the hypertensive crisis resulting from the ingestion of tyramine-containing foods by patients treated with monoamine oxidase inhibitors (Sapeika, 1969).

2.7 PATIENT COMPLIANCE

The degree to which a patient will comply with his prescribed regimen is nearly impossible to judge. Stewart and Cluff (1972) reviewed several prospective studies and found that the percentage of patients failing to take their medication as directed, with few exceptions, ranged from 20 to 82%. This factor should be carefully considered when designing drug interaction studies in ambulant populations, and methods should be developed to ensure that the patient actually receives the drugs under investigation.

Ironically, it seems that patients will use many drugs that have not been prescribed. Therefore, it is desirable to instruct the patient about the importance of not using other drugs during a drug interaction study. If possible, a urine screen for drugs should be conducted during the course of any study.

2.8 DISEASE STATE

Another important factor to consider when analyzing drug interactions is whether the response observed results from interaction of drug combinations or from a disease–drug phenomenon. The influence diseases have on the response to drugs cannot be treated here comprehensively, therefore, only a few examples will be reviewed. Clearly, however, variations in pharmacological response or its absence can result from alteration of metabolism or other pathological states, and may profoundly affect drug interactions.

Smith et al. (1966) found sedative and diuretic drugs produced adverse effects more than four times as often in patients with decreased as in patients with normal renal function. So significant is the importance of impaired renal function in therapy that Bennett et al. (1970) and McHenry et al. (1971) have prepared practical guides to assist in adjusting therapy.

Ampicillin has been shown by Speck (1971) to produce a much higher incidence of rash in patients with infectious mononucleosis. In a report by Patel (1967) skin rash occurred in all 13 children with infectious mononucleosis beginning 5–8 days after ampicillin administration. It is common knowledge that atropine type drugs may produce attacks of glaucoma, however, Kalow (1962) found that anticholinergic drugs precipitate glaucoma only in narrow angle disease. The use of barbiturates and sulphonamides has been shown to be hazardous in patients with a history of intermittent acute (hepatic) porphyria since these drugs can precipitate acute exacerbations of the disease (Rosenthal and Schmid, 1970). Thiazide diuretics (Monroe and Cluff, 1968) decrease uric acid excretion in man and have produced attacks of gouty arthritis in predisposed patients. The progressive weakness and paralysis of myasthenia gravis can be accentuated by agents which exert a blocking effect at the neuromuscular junction. Aminoglycoside antibiotics (e.g., kanamycin and streptomycin) and quinidine act as neuromuscular blocking agents and aggravate this disease. Diseases associated with hyperthermia may be unusually sensitive to salicylates, and patients may not only defervesce, but go into shock after aspirin therapy.

2.9 MULTIPLE DRUG THERAPY

When evaluating drug interactions it is imperative that one considers all drugs reaching the patient. This variable may be easily controlled in laboratory animals but it is difficult to control in hospitalized patients and is an enormous challenge in outpatient populations.

Hospitalized patients are given many therapeutic and diagnostic agents which may interact. In studies at Johns Hopkins, Seidl et al. (1966) found patients who experienced adverse effects of drugs received an average of 14 drugs. Cluff and Stewart (L. E. Cluff and R. B. Stewart, 1972, unpublished data) have found the average patient admitted to the medical ward of the University of Florida's Shands Teaching Hospital receives 9.5 drugs during their hospitalization, and pediatric patients in the same institution receive 4.5 drugs. In a study of drug utilization in 6 hospitals Jick et al. (1970) found the average number of exposures to be 8.4 drugs.

Patients are also exposed to numerous diagnostic and therapeutic agents which may or may not be included in normal drug utilization data collected in hospital monitoring programmes. A physician performing an examination of the ocular fundus may employ a drop of phenylephrine ophthalmic solution as a mydriatic and then on completion he may instill pilocarpine to reverse the mydriasis. He considers this routine evaluation, therefore, the drugs may not be included in the list of drugs administered to his patient. Similarly, tonometry may be performed with the use of a local anaesthetic or procedures such as lumbar puncture, renal and liver biopsies may be performed with the aid of local anaesthetics which are not considered drug therapy. Information on drugs administered in diagnostic clinics removed from the hospital ward such as barium, cardiac dyes, and preoperative medications is often difficult to obtain. Many procedures performed on the ward such as renal and liver function studies require administration of diagnostic agents often disregarded as drug therapy. It is doubtful that drug exposures of this nature are included in statistics of the studies cited above. Nonetheless, these 'non-therapeutic' drug exposures must be considered when studying drug interactions.

In drug interaction studies conducted among outpatient populations the difficulty of obtaining complete drug exposure information is compounded to truly monumental proportions. It has often been stated that every patient has at least two prescribers, his doctor and himself and often the patient's friends constitute a third prescriber. Information relative to medication utilization practices of ambulant patients has been sketchy but recent studies have shed some light on the multiplicity of drugs used by outpatients. Latiolais and Berry (1969), studied ambulant patients from a university hospital and found the average patient took 2.3 prescribed medications.

They also found 55% of the patients using over-the-counter drugs concurrently with prescribed medications. An interesting approach to the study of self-medication was employed by Bleyer et al. (1970), in a maternal care clinic. A maternal diary composed of a day-by-day medication record maintained by 67 patients during the last trimester of pregnancy revealed that patients took an average of 8.7 medications during the study period. An average of 6.9 (80%) of the drugs were taken without medical supervision or knowledge while only 20% were specifically ordered by the physician. Aspirin, thiazide diuretics, and antibiotics were used by 69, 30 and 16% of the patients respectively.

Stewart and Cluff (1971) studied drug utilization characteristics in a university outpatient clinic and found the average patient had used 3.2 prescription and 2.9 non-prescription drugs within a 30-day period prior to the clinic appointment. In a group of 60 patients using prescribed drugs 26 patients (43%) were taking drugs from more than one physician. Considering the ingredients contained in the combination drug products the average patient had ingested 9.5 different chemicals in the month preceding clinic visitation.

One problem of multiple drug administration is that the rate of adverse effects observed increases disproportionately with an increase in the number of drugs given to the patient. In one study (Smith et al. 1966: see fig. 1) an adverse reaction rate of 40% was seen in patients given 16–20 drugs compared with a rate of 7% in those given 6–10 drugs.

The frequency of adverse reactions to drugs in all prospective reaction studies as observed by Gardner and Cluff (1970) has been directly related to the number of drugs administered. One can speculate that the increase is in part due to the effect of interaction between the drugs.

3 Methods of investigating drug interactions

3.1 SPONTANEOUS REPORTING

Voluntary or spontaneous reporting of individual suspected cases of adverse drug reactions or drug interactions is a valuable and effective method and this form of reporting of possible drug–drug interactions is a technique that must be encouraged. Although there are obvious problems of individual reporting systems this method has valuable characteristics not found in other systems. This type of reporting has been used for many years in studying adverse drug reactions and it must be improved and expanded to include the study of drug interactions.

3.1.1 *Value of spontaneous reporting*

Spontaneous reporting provides a mechanism for surveillance of wide geo-

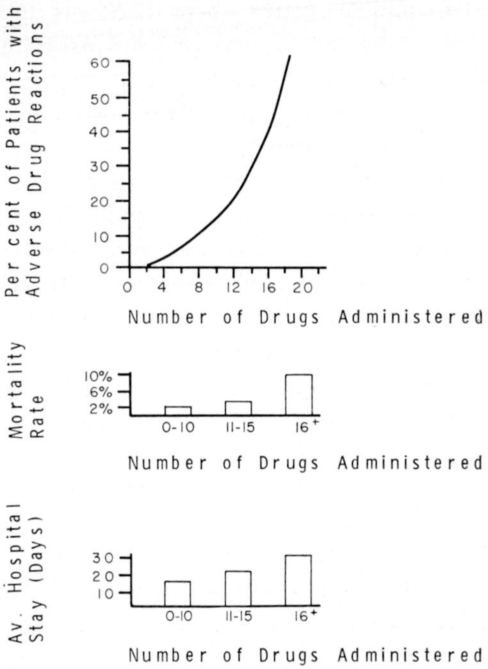

Fig. 1[a]. The relationship of rate of adverse drug reactions to: (1) number of drugs administered; (2) mortality rate; (3) duration of hospitalization.

graphical locations. By virtue of this characteristic patients exposed to nearly every drug combination and receiving treatment from every type of specialist are under surveillance. In the United States alone, there are several hundred thousand potential observers monitoring two hundred million patients.

Voluntary reporting provides advantages difficult to build into a study designed in a teaching institution since most teaching hospitals employ a drug formulary system and there is little utilization of combination drug products. In addition, patients in the institutional environment are closely monitored and generally are not allowed to self-medicate, consume alcohol or engage in daily habits that may precipitate drug interactions. Voluntary case reports from those whose practice is primarily outside hospitals adds an additional dimension of patients being treated for extended periods of time.

It is in this group of patients that one may see the occurrence of slowly developing or delayed drug interactions. The story is told of the drunk searching for his keys under the street light rather than in the dark where he

[a] Findings of Smith et al. (1966).

had lost them, as he could see better where there was light illustrating the fallacy of looking for drug interactions only in places that can be easily studied and carefully controlled. Drug interactions must be studied in diverse populations exposed to numerous types of therapeutic agents, and spontaneous reporting provides that capability.

One must recognize the value of spontaneous reporting. Strong evidence of the importance of casual observation and spontaneous reporting in recognition of previously unsuspected drug reactions, was observed in the study of 850,000 patients over 6 years undergoing anaesthesia with halothane. Inconclusive evidence of halothane liver toxicity resulted from the study, but subsequently it was demonstrated by casual observation of two anaesthesiologists. One must face the fact that nearly all new previously unrecognized adverse effects and drug interactions have been identified by casual observation and not by intensive monitoring programmes.

Admittedly, this method has many shortcomings and is in need of improvement. Spontaneous reporting is erratic, incomplete and not always reliable. It requires that the physician be familiar with the concepts of drug interactions and recognize that an interaction has occurred. Another disadvantage of this reporting system is that little or no denominator data (patients at risk) may be available.

A major defect in individual reporting systems is under-reporting. Under-reporting may result from a number of factors including uncertainty of what to report, lack of information on where the report should be directed and fear of medico–legal action. Erratic or incomplete reporting in addition to underestimating the problem, may lead to fad reporting and introduce bias into the system.

In a voluntary reporting system a physician must know what to report (Westerholm, 1972). One must have a reasonable degree of suspicion that an interaction or adverse reaction has occurred and therefore if a physician is not familiar with a potential interaction it is unlikely to be reported.

Lack of denominator data provides additional difficulties in interpreting data collected. A cluster of reports linking a drug or drug combination with an adverse drug reaction may simply be a reflection of increased utilization of the drug or changes in the method of administration. The same problem of interpretation would exist if an increased number of reports were observed regarding a specific brand of a drug.

Voluntary reporting also stimulates the pursuit of many false leads and blind alleys, but without more sophisticated systems than now available, is essential for identifying potential problems. These reports provide clues which can be investigated in the laboratory or in the clinic to identify and document those of significance and discard others.

3.2 EPIDEMIOLOGICAL METHODS

Epidemiology is the study of patterns of occurrence of disease in populations or groups of people. This method may also be applied to determine the incidence and significance of drug interactions. Studies have been conducted employing both prospective and retrospective design and have included hospitalized and out of hospital patients. Studies can be designed utilizing vital statistics or isolated population groups or may include the study of broad drug categories, single drugs or specific diseases. In nearly every type of epidemiological investigation computer assistance is usually required to handle the data.

3.3 PROSPECTIVE INSTITUTIONAL STUDIES

A prospective study (i.e. one designed to identify interactions as they occur) is much more valuable since it usually facilitates more complete documentation. An additional advantage to the prospective study is that interactions or adverse reactions may actually be prevented if detected early in the patient's treatment.

Therapeutic regimens of patients in fourteen nursing homes were reviewed by Lang and Kabat (1970) to determine if drug interactions were occurring within the patients' prescription medications. The names, strength and frequency of administration of all prescription drugs were obtained at the nursing station of each nursing home by reviewing nurses' cardexes and this therapy was checked against published reported drug interactions. An interaction was defined as 'when the effectiveness of one drug is adversely modified by the concurrent administration of another drug'. Interactions were included in the study if they: altered drug absorption; displaced drugs from receptor sites; altered metabolism or excretion. Medications of 151 patients were reviewed and 128 possible interactions were observed.

Pucket and Visconti (1971) have described a study employing prospective epidemiological methods utilizing a pharmacist monitor and computer techniques to assess the clinical significance of drug–drug interactions. The investigation was performed over a 2-month period in a private, community hospital. An interaction was defined as the undesired phenomenon which occurred in the body when the effects of one drug were modified by the concurrent or prior administration of another drug. Interactions included in the computer programme were those manifestations which could be detected from the patient's chart, such as effects on laboratory values, vital signs, and course of therapy, etc. The patient's daily medication orders were processed by the computer and compared with previous drug orders using data processing cards. A daily 'Drug Interaction Report' was printed-out by the computer.

Charts of patients listed in the 'Drug Interaction Report' were reviewed each day to verify the administration of potentially interacting drugs. Charts were followed daily during administration of potentially interacting drugs and then for a week after an interacting drug was discontinued. The purpose of the chart review was to identify drug interactions responsible for changes in the patient's condition, diagnostic or laboratory test values, vital signs, or clinical course. Before an adverse drug interaction was recorded the attending physician had to verify that the suspected interaction was taking place or had taken place and that it had clinically significant effects on his patient.

During the study, 2422 patients were screened for potential drug–drug interactions, representing 25,005 days of hospitalization. Of the patients studied, 113 (4.7%) were found to have received interacting drug combinations. Signs of drug interaction were identified in 7 (6.2%) of these patients, and 0.3% of the population surveyed.

Several limitations of the methods employed in the study were cited by the investigators. The 108 interactions actually represented a small percentage of those that have been reported and in addition the patient's chart was heavily relied upon to reveal the existence of an interaction. Also, laboratory tests often were not ordered for patients on drugs whose effects are monitored by these means, and finally physician and pharmacist judgement was used to detect and classify the interactions.

Drug interactions occurring during anticoagulant therapy have been studied by Ku et al. (1970) using epidemiological methods. Ninety-five patients taking Warfarin and 12 patients taking *bis*hydroxycoumarin were monitored by prospective epidemiological methods. Specially designed profile cards were used to study drugs given to patients while receiving anticoagulants. Factors which could alter prothrombin-time were entered on the profile card including pre-admission medications, diagnosis, blood transfusions and operations, etc. Interacting drugs were analyzed to see if their reported effects could be observed by changes in Warfarin dosage or by drastic changes of prothrombin-time. It was concluded that drugs reported to potentiate or inhibit prothrombin-times did in fact result in either the lowering or elevation of average daily maintenance doses of Warfarin, respectively.

Several intensive monitoring programmes have been conducted in the past few years. Although the main objective of these programmes has been the study of drug utilization and adverse drug reactions, the problem of drug interactions has also been investigated.

At the University of Florida an extensive computerized review of adverse drug reactions, drug utilization and drug interactions is being conducted.

This is a continuation of work previously conducted by Cluff et al. (1964). This epidemiological study is designed to provide data on rates of adverse reactions to drugs, and information useful in preventing adverse reactions and drug interactions.

Computerized records are maintained on all drugs and doses administered to patients admitted to a 65-bed general medical ward and a 50-bed paediatric ward. A master patient profile is created for each patient, containing information on sex, race, marital status, age, drugs, diagnoses, laboratory and diagnostic procedures and is processed for computer storage. Information collected on adverse reactions is also processed for storage into the computer in the format established by the Food and Drug Administration (1970). Epidemiological data has been collected on over 12,000 patients.

Adverse drug reactions resulting from drug interactions have been studied through the aid of a specially designed computer programme (Table II).

TABLE II

Drug interaction analysis report

Adverse reaction – gastrointestinal haemorrhage

Patients having this reaction	Drugs received by all patients in order of frequency prior to or at the time of reaction						
126622	Dextrose	Heparin	KCl	Chloral hydrate	Darvon	Digoxin	
127734	Dextrose	Heparin	KCl				Aluminium hydroxide
129542	Dextrose	Heparin	KCl	Chloral hydrate	Darvon	Digoxin	
163422	Dextrose	Heparin					
135291	Dextrose		KCl	Chloral hydrate	Darvon		Aluminium hydroxide
128432	Dextrose	Heparin			Darvon	Digoxin	
132332	Dextrose	Heparin	KCl	Chloral hydrate			
145332	Dextrose	Heparin	KCl		Darvon		Aluminium hydroxide
127449			KCl	Chloral hydrate			
135555	Dextrose	Heparin		Chloral hydrate		Digoxin	

Three most common drugs	Number of gastrointestinal haemorrhage patients taking drug	Percent of all patients taking drugs
Dextrose	9	21
Heparin	8	10
KCl	7	23

This programme identifies all patients who have had a particular adverse reaction, such as gastrointestinal haemorrhage and then drug records of all patients experiencing this reaction are screened. The programme lists in order of frequency the drugs given prior to or at the time of the reaction. The computer then prints out a listing of all patients experiencing the adverse reaction and the drugs most commonly received by those patients. This programme should provide useful information which will allow one to correlate adverse drug reactions resulting from drug interactions.

The 'Boston Collaborative Drug Surveillance Program' has been in operation since 1966 and is primarily concerned with collection and analysis of drug experience data in humans (Borda et al., 1968; Slone et al., 1969). Data are collected by specially trained nurse-monitors in inpatient wards, from nine hospitals in the United States and abroad. Data collected include demographic information, details of drugs administered to each patient, and a record of adverse effects considered by the attending physician to be drug related.

In this study the computer scans the data for adverse reactions or abnormal laboratory results that may be associated with administration of a single drug or drug combination. Several interactions have been detected by this method including an interaction between chloral hydrate and Warfarin, and a tetracycline-induced rise in blood urea nitrogen levels (Boston Collaborative Drug Surveillance Program, 1972a, and Boston Collaborative Drug Surveillance Program, 1972b).

3.4 RETROSPECTIVE STUDIES

This type of study involves the review of a patient's medical record after discharge. A disadvantage of this method of investigation is that necessary data needed to confirm the presence of an adverse effect or interaction are usually lacking.

Retrospective epidemiological studies of anticoagulant drug interactions have not found clinically significant drug interactions to be common. A chart review technique was employed by Kleinman and Griner (1970) on a sample of medical records of adult inpatients receiving Warfarin. Daily Warfarin doses and prothrombin times were recorded as well as the presence of bleeding or thromboembolic complications. Drugs having potential for interaction were recorded if administered for at least 72 hr. A definite interaction was identified in only one instance thus leading the authors to conclude that clinically significant interactions in hospitalized patients treated with Warfarin are uncommon.

3.5 PROSPECTIVE OUTPATIENT STUDIES

Studying drug interactions in outpatient populations is more difficult as a result of the multiple sources from which a patient may obtain drugs. Stewart and Cluff (1971) conducted a study to determine the frequency with which outpatients take drugs with a potential for interaction. Seventy-five patients receiving treatment in a university medical clinic were interviewed by a pharmacist-investigator to determine all prescription and non-prescription medication taken by patients in the month preceeding their visit.

Patients were interviewed at the time of their visit and a checklist of symptoms frequently treated with non-prescription drugs (See Table III) was used to stimulate recall of additional medications. Verification of the prescription-medication information was accomplished by telephoning pharmacies that had filled each of the patients prescriptions.

TABLE III
Medication history checklist

The following list will be used to stimulate recall of patient medications	
Cold (cough)	Weight control (diet pills)
Stomach (antacid)	Nerves
Laxatives (constipation)	Vitamins
Pain (headache)	Menstrual discomfort (periods)
Sleep	Oral contraceptives (birth control pills)
Eye drops or ointments	Ointments for skin
Ear drops	Worm medications

Three drug interaction definitions were used in this study: (1) therapeutic duplication – occurring when two or more drugs with the same pharmacological effect were administered by separate dosage forms from one prescriber, multiple prescribers, or other sources; (2) therapeutic antagonism – occurring when two or more drugs with the opposite pharmacological effect were administered by separate dosage forms from one prescriber, multiple prescribers, or other sources; (3) therapeutic contraindication – occurring when one or more drugs were administered to a patient with a disease or condition in which the use of that drug is generally contraindicated, or when two drugs which decrease or increase their respective activity were administered concurrently.

Thirty-one (51.7%) patients were taking prescription medication with a potential for interaction as defined above. Nine (12%) patients had taken prescription medication, during the month, which had been borrowed from friends or relatives. All but one of the 60 patients taking prescribed medications were also treating themselves with over-the-counter medications. The most common interaction observed in this study was duplication of agents in the same pharmacological class as a result of taking drugs from multiple sources.

The Kaiser-Permanente Drug Reaction Monitoring System is an epidemiological adverse drug reaction study which systematically monitors ambulant patients (Friedman et al., 1971). Data on drug utilization in this system are collected through outpatient pharmacies by means of electric typewriters connected to a central computer. While this system is designed primarily for studying adverse reaction, the method could be adopted for the study of drug interactions.

3.6 OTHER METHODS

Every investigative epidemiological technique employed in the study of adverse drug effects or drug interactions will have limitations. Therefore, all potential sources of information should be employed including vital statistics or morbidity and mortality reports, population monitoring of hospital or clinic patients and records of drug utilization from countries developing national plans for supplying drugs to patients.

3.7 COMPUTER NEEDS

Epidemiological methods such as population monitoring necessitate advanced computer technology to store large amounts of data. Rapid advances are being made in electronic processing of patient records, presenting unusual opportunity to develop drug monitoring systems. Only through the capability of storing and retrieving large amounts of data can detection of rare adverse effects or interactions (1 in 10,000–50,000) be accomplished.

Sophisticated analytical programmes must be designed to identify associations that may result from drug–drug interactions. Computer programmes are currently available which will analyze associations between drugs received by patients and the occurrence of adverse effects and compute the chi-square (Gaetano and MacLaughlin, 1971). This system provides clues to researchers which can in turn be used to plan intensive investigation.

4 Clinical investigation of specific drug interactions

4.1 GENERAL

Spontaneous reporting of chance observations and prospective epidemiological studies for identifying drug interactions can be very useful in providing clues for further investigation. Once the possibility of a drug interaction has been identified it may deserve additional study to elucidate the mechanism of interaction. Verification and quantitation of drug interactions can be accomplished by controlled studies in a small number of volunteers as patients. In general, drug interactions result either from alterations in absorption, metabolism, excretion or distribution. Therefore methods will be described that have been used to study the clinical significance of interactions occurring at these points.

The physiological impact of a drug's ability or inability to be absorbed from the gastrointestinal tract is obvious. If one drug can alter absorption of another then the potential for interaction exists and may result in either an increase or decrease in the relative rate of absorption or the total amount of the drug absorbed. Investigations of absorption interactions have been conducted by administering a single drug to patients thus establishing a baseline pattern of absorption. Then other drugs are administered concomitantly with the index drug to determine their effect on absorption rates. Robinson et al. (1971) employed this method to investigate the possible interaction of Warfarin with the non-systemic gastrointestinal drugs, cholestyramine, magnesium and aluminium hydroxide and psyllium hydrophyllic mucilloid. In this study only cholestyramine was found to significantly decrease mean plasma Warfarin levels.

A similar technique has been employed by Neuvonen et al. (1970) to show that orally administered ferrous sulfate can impair the absorption of simultaneously administered tetracyclines. Great reductions (40–85%) of oxytetracycline, methacycline and doxycycline blood levels were obtained when these drugs were given concomitantly with ferrous sulfate. Hall and Davis (1969) studied the effect of a non-absorbable alkali (magnesium trisilicate) on iron absorption and found that magnesium trisilicate significantly reduced the amount of iron absorbed.

Although animal studies have shown hundreds of compounds with the ability to induce enzymes in the endoplasmic reticulum of liver, few investigations have been carried out in humans. Studies that have been conducted usually measure the change in rate of metabolism of a key drug that occurs when patients are pre-treated or are treated simultaneously with other drugs.

Christensen and Skovsted (1969) found chloramphenicol retarded the metabolic transformation of tolbutamide, diphenylhydantoin and dicoumarol in man. The method used to study this interaction has been employed in many other metabolic interaction studies. Serum half-lives of the 3 drugs were first determined, then patients were given therapeutic doses of tolbutamide and diphenylhydantoin for 4 days. When chloramphenicol (2 g/day) was also given, a considerable elevation in the serum level of tolbutamide and diphenylhydantoin was observed in all patients. The half-life of dicoumarol showed a similar prolongation resulting from chloramphenicol administration.

Allopurinol and nortriptyline has been shown by Vesell et al. (1970) to inhibit drug metabolism. To determine the effect of these drugs on metabolism, a single oral dose of antipyrine or *bis*hydroxycoumarin was given before allopurinol or nortriptyline was started and 24 hr after the last dose of these drugs. It was observed that therapy with nortriptyline or allopurinol increased the half-lives of antipyrine and *bis*hydroxycoumarin. Similar methods have been used by Hansen et al. (1971) and Robinson and Sylwester (1970) to demonstrate accelerated metabolism resulting from drug interactions.

Alterations in drug distribution can result from drug–drug interactions, and can be demonstrated by titrating patients on a standard dose of one drug and then producing increases or decreases in serum levels by administration of a second drug. Sellers and Koch-Weser (1970b) found chloral hydrate increased free-plasma Warfarin levels when administered to anticoagulated subjects. Chloral hydrate was believed to displace Warfarin from binding sites on plasma albumin and thereby potentiate the depression of vitamin K-dependent clotting factor synthesis in the liver (see Chapter 7, p. 122). Similar methods have been used by O'Reilly and Levy (1970) and Field et al. (1967) to demonstrate alterations of drug distribution in the body as a result of drug interactions.

Since most drugs are partially or totally dependent upon elimination by renal excretion, agents which alter renal output or urinary pH have often been implicated in drug interactions. For example, Gerhardt et al. (1969) found the renal clearance of quinidine is reduced to one tenth the normal level when urinary pH is increased from 6.0 to 7.5, and Skeith et al. (1968) used labelled indomethacin to show that renal excretion of that drug is inhibited by probenecid. [2-^{14}C] Indomethacin was administered to human volunteers and its renal excretion was measured with and without concurrent administration of probenecid. These studies showed when patients were taking probenecid, blood levels of indomethacin were 6-fold the control values and 15% of peak values at 48 hr. Champion et al. (1972) employed a similar methodology to study the possible interaction between aspirin on serum indomethacin. Utilizing spectrofluorometric techniques they found serum concentrations of indomethacin unaffected by aspirin administration.

4.2 ANIMAL STUDIES

The observation that one drug could alter the metabolism of another by inducing liver enzyme systems was made first in laboratory animals by Conney and Burns (1962) and Remmer (1962). These findings led to further investigations of similar effects in humans by Cucinell et al. (1965) and have subsequently had a major impact on therapy in man. While animal studies have provided useful information concerning drug–drug interactions many feel that their value may be limited.

Goodman (1964) has stated . . . "at best, animal pharmacology provides only paradigms and analogies, the clinical predictive value of which remains to be demonstrated. The best model for a cat is another cat. The best model for man is man himself. I have said before, and repeat here, that animal pharmacology, except for veterinarians and except for its intrinsic and heuristic and aesthetic values, and except for providing a livelihood for a segment of the scientific population, including the author is mainly a prelude to human pharmacology". Similar limitations of animal studies have been cited by others such as Macgregor (1965), Brodie (1962) and Modell (1964). It would seem then that the most fruitful approach to the study of drug interactions in man is to employ that species.

4.3 IN VITRO STUDIES

Unfortunately, recognition of drug interactions has often had to wait on observations by an astute clinician. Therefore, an interaction may be uncovered only after long clinical experience with the drug and often at a cost of severe morbidity to patients. Several investigators have attempted to predict clinically important drug interactions by demonstrating them in the laboratory.

4.4 PROTEIN DISPLACEMENT

One important class of drug interaction results from displacement of drugs bound to plasma proteins. Displacement of drugs from binding sites on plasma proteins increases the concentration of the free bioactive form, resulting in increased pharmacological effect, rate of metabolism and renal clearance.

Sellers and Koch-Weser (1970a) have developed a method to determine the relative potency of displacing agents in vitro. Competitive binding of Warfarin to human albumin was studied by equilibrium dialysis. The relative potency of the drugs studied was, in decreasing order, mefenamic acid, ethacrynic acid, diazoxide and nalidixic acid (see Chapter 7, p. 122). A method has also been described by Solomon and Thomas (1971) to estimate drug–albumin affinity constants in human plasma. This method of studying displacing potency represents a valuable tool for identification of drugs with this interaction potential.

4.5 INTERACTIONS OF PARENTERAL MEDICATIONS

Much attention has been directed at the problem of interactions which occur after drugs are administered to patients. A clinically significant interaction between drugs may also result when drugs are admixed to intravenous fluids prior to administration. Investigations have shown that many drugs are chemically or physically incompatible in solution and cannot be safely admixed for intravenous administration. Intravenous incompatibility studies have been concerned with areas such as physical incompatibility, chemical incompatibility, and stability after reconstitution of drugs.

Thirty-four drugs intended for intravenous administration were tested for physical incompatibility by Misgen (1965). In this study inspection for particulate matter was made after various drug combinations were prepared. Parker (1967) studied chemical incompatibilities of some intravenous admixtures which do not produce visual changes in the solution. He studied 8 common drug products used in parenteral fluids and found significant decomposition in half of the drugs. Shoup et al. (1964) studied the stability of 156 drugs with regard to their stability after reconstitution. For a more detailed review of incompatibility involving intravenous admixtures reference should be made to the publications of Bair (1966), Fowler (1967) and Webb (1969).

In an effort to prevent this type of drug interaction the responsibility for admixing drugs for intravenous use has in many institutions been assumed by the hospital pharmacy. Centralizing the responsibility for intravenous admixture services insures better control of these preparations since they can be prepared by pharmacists specializing in the prevention of incompatibilities.

5 Future approaches to the problem of drug interactions

5.1 INTRODUCTION

The drug interaction problem is of sufficient magnitude to require concerted effort on the part of all health professionals and national health agencies. Methods must be developed to identify previously unsuspected interactions between drugs and to prevent the occurrence of well-documented interactions.

5.2 NEED FOR A COORDINATING CENTRE

A national coordinating centre should be established to develop an organized approach to the study and prevention of drug interactions. The primary objectives of such a centre would be to collate information derived from voluntary reporting, attempt to document drug–drug interactions and develop educational programmes for the medical community concerning methods of preventing drug interactions.

Voluntary reporting systems generate tremendous amounts of data. During a 10-yr period the 'United States Food and Drug Administration's Hospital Reporting Program' received over 100,000 reports (Esch, 1972). A national centre similar to the 'Center for Disease Control' (CDC) in the United States could serve to collect, classify, and quantify reports. Such a centre could identify high priority interactions representing serious risk to the public and requiring immediate attention.

Reports collected by this centre could be grouped by probable mechanism of interaction and forwarded to investigators equipped to study the interaction. For instance, several institutions have programmes investigating protein binding, others enzyme induction and others gastrointestinal absorption etc.

A listing of reported interactions by mechanism could be made available to respective institutions for further evaluation. Still other reports might be best confirmed by comprehensive monitoring programmes.

Education is a vital function of a national centre. Once an interaction has been validated the information must be disseminated to practicing physicians and pharmacists. Feed-back of this information may be accomplished by many forms such as direct mailing of circulars to health professionals, through scientific journals and by periodic educational programmes.

Creation of a position concerned with drug utilization control in large medical institutions is another method which should be considered. This professional, comparable to an Infections Control Officer, would have the responsibility to monitor adverse drug reactions, drug interactions, and drug utilization and present feed-back information to the medical staff, thereby improving the quality of prescribing.

5.3 LINKING INTENSIVE MONITORING PROGRAMMES

To complement spontaneous voluntary reporting, improved methods of intensive monitoring must be developed. The intensive monitoring approach for studying drug interactions is expensive, requiring automatic data processing facilities and skilled personnel. Since intensive monitoring programmes only monitor a relatively small number of patients, record linkage is essential to coordinate data collected in different locations and available from different sources. Take for example a programme following only 4000 patients per year. Let us assume an interaction between 2 widely-used drugs, digoxin and amitriptyline is to be studied. Approximately 20% of patients admitted to medical wards may have received digoxin, which is not bad, we have 800 patients. Amiptriptyline, on the other hand, is used by only about 5% of the patients (i.e. 200 patients). Unfortunately when one looks for patients receiving both drugs concurrently probably only 20 patients (0.5%) will be identified. This sample size is obviously too small to draw meaningful conclusions. Therefore, even highly used drugs are difficult to study, necessitating cooperation and data sharing between monitoring programmes. Linkage of different records, however, require some standardization of information for storage and retrieval to allow for automatic integration of data relevant to drug monitoring. This too could be a responsibility of a national centre.

5.4 COMPUTERIZED MONITORING PROGRAMMES IN THE COMMUNITY

Drug utilization review programmes should be developed to improve prescribing and usage in the community. Methods should be developed to collect information on prescriptions filled at pharmacies as well as information on routine use of over-the-counter medications by patients. A central computer centre would store this information and make it available on request to the patient's physician or pharmacist. Such a system could be designed to provide the physician review capabilities of a patient's medication file to insure that current therapy is appropriate and any additional therapeutic measures will not duplicate or antagonize existing medications. Additionally, epidemiological data on a large segment of the population would be generated from this programme. This would facilitate studies concerned with drug exposure such as frequency rates of adverse reactions, studies on significance of interactions, and analysis of congenital birth defects to determine potential associations with drugs taken by mothers.

6 Summary

Striking changes in availability and use of drugs have occurred over the past 30 years. Adverse reactions to drugs and drug interactions were less of a problem when few drugs were at hand, but have become a more serious problem recently, partly because of the large number and potency of our present medications. In the study of adverse drug reactions one looked primarily for deleterious responses from drug therapy, now a new dimension has been added with drug–drug interactions and we must look also for lack of therapeutic response resulting from multiple drug therapy.

No single approach will unveil the complexities of drug interactions. A multidisciplinary cooperative effort from private practitioners, clinical investigators, researchers in the laboratories, and teachers of pharmacology and therapeutics will be required. Old approaches to new complex problems will not be sufficient. Imaginative investigation and application of new sophisticated technologies including computers must be developed.

References

Bair, J. N. (1966): A brief review of drug compatibility and stability literature. *Amer. J. Hosp. Pharm.*, **23**, 344.

Bennett, W. M., Singer, I. and Coggins, C. H. (1970): A practical guide to drug usage in adult patients with impaired renal function. *J. Amer. med. Assoc.*, **214**, 1468.

Bleyer, W. A., Au, W. Y., Lange, W. A. and Raisz, L. G. (1970): Studies on the detection of adverse drug reactions in the newborn. I. Fetal exposure to maternal medications. *J. Amer. med. Assoc.*, **213**, 2046.

Borda, I. T., Slone, D. and Jick, H. (1968): Assessment of adverse reactions within a drug surveillance program. *J. Amer. med. Assoc.* **205** 645.

Boston Collaborative Drug Surveillance Program (1972a): Interaction between chloral hydrate and Warfarin. *New Eng. J. Med.*, **286**, 53.

Boston Collaborative Drug Surveillance Program (1972b): Tetracycline and drug attributed rises in blood urea nitrogen. *J. Amer. med. Assoc.*, **220**, 377.

Brodie, B. B. (1962): Difficulties in extrapolating data on metabolism of drugs from animals to man. *Clin. Pharmacol. Therap.*, **3**, 374.

Champion, G. D., Paulus, H. E., Mongan, E., Okun, R., Pearson, C. M. and Sarkissian, E. (1972): The effect of aspirin on serum indomethacin. *Clin. Pharmacol. Therap.*, **13**, 239.

Christensen, L. K. and Skovsted, L. (1969): Inhibition of drug metabolism by chloramphenicol. *Lancet*, **2**, 1397.

Cluff, L. E., Thornton, G. F. and Seidl, L. G. (1964): Studies of the epidemiology of adverse drug reactions, I. Methods of surveillance. *J. Amer. med. Assoc.*, **188**, 976.

Conney, A. H. and Burns, J. J. (1962): Factors influencing drug metabolism. *Advan. Pharmacol.*, **1**, 31.

Cucinell, S. A., Conney, A. H., Sansur, M. and Burns, J. J. (1965): Drug interactions in man. I. Lowering effect of phenobarbital on plasma levels of bishydroxycoumarin (Dicoumarol) and diphenylhydantoin. *Clin. Pharmacol. Therap.*, **6**, 240.

Esch, A. F. (1972): The planning of a national drug monitoring system, International Drug Monitoring: The Role of National Centers, No. 498, p. 44, WHO, Geneva, Switzerland.

Evans, D. A. P., Manley, K. A. and McKusick, V. A. (1960): Genetic control of isoniazid metabolism in Man. *Brit. med. J.*, **2**, 485.

Ewy, G. A., Kapadia, G. G., Yao, L., Lullin, M. and Marcus, F. I. (1969): Digoxin metabolism in the elderly. *Circulation*, **39**, 449.

Field, J. B., Ohta, M., Boyle, C. and Remmer, A. (1967): Potentiation of Acetohexamide hypoglycemia by phenylbutazone. *New. Engl. J. Med.*, **277**, 889.

Fingl, E. and Woodbury, D. M. (1971): General principles. In: *The Pharmacologic Basis of Therapeutics, 4th ed.*, p. 23. Editors: L. Goodman and A. Gilman. MacMillan, New York, N.Y.

Food and Drug Administration (1970): National Adverse Drug Reaction Directory, Rockville, Maryland.

Fowler, T. J. (1967): Some incompatibilities of intravenous admixtures, *Amer. J. Hosp. Pharm.*, **24**, 450.

Friedman, G. D., Collen, M. F., Harris, L. E., Van Brunt, E. E. and Davis, L. S. (1971): Experience in monitoring drug reactions in outpatients. *J. Amer. med. Assoc.*, **217**, 567.

Gaetano, L. F. and MacLaughlin, D. S. (1971): Data processing aspects of the Boston Collaborative Drug Surveillance Program, *Drug Information Bulletin*, p. 40.

Gardner, P. and Cluff, L. E. (1970): The epidemiology of adverse drug reactions; a review and perspective. *Johns Hopkins med. J.*, **126**, 77.

Gerhardt, R. E., Knouss, R. F., Thyrum, P. T., Luchi, R. J. and Morris, J. J. (1969): Quinidine excretion in aciduria and alkaluria. *Ann. Intern. Med.*, **71**, 927.

Glazko, A. J., Kindel, A. W., Alegnani, W. C. and Holmes, E. L. (1968): An evaluation of the absorption characteristics of different chloramphenicol preparations in normal human subjects, *Clin. Pharmacol. Therap.*, **9**, 472.

Goldstein, A., Aronow, L. and Kalman, S. (1968): Drug metabolism. In: *Principles of Drug Action*, p. 270. Harper & Rowe, New York, N.Y.

Goodman, L. S. (1964): The problem of drug efficacy: an exercise in dissection. In: *Drugs in Our Society*, p. 53. Editor: P. Talalay. The Johns Hopkins Press, Baltimore, Maryland.

Hall, G. J. L. and Davis, A. E. (1969): Inhibition of iron absorption by magnesium trisilicate. *Med. J. Aust.*, **2**, 95.

Hansen, J. M., Siersbaek-Neilsen, K. and Skovsted, L. (1971): Carbamazepine-induced acceleration of diphenylhydantoin and warfarin metabolism in man. *Clin. Pharmacol. Therap.*, **12**, 539.

Hughes, H. B., Biehl, J. P., Hones, A. P. and Schmidt, L. H. (1954): Metabolism of isoniazid in man as related to the occurrance of peripheral neuritis. *Amer. Rev. Tubercul.*, **70**, 266.

Jick, H., Slone, D., Borda, I. T. and Shapiro, S. (1968): Efficacy and toxicity of heparin in relation to age and sex. *New Engl. J. Med.*, **279**, 284.

Jick, H., Miettinen, O. S., Shapiro, S., Lewis, G. P., Sisking, V. and Slone, D. (1970): Comprehensive drug surveillance. *J. Amer. med. Assoc.*, **213**, 1455.

Kalow, W. (1962): Heredity and the response to drugs. In: *Pharmacogenetics*. W. B. Saunders, Philadelphia, Pa.

Kleinman, P. D. and Griner, P. F. (1970): Studies of the epidemiology of anticoagulant–drug interactions. *Arch. intern. Med.*, **126**, 522.

Ku, L., Ward, C. O. and Durgin, J. M. (1970): A clinical study of drug interaction and anticoagulant therapy. *Drug Intelligence clin. Pharm.*, **4**, 300.

Kunin, C. M. and Finland, M. (1961): Clinical pharmacology of the tetracycline antibiotics. *Clin. Pharmacol. Therap.*, **2**, 51.

Lang, L. A. and Kabat, H. F. (1970): Drug interactions in nursing home patients. *Amer. Pharm. Assoc., NS10*, 674.

Latiolais, C. H. and Berry, C. C. (1969): Misuse of prescription medications by outpatients. *Drug Intelligence clin. Pharm*, **3**, 270.

Lewis, R. J., Spivack, M. and Spaet, T. H. (1967): Warfarin resistance. *Amer. J. Med.*, **42**, 620.

Lindenbaum, J., Mellow, M. H., Blackstone, M. O. and Butler, V. P. (1971): Variation in biologic availability of digoxin from four preparations. *New. Engl. J. Med.*, **285**, 1344.

Loewe, S. (1953): The problem of synergism and antagonism of combined drugs. *Arzneimittel-Forsch.*, **3**, 285.

Lowe, C. U. (1968): Pediatric pharmacology. *J. clin. Pharmacol.*, **8**, 31.

Macgregor, A. G. (1965): Review of points at which drugs can interact. *Proc. Roy. Soc. Med.*, **58**, 945.

McHenry, M. C., Gaven, T. L., Gifford, R. W., Jr., Geurkink, N. A., Van Ommen, R. A., Town, M. A. and Wagner, J. G. (1971): Gentamycin dosages for renal insufficiency. Adjustments on endogenous creatinine clearance and serum creatinine concentration. *Ann. Intern. Med.*, **74**, 192.

Medical Letter (1971): Vitamin C – were the trials well controlled and are large doses safe? *Med. Letter Drugs Therap.*, **13**, 48.

Meyler, L. (1968): In: *Drug-Induced Diseases, Vol. 3*, p. 1. Editors: L. Meyler and H. M. Peck. Excerpta Medica, Amsterdam.

Misgen, R. (1965): Compatibilities and incompatibilities of some intravenous solution admixtures. *Amer. J. hosp. Pharm.*, **22**, 92.

Modell, W. (1964): The Extraordinary side effects of drugs. *Clin. Pharmacol. Therap.*, **5**, 265.

Monroe, J. F. and Cluff, L. E. (1968): Problems with multiple drugs. In: *Pharmacology for the Preoperative Visit, Vol. 6*, p. 19. Editor: J. S. Gravenstein. Little, Brown, Boston, Mass.

Neuvonen, P. J., Gothoni, G., Hackman, R. and Bjorksten, K. (1970): Interference of iron with the absorption of tetracycline in man. *Brit. med. J.*, **4**, 532.

O'Reilly, R. A., Aggeler, P. M., Hoag, M. S., Leong, L. S. and Kropatkin, M. L. (1964): Hereditary transmission of exceptional resistance to coumarin anticoagulant drugs. *New Engl. J. Med.*, **271**, 809.

O'Reilly, R. A. and Levy, G. (1970): Pharmacokinetic analysis of potentiating effect of phenylbutazone on anticoagulant action of Warfarin in man. *J. pharmac. Sci.*, **59**, 1258.

Parker, E. A. (1967): Solution additive chemical incompatibility study, *Amer. J. Hosp. Pharm.*, **24**, 434.

Patel, B. M. (1967): Skin rash with infectious mononucleosis and ampicillin, *Pediatrics*, **40**, 910.

Puckett, W. H. and Visconti, J. A. (1971): An epidemiological study of the clinical significance of drug-drug interactions in a private community hospital, *Amer. J. Hosp. Pharm.*, **28**, 247.

Remmer, H. (1962): Drugs as activators of drug enzymes. In: *Proceedings of First International Pharmacologic Meeting, Vol. 6*, p. 235. Editors: B. Brodie and E. G. Erdos. MacMillan, New York, N.Y.

Robinson, D. S. and Sylwester, D. (1970): Interaction of commonly prescribed drugs and Warfarin. *Ann. Intern. Med.*, **72**, 853.

Robinson, D. S., Benjamin, D. M. and McCormack, J. J. (1971): Interaction of Warfarin and non-systemic gastrointestinal drugs. *Clin. Pharmacol. Therap.*, **12**, 491.

Rosenthal, I. M. and Schmid, R. (1970): Disorders of porphyrin and hemoglobin metabolism. In: *Current Pediatric Therapy, 4th ed.*, p. 528. Editors S. Gellis and B. Kagan. Saunders, Philadelphia, Pa.

Sapeika, N. (1969): Foods of animal origin. In: *Food Pharmacol.*, p. 93. Thomas, Springfield, Ill.

Seidl, L. G., Thornton, G. F., Smith, F. W. and Cluff, L. E. (1966): Studies on the Epidemiology of adverse drug reactions. *Bull. Hopkins Hosp.*, **119**, 299.

Sellers, E. M. and Koch-Weser, J. (1970a): Displacement of Warfarin from human albumin by diazoxide and ethacrynic, mefenamic, and nalidixic acids. *Clin. Pharmacol. Therap.*, **11**, 524.

Sellers, E. M. and Koch-Weser, J. (1970b): Potentiation of Warfarin-induced hypoprothrombinemia by chloral hydrate. *New Engl. J. Med.*, **283**, 827.

Shoup, L. K., Anderson, R. D. and Latiolais, C. J. (1964): Stability of drugs after reconstitution. *Amer. J. Hosp. Pharma.*, **21**, 118.

Skeith, M. D., Simkin, P. A. and Healey, L. A. (1968): The renal excretion of indomethacin and its inhibition by probenecid. *Clin. Pharmacol. Therap.*, **9**, 89.

Slone, D., Gaetano, L. F., Lipworth, L., Shapiro, S., Lewis, G. P. and Jick, H. (1969): Computer analysis of epidemiologic data on effects of drugs on hospital patients. *Publ. Hlth Reports*, **84**, 39.

Smith, J. W., Seidl, L. G. and Cluff, L. E. (1969): Studies on the epidemiology of adverse drug reactions. V. Clinical factors influencing susceptibility. *Ann. intern. Med.*, **65**, 629.

Solomon, H. M. and Thomas, G. B. (1971): A rapid method for the estimation of drug–albumin affinity constants in human plasma. *Clin. Pharmacol. Therap.*, **12**, 445.

Speck, W. T. (1971): High frequency of ampicillin rashes in infectious mononucleosis. *Clin. Pediat.*, **10**, 59.

Stewart, R. B. and Cluff, L. E. (1971): Studies on the epidemiology of adverse drug reactions. VI. Utilization and interactions of prescription and non-prescription drugs in outpatients. *Johns Hopkins med. J.*, **129**, 319.

Stewart, R. B. and Cluff, L. E. (1972): A review of medication errors and compliance in ambulant patients. *Clin. Pharmacol. Therap.*, **13**, 463.

Taussig, H. B. (1962): A study of the German outbreak of phocomelia. *J. Amer. med. Assoc.*, **180**, 1106.

Vessell, E. S., Passananti, G. T. and Greene, F. E. (1970): Impairment of drug metabolism in man by allopurinol and nortriptyline. *New Engl. J. Med.*, **283**, 1484.

Wagner, J. G. (1971): Generic equivalence and inequivalence of oral products. *Drug. Intell. Clin. Pharm.*, **5**, 115.

Webb, J. W. (1969): A pH pattern for i.v. additives. *Amer. J. hosp. Pharm.*, **26**, 31.

Westerholm, B. (1972): The Swedish drug monitoring system. International Drug Monitoring: The Role of National Centers, No. 498, p. 27. WHO, Geneva, Switzerland.

Woodbury, D. M. (1971): Analgesics–antipyretics, anti-inflammatory agents, and inhibitors of uric acid synthesis. In: *The Pharmacologic Basis of Therapeutics, 4th ed.*, p. 314. Editors: L. Goodman and A. Gilman. MacMillan, New York, N.Y.

CHAPTER 4

Pharmacokinetic aspects of drug interactions

L. DETTLI

Pharmacokinetics may be defined as the discipline which describes concentration changes of drugs in the organism as a function of time. Since the present volume is intended for the interested physician, the above definition poses a serious problem because physicians are not primarily interested in going deeply into mathematics. Still worse, the mathematics of interaction kinetics is even more complex than most equations describing the kinetics of a single drug because so-called 'non-linear' processes (Wagner, 1971) are involved in most cases. On the other hand, it is impossible to avoid the mathematical tool. However, for the reasons just outlined, approximations, simplifications and semiquantitative analogies will be extensively used and only the very simplest equations will be presented in order to demonstrate some of the factors responsible for drug interaction on a kinetic level. The discussion will be restricted to the following topics: (i) some basic concepts which allow description of quantitative or conceptual characteristics of drug interaction kinetics, and (ii) some clinically important pharmacokinetic consequences of drug interactions.

1 Pharmacokinetic bases of drug interactions

1.1 DRUG ELIMINATION

In this context the term 'elimination' denotes the sum of all processes resulting in a decreased amount of unchanged drug in the organism (Dettli and Spring, 1968a; Dost, 1968). For the sake of simplicity, it is assumed in this section that the drug is not bound to the plasma proteins and that its elimination kinetics can be described by a one-compartment model.

1.1.1 *The concept of 'first-order kinetics'*

The most important tools of pharmacokinetics are equations describing the concentration or amount of drug in the organism as a function of time. Thus, the decline of the plasma concentration, *c*, of many drugs can be described with sufficient approximation by the following equation:

$$\frac{-\mathrm{d}c}{\mathrm{d}t} = k \times c, \tag{1}$$

where *k* is called the 'elimination rate constant'. The minus sign signifies that *c* decreases with time. Eq. 1 states that the *change* of the variable per unit of time ($-\mathrm{d}c/\mathrm{d}t$) is proportional to the *value* of the variable (c) or, in other words, that $-\mathrm{d}c/\mathrm{d}t$ is a constant fraction (k) of c:

$$\frac{-\mathrm{d}c/\mathrm{d}t}{c} = k. \tag{2}$$

Any process which can be described in this way is called a *'first-order process'* because the exponent of the variable on the right side of eq. 1 is unity ($c = c^1$). The expression *'linear kinetics'* is also used because the concentration–time curve is a straight line when plotted semilogarithmically. In the linear plot the negative slope decreases with decreasing values of *c* (see fig. 1).

Fig. 1. Concentration–time curves of two hypothetical drugs during the elimination process. a) semi-logarithmic plot; b) linear plot. *Curve 1:* First-order elimination according to eq. 1. *Curve 2:* Capacity-limited elimination according to eq. 16 and 19. Note the transition from apparent zero-order to apparent first-order kinetics. For further explanations see text and Table II.

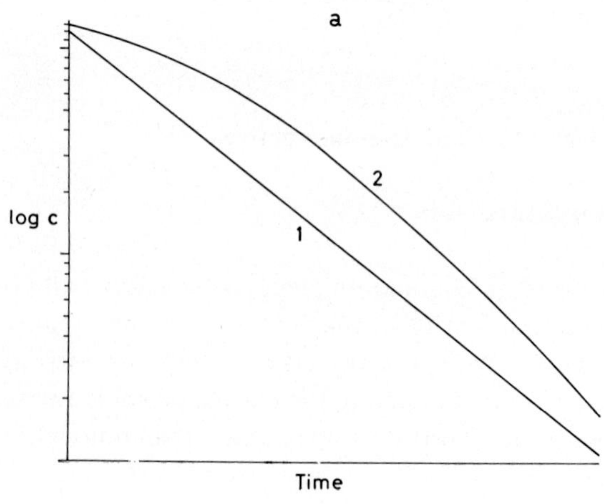

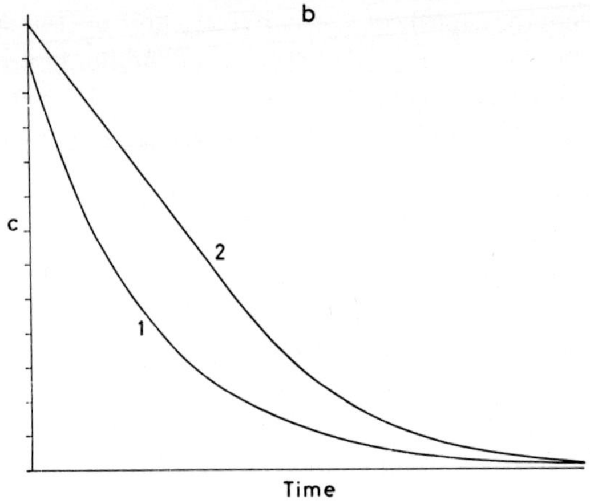

It is evident that eq. 1 tells nothing of the factors influencing the elimination process and contains therefore no element indicating the possibility of drug interactions. Since first order processes are very common in nature, the problem can be discussed using a much simpler analogous example (Dettli and Spring, 1970).

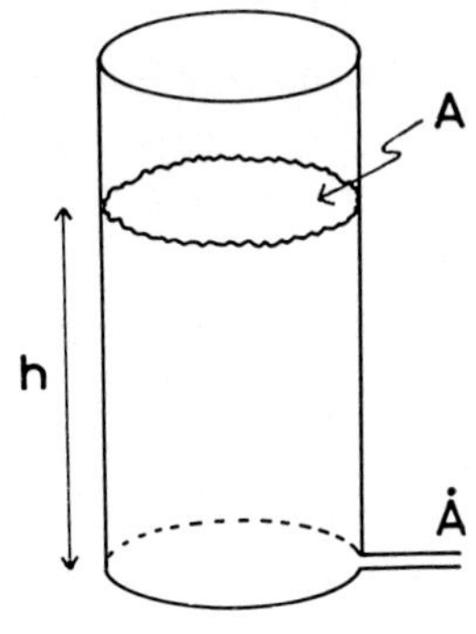

Fig. 2. A hydrokinetic first-order 'elimination' process: The water in the vessel with the cross sectional area *A* empties through a capillary at the bottom. When the flow in the capillary is laminar the decline of the height of the water-level, *h*, with time is a first order process described by eq. 3 and will be proportional to the conductivity of the capillary, *A*, of the vessel. For further explanations see text.

The water in the vessel depicted in fig. 2 empties through a narrow capillary at the bottom. When the flow in the capillary is laminar the decline of the height, h, of the water level with time is a first order process:

$$-\mathrm{d}h/\mathrm{d}t = k \times h. \qquad (3)$$

Again, eq. 3 tells nothing of the factors influencing the emptying process. However, by varying the experimental conditions, Poiseuille demonstrated that the rate constant (k) depends on the following factors: on the radius, r

(cm), and the length, l (cm), of the capillary, and on the specific gravity, ρ (g*/cm³), and the viscosity, η (g*min/cm²), of the fluid. Furthermore, it is evident that k must be inversely proportional to the cross-sectional area, A (cm²), of the vessel. As a result, Poisseuille obtained the following expression (Poisseuille's law):

$$k = \frac{r^4 \times \pi \times \rho}{8\eta \times l \times A}. \tag{4a}$$

By introducing eq. 4a in eq. 3 one finds:

$$-\mathrm{d}h/\mathrm{d}t = \left(\frac{r^4 \times \pi \times \rho}{8\eta \times l \times A}\right) \times h. \tag{4b}$$

It is now clear from eq. 4b that any change in one of the factors between the brackets will influence k. For example, the addition of glycerol would change the values of ρ and η and may be taken as an analogue of a 'drug' interaction. It should be noted that in this case only the *value* of k is changed whereas the emptying process still obeys first-order kinetics.

However, the system can be influenced in such a way that the emptying process no longer obeys first-order kinetics. For example, when only a small amount of water is used resulting in a much lower height of the water level, it turns out that $-\mathrm{d}h/\mathrm{d}t$ is no longer proportional to h as indicated in eq. 2 but rather to the square root of h (Torricelli's law). On the other hand, when the water level is very high and when the capillary has some critical diameter, flow will become turbulent. As a result, the relation of —$\mathrm{d}h/\mathrm{d}t$ to h will become highly complex. Since these profound kinetic changes of the emptying process were brought about by simply changing the 'dose' of water, one could speak of 'dose-dependent' kinetics.

The following conclusions which are valid for any kinetic process may be drawn from these facts: a pharmacokinetic equation is no more than a mathematical description of a process and tells nothing of its 'real' nature. In order to find the factors which may possibly interact with the process, the equations must be interpreted in the light of established physico-chemical and biological knowledge. In pharmacokinetics, the problem is to describe the transport and the transformation of substances in molecular dispersion. In the living organism the following processes are involved: macroscopic flow; ultrafiltration; diffusion; metabolic transformation; 'active' transport; and macromolecular binding of drug molecules. Consequently, the equations must be discussed in the light of our present knowledge in these fields. When a process is found to obey first-order kinetics, this may be true only under certain experimental conditions. It appears therefore appropriate to use the term '*apparent*' first-order kinetics. Insight into the true nature of the process may be gained by varying the experimental conditions such as the dosage range. With these considerations in mind, some aspects and consequences of drug interaction kinetics will be discussed in the following sections.

1.1.2 *Glomerular filtration*

In order to discuss glomerular filtration of drugs, we introduce the clearance concept as follows: the constants r, ρ, η and l in eq. 4 describe the interaction between the fluid and the capillary, in other words, these constants characterize the *conductivity* of the system and may therefore be combined into one single *conductivity constant*, $\dot{A}$. On the other hand, the cross-sectional area, $A = m/h$, is a *capacity constant* because it characterizes the capacity of the system and relates the height h of the water level to the amount m of water in the vessel. It follows from eq. 4 that:

$$k = \frac{\dot{A}}{A} \tag{5}$$

According to eq. 5 the rate constant is proportional to the conductivity, $\dot{A}$, and inversely proportional to the capacity, A, of the system.

In pharmacokinetics, the 'conductivity' constant, $\dot{V}$, of the drug-eliminating organs is called '*clearance*', and the capacity constant, $V = m/c$, relating the amount of drug, m, in the organism to its plasma concentration, c, is called '*distribution volume*'. In analogy to eq. 5 one can write

$$k = \frac{\dot{V}}{V}. \tag{6}$$

Introducing eq. 6 in eq. 1 results in

$$-\mathrm{d}c/\mathrm{d}t = \frac{\dot{V}}{V} \times c. \tag{6a}$$

When eq. 6a is multiplied by V, one obtains

$$-\mathrm{d}m/\mathrm{d}t = \dot{V} \times c, \tag{6b}$$

i.e. the amount of drug eliminated per unit of time.

In the glomeruli of the kidneys, a certain fraction – the so-called *filtration fraction,p* – of the plasma flow, $\dot{F}$, is ultrafiltered into the tubular lumen:

$$\dot{V} = \dot{F} \times p. \tag{7}$$

Combining eqs. 1, 6 and 7, results in

$$-\mathrm{d}c/\mathrm{d}t = \frac{\dot{F} \times p}{V} \times c = k \times c. \tag{8}$$

Eq. 8 indicates that the elimination of a drug by glomerular filtration is a first-order process. Based on the well-known physico-chemical rule that the filtration or diffusion of one molecular species is usually not influenced by the presence of another molecular species, it may be predicted that direct drug interactions are unlikely to occur in glomerular filtration. However, as indicated in eq. 8 the process depends on the plasma flow, $\dot{F}$, through the glomeruli and on the filtration fraction, p, which is influenced by the intra-glomerular pressure and by the contact time. It is therefore to be expected that any drug influencing intraglomerular flow or pressure may influence the elimination of itself and of other drugs. Examples are blood pressure lowering agents and thiazide diuretics.

1.1.3 *Tubular 'reabsorption'*

About 99% of the water filtered through the glomerular membrane is 'actively' reabsorbed by the tubular cells. As a consequence, the concentration of a filtered drug will increase in the tubular lumen and will exceed greatly the drug concentration in the peritubular capillaries. The drug molecules in the tubular fluid tend therefore to diffuse back into the peritubular capillaries. This process is usually called 'tubular reabsorption'. It should be emphasized however, that no 'active' transport is usually involved in the case of substances foreign to the body. It appears therefore reasonable to assume that tubular 'reabsorption' of drugs may be adequately described by the rules governing passive diffusion of small molecules through cellular membranes. As in the case of filtration, direct interactions between different molecules are unlikely to occur. However, one of these rules – the so-called 'non-ionic partition theory' – states (Milne et al., 1958) that cellular membranes are much more permeable to nonpolar ('lipid-soluble') than to polar ('water-soluble') molecules. When a drug is an acid or a base, it will undergo hydrolytic dissociation. The ionized moiety is usually much more polar than the neutral molecule and will therefore permeate much less through the tubular cells. It follows that the extent of tubular 'reabsorption' depends on the degree of ionization of the drug in the tubular fluid. According to the law of mass action, the fraction of neutral molecules, φ, depends on the pH of the solvent. The administration of acidifying or alkalinizing agents will therefore influence the elimination rate of acidic and basic drugs.

In the following discussion an acidic drug, SH, which dissociates according to the scheme $SH \rightleftharpoons S^- + H^+$ is taken as an example. The fraction of neutral molecules, $\varphi = SH/(S^- + SH)$, depends in the following way on the hydrogen ion concentration (H^+) and on the apparent acid dissociation constant (K_a) of the drug: according to the law of mass action one has to write $(S^-) \times (H^+) = K_a \times (SH)$. By rearrangement one finds

$$\frac{(S^-)}{(SH)} = \frac{K_a}{(H^+)} \tag{9a}$$

Adding (SH)/(SH) = 1 on the left side and $(H^+)/(H^+) = 1$ on the right side of eq. 9a yields:

$$\frac{(S^-) + (SH)}{(SH)} = \frac{(H^+) + K_a}{(H^+)}. \tag{9b}$$

The reciprocal value of eq. 9b is

$$\varphi = \frac{(SH)}{(S^-) + (SH)} = \frac{(H^+)}{(H^+) + K_a} = \frac{1}{1 + K_a/(H^+)} = \frac{1}{1 + 10^{pH - pK_a}}. \tag{9c}$$

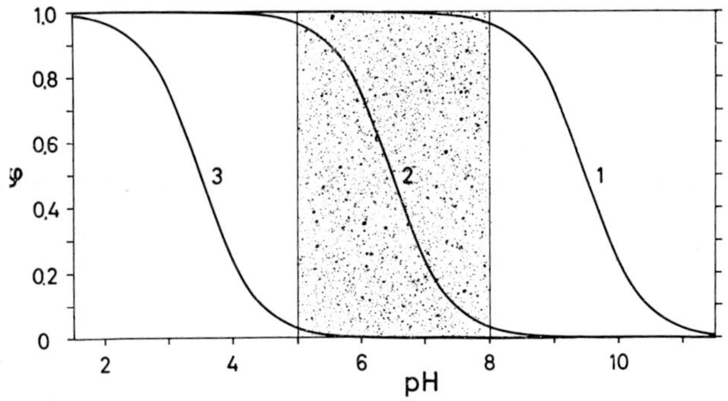

Fig. 3. The fraction of neutral molecules of three hypothetical acidic drugs with different pK_a-values as a function of the pH of the solvent according to eq. 9c. The shaded area represents the physiological range of the urine pH. When the pK of the drug is above the physiological pH-range of the urine (*curve 1*, $pK_a = 9.5$) the fraction and the concentration of neutral diffusible molecules, φ, will be high in the alkaline as well as in the acid urine. When the pK_a of the drug lies within the physiological range of the urine pH (*curve 2*, $pK_a = 6.5$), φ is small in the alkaline and much greater in the acid urine. When the pK_a of the drug lies below the physiological range of the urine pH (*curve 3*, $pK_a = 3.5$), the concentration of neutral molecules is low both in the alkaline and in the acid urine. The consequences of these facts are predicted by eq. 10 and discussed in the text.

K_a characterizes the strength of the acid, i.e. the affinity between ionized molecules (S^-) and hydrogen ions (H^+). Its value decreases with increasing strength of the acid. When $K_a = (H^+)$ one finds $\varphi = 0.5$. K_a may therefore be defined as the hydrogen ion concentration where half of the drug molecules are ionized. pH and pK_a are the negative logarithms of (H^+) and K_a respectively. Fig. 3 shows the values of φ as a function of the urine pH for three hypothetical acidic drugs with different pK_a values. As can be seen, the fraction, φ, of neutral diffusible molecules decreases with increasing pH values of the urine. It follows that the renal elimination of acidic drugs will be faster in the alkaline than in the acidic urine. When the urine pH is raised from $pH_1 = 5$ to $pH_2 = 8$ by the administration of alkali, the ratio, $G = \varphi_1/\varphi_2$ between the corresponding φ values can be described by the following equation:

$$G = \varphi_1/\varphi_2 = \frac{\dfrac{1}{1+10^{pH_1 - pK_a}}}{\dfrac{1}{1+10^{pH_2 - pK_a}}} = \frac{1+10^{pH_2 - pK_a}}{1+10^{pH_1 - pK_a}} = \frac{1+10^{8 - pK_a}}{1+10^{5 - pK_a}} \tag{10}$$

According to eq. 10, the influence of alkali administration on the value of G decreases with increasing values of its pK_a and is negligible in the case of very weak acids (p$K_a > 8$). However, as can be concluded from fig. 3, the concentrations of neutral drug molecules become very small in both alkaline and acid urine when the pK_a of the drug lies markedly below the physiological pH range of the urine. The same must be true for the concentration *differences* between the intratubular and the peritubular fluid. Since this concentration difference is the 'driving force' of tubular 'reabsorption', it follows that the influence of alkali administration on the elimination rate of acidic drugs reaches a maximum when the pK_a of the drug lies in the lower physiological pH range of the urine or somewhat below. Table I shows how the elimination rate of different sulphonamides could be increased by the concomitant administration of sodium bicarbonate (Dettli and Spring, 1968a, b). As predicted by eq. 10, the effect of alkalinisation increases with decreasing pK_a values of the drug.

Sulphamethoxazole is an exception to this rule: Despite its relatively low pK_a, the elimination rate increases only slightly. This is due to the fact that sulphamethoxazole is so extensively metabolized that only a small fraction of the dose is eliminated unchanged in the urine. The overall elimination rate constant, k, is therefore the sum of the renal elimination rate constant, k_I, and the metabolic elimination rate constant, k_{II}:

$$k = k_I + k_{II}. \tag{11}$$

TABLE I

The influence of alkali administration and of sleep on the elimination rate of five sulphonamides with different pK_a values

Compound	pK_a	Q_{pH}	$Q_{n/d}$
Sulphisoxazole	4.9	2.0	2.5
Sulphasymazine	5.5	2.4	2.9
Sulphamethoxazole	5.6	1.4	1.5
Sulphasomidine	7.4	1.2	1.4
Sulphanilamide	10.5	1.0	1.1

The quotient Q indicates how many times the elimination rates of the drugs increased during concomitant alkali administration (Q_{pH}) or after the transition from sleep to wakefulness ($Q_{n/d}$). For the discussion of the results see text.

For drugs which are eliminated by two different pathways, I and II, with the rate constants k_{I} and k_{II}, respectively, the following rule of general validity may be derived from eq. 11: when an interacting substance influences only one of several elimination rate constants, e.g. k_{I}, the influence on the overall elimination rate constant, k, will hardly be of practical significance, when $k_{\mathrm{I}} \ll k_{\mathrm{II}}$. For example, when only 10% of a drug is eliminated by the kidneys ($k_{\mathrm{I}}=0.1\ k$) and 90% by hepatic metabolism ($k_{\mathrm{II}}=0.9\ k$), the overall elimination rate constant, k, will increase only by 10% when k_{I} increases by 100%. In contrast, when 90% of a drug is eliminated by the kidneys ($k_{\mathrm{I}}=0.9\ k$) k will increase by 90% when k_{I} increases by 100%.

An interesting consequence of non-ionic tubular drug reabsorption is the finding that the renal elimination of acidic drug decreases during sleep (Dettli and Spring, 1966). The phenomenon is caused by the slight acidosis elicited by sleep. Table I shows the influence of sleep on the elimination of different sulphonamides. As in the case of alkali administration, the elimination rate is influenced most when the pK_a of the drug is in the lower physiological range of the urine pH. It may be concluded from these facts that the administration of an anesthetic or of a strong hypnotic may influence the renal elimination of ionized drugs.

The same considerations apply to the interaction of acidifying and alkalinizing substances with the renal elimination of alkaline drugs. In this case the fraction of neutral molecules depends in the following way on the pH of the urine:

$$\varphi = \frac{(\mathrm{SOH})}{(\mathrm{S}^+)+(\mathrm{SOH})} = \frac{{}^{\mathrm{ɐ}}K\ \mathrm{H}^+}{K_a+(\mathrm{H}^+)} = \frac{1}{1+10^{\mathrm{p}K_a-\mathrm{pH}}} \tag{12}$$

It follows from eq. 12 that the renal elimination of alkaline drugs such as amphetamine (Rowland et al., 1965) is decreased by the concomitant administration of alkalinizing agents and increases during sleep.

The renal clearance of substances such as inulin is independent of urine flow within wide limits. This is not true for drugs undergoing tubular 'reabsorption', because when a great amount of water or a strong diuretic is administered concomitantly with such drugs, the extent of tubular water reabsorption and consequently the increase in intratubular drug concentration will be smaller. As a consequence of the smaller 'driving force' the extent of tubular reabsorption will decrease resulting in a faster elimination of the drug. In addition, the increased urine flow decreases the contact time of the drug with the tubular wall and may thus further diminish tubular reabsorption.

These kinetic factors should be considered when patients with drug intoxication are to be treated by forced diuresis and the administration of acidifying or alkalinizing agents.

1.1.4 *Tubular secretion*

Many organic acids and bases in therapeutic use are eliminated in the kidneys by 'active' tubular secretion (Milne et al., 1958; Weiner and Mudge, 1964). Most authors assume that this transport process is mediated by reversible binding of drug molecules to carrier macromolecules in the tubular cell wall. When reversible binding of molecules is involved it appears probable that the process may be described by the law of mass action. Under the reasonable assumption that the rate of drug transport, $v = -\mathrm{d}m/\mathrm{d}t$, is proportional to the fraction of binding sites occupied by drug molecules, b, one may write:

$$v = -\mathrm{d}m/\mathrm{d}t = k' \times n \times b, \tag{13}$$

where n is the number of binding sites of the carrier molecules. The transport system is saturated and the transport rate reaches its maximum, $v_{\max}$, when all binding sites are occupied, i.e. when $b = 1$. It follows that

$$v_{\max} = k' \times n. \tag{14}$$

Using for b the same expression as for φ in eq. 9c and introducing eq. 14 into eq. 13 results in

$$v = -\mathrm{d}m/\mathrm{d}t = v_{\max} \times b = v_{\max} \times \frac{c}{c + K'} \tag{15}$$

In eq. 15, K' is the dissociation constant of the drug–carrier complex characterizing the affinity of the drug molecules to the carrier molecules, and c is the drug concentration in the plasma*. In order to demonstrate how the elimination rate ($-\mathrm{d}m/\mathrm{d}t$) is related to the plasma concentration (c) of the drug, we consider the following hypothetical example (see Table II): Let $v_{max}=10$ mass units per time unit and $K'=100$ concentration units. The elimination rate, $-\mathrm{d}m/\mathrm{d}t$, is now calculated according to eq. 15 for a concentration range between 10^{-2} and 10^5 concentration units. As can be seen from the results in column B of Table II the elimination rate of the drug increases in proportion to the drug concentration in the plasma when $c \ll K'$. However, with increasing values of c, the elimination rate increases less than proportional and approaches the constant maximum value, $v_{max}=10$.

TABLE II

Capacity-limited elimination kinetics

A	B	C	D
c	$-\mathrm{d}m/\mathrm{d}t$	$-\mathrm{d}c/\mathrm{d}t$	k
10^{-2}	10^{-3}	10^{-4}	10^{-2}
10^{-1}	10^{-2}	10^{-3}	10^{-2}
1	10^{-1}	10^{-2}	10^{-2}
10	9.1×10^{-1}	0.9×10^{-1}	0.9×10^{-2}
10^2	5.0	0.5	0.5×10^{-2}
10^3	9.1	0.9	0.9×10^{-3}
10^4	10	1.0	10^{-4}
10^5	10	1.0	10^{-5}

Based on a hypothetical example it is demonstrated how the elimination rate ($-\mathrm{d}m/\mathrm{d}t$ and $-\mathrm{d}c/\mathrm{d}t$) and the elimination rate constant (k) depend on the plasma concentration (c). The results which have been calculated according to eqs. 3, 15 and 16 are discussed in the text.

When a process is described by eq. 15 we speak of a saturable or capacity-limited process. The corresponding equation describing the concentration curve in the plasma is found by dividing eq. 15 through the distribution volume, V, of the drug:

$$-\mathrm{d}c/\mathrm{d}t = \frac{-\mathrm{d}m/\mathrm{d}t}{V} = \frac{v_{max}}{V} \times \frac{c}{c+K'} \qquad (16)$$

* Note that the binding affinity increases with *decreasing* values of the dissociation constant and vice versa.

It is evident that eq. 16 is not a first-order process because $-\mathrm{d}c/\mathrm{d}t$ is not simply proportional to c.

Assuming a value of $V=10$ volume units we calculate values of $-\mathrm{d}c/\mathrm{d}t$ for our hypothetical example. From the results in column C of Table II it is evident that $-\mathrm{d}c/\mathrm{d}t$ increases also in proportion to c when $c \ll K'$. With increasing values of c, the increase in $\mathrm{d}c/\mathrm{d}t$ is again less than proportional and approaches the maximum value $-\mathrm{d}c/\mathrm{d}t = v_{\max}/V = 1.0$. When the elimination rate constant, k, is calculated according to eq. 2 the results listed in column D of Table II are found. As can be seen, k is also a constant when $c \ll K$. With increasing values of c, the values of k no longer remain constant but decline steadily. Since k describes the negative slope of the concentration–time curve in the semilogarithmic plot during the elimination process, it follows from these results that the semilogarithmically plotted concentration–time curve will not be linear. Instead, immediately after the absorption of a high dose, the slope of the curve is small and then increases steadily with decreasing values of c until a constant value is approached in the lowest concentration range resulting in 'apparent' first-order kinetics (see fig. 1). With a lower dose the curve would follow first-order kinetics during the whole period of elimination. We speak therefore of '*dose-dependent kinetics*'.

The existence of capacity-limited tubular drug transport processes which can be described by the law of mass action constitutes the basis for possible kinetic drug interactions. Based on the well established fact that a great number of organic anions undergo tubular secretion, the assumption appears reasonable that all these drugs are bound and transported by the same carrier molecules. This lack of specificity of the transport mechanism combined with its saturable nature opens up the possibility that the secretion of a drug is competitively inhibited by a second drug. It is intuitively clear that the inhibitory effect of an interacting drug will increase with its increasing plasma concentration and with its increasing affinity to the carrier molecules (i.e. with decreasing values of K'). In mathematical terms this results in the following equation:

$$-\mathrm{d}c_{\mathrm{I}}/\mathrm{d}t = \frac{v_{\mathrm{I}\,\max}}{V_{\mathrm{I}}} \times \frac{c_{\mathrm{I}}}{c_{\mathrm{I}} + K'_{\mathrm{I}} \times (1 + c_{\mathrm{II}}/K'_{\mathrm{II}})} \qquad (17)$$

The symbols of eq. 17 have the same meaning as in eq. 16. The only difference is that the subscript I refers to an inhibited drug I and subscript II to an inhibiting drug II. When the lack of specificity of the transport system involved is considered, it must be concluded that such kinetic drug interactions must occur rather frequently at the tubular level. The well known inhibition of the renal secretion of penicillin by probenecid is just one of many examples. According to eq. 17 a competitive inhibition results in an increased value of the denominator of the right-hand term of eq. 17 and consequently a decreased slope, $-dc_I/dt$, of the time–concentration curve of drug I in the plasma. However, in many instances the conditions $c_{II} \ll K'_{II}$, $K'_{II} \gg K'_I$, and/or $c_{II} \ll c_I$ are fulfilled. Under these conditions, the inhibitory effect may be so small that it remains undetected and is of no practical significance. However, when $c_I \ll K'_I$ it follows that $c_I + K'_I \times (1 + c_{II}/K'_{II}) \simeq K'_I \times (1 + c_{II}/K'_{II})$. Combining the three constants $v_{I\,max}$, V_I and K'_I into one single rate constant, $k = v_{max}/(V_I \times K'_I)$, results in the following expression:

$$-dc_I/dt = k \times \frac{c_I}{1 + c_{II}/K'_{II}}. \tag{18}$$

When drug II is administered by continuous infusion, c_{II} will approach a constant steady-state value. Eq. 18 predicts under these circumstances that the elimination rate of drug I will be slower than normal by a factor $(1 + c_{II}/K'_{II})$ but the elimination will still follow first order kinetics.

1.1.5 *Biliary excretion*

Many drugs are secreted into the bile by an active, saturable and unspecific transport system. Therefore, as far as drug interactions at this level are concerned, very similar considerations apply as in the case of tubular secretion, although the process may be complicated by the huge storage capacity of the liver for some drugs. A typical example are the rifamycin antibiotics which inhibit the biliary excretion of bilirubin and of bromsulfalein (Acocella et al., 1965). A bromsulfalein test performed during rifamycin administration will therefore yield pathological results. This should not be interpreted as a sign of liver toxicity due to rifamycin but rather as the consequence of a mutual biliary transport inhibition.

1.1.6 *Metabolism*

Until recently, it was generally accepted that the metabolic transformations of all substances foreign to the body with the notable exception of ethyl alcohol, follow first-order kinetics (Dost, 1968). However, drug transformations are enzymatic processes involving the reversible binding of drug molecules to a limited number of enzyme molecules. It appears therefore reasonable to assume that the kinetics of drug transformations may be described by the law of mass action, i.e. that eqs. 15 and 16 are valid*. Whether or not saturation phenomena occur to a clinically significant extent depends again on the relation of K to c. Thus, $K' \gg c$ will result in apparent first-order kinetics. In contrast, when $K' \ll c$ it follows from eq. 16 that $c/(K'+c)=1$. The remaining constants, v_{max} and V, may be combined into a single constant, $k^* = v_{max}/V$, and eq. 16 will then be reduced to

$$-\mathrm{d}c/\mathrm{d}t = k^*. \qquad (19)$$

Eq. 19 describes a *zero-order process* because the exponent of the variable is zero ($c^0=1$). The concentration–time curve corresponding to eq. 19 is not linear in a semi-logarithmic but rather in a linear plot (see fig. 1). It is well known from forensic medicine that this is characteristic for ethyl alcohol in man. It follows from these considerations that metabolic zero-order and first-order processes should be interpreted as special cases of capacity-limited or Michaelis–Menten kinetics. This statement is corroborated by the fact that alcohol elimination becomes a first-order process in the very low concentration range. Such a behaviour is predicted by eq. 16 because the condition $K' \ll c$ is no longer fulfilled (see fig. 1).

Moreover, it is well known that most drug metabolizing enzymes are highly unspecific. As a consequence, the possibility of metabolic drug interactions must be postulated. This would mean that eq. 17 with all its consequences is also valid for metabolic drug transformations.

The validity of these concepts has been proven beyond doubt during recent years. For example, the kinetics of salicylic acid metabolism exhibit saturation phenomena even in the low therapeutic concentration range. As a consequence, the elimination rate of salicylic acid decreases almost 10-fold when the dose is increased from 0.25 to 10–20 g. In a series of elegant experiments, Levy (1968) was able to show that it is notably the conjugation of salicylic acid with glycine which has a very limited capacity in man, and that the deviations from apparent first-order kinetics can be adequately described by Michaelis–Menten kinetics. Moreover, several cases of unequivocal competitive metabolic drug interactions could be demonstrated. For example, the conjugation of salicylic acid with glucuronic acid is competitively inhibited by salicylamide. Salicylamide is a drug which is also partly conjugated with glucuronic acid in man (Levy and Matsuzawa, 1967).

* In enzyme kinetics the terms 'capacity-limited kinetics' or 'dose-dependent kinetics' are replaced by the term Michaelis–Menten kinetics and the dissociation constant is called Michaelis–Menten constant.

Similarly, the transformation of salicylic acid to salicyluric acid by the conjugation with glycine is competitively inhibited by the concomitant administration of benzoic acid, a drug which is transformed to hippuric acid by the conjugation with glycine. In these cases it could be shown that the concomitantly administered drugs compete for a limited number of enzymatic binding sites.

Another type of kinetic drug interaction has been observed between high doses of benzoic acid and glycine. In this case the capacity-limiting step in the formation of hippurate from benzoate is not the limited amount of enzyme but rather the availability of glycine (Levy and Amsel, 1966). The rate of hippurate formation can therefore be increased by co-administration of glycine.

Competitive kinetic drug interactions may be of therapeutic importance. An example is the administration of ethyl alcohol in cases of acute ethylene glycol intoxication. The toxicity of ethylene glycol is mainly due to its metabolic transformation to oxalic acid resulting in fatal crystalluria. This metabolic process is competitively inhibited by ethyl alcohol and ethylene glycol is slowly eliminated unchanged (Wacker et al., 1965).

There is little doubt that many similar examples of saturation kinetics and drug interactions will be found in the future. As a prerequisite, kinetic studies should be performed after the administration of widely different doses and of different drug combinations.

A special characteristic of drug metabolism is the possibility of *enzyme induction* (Conney, 1967) caused by coadministration or pre-treatment with a second drug. In terms of eqs. 13 and 16 this means an increase in the number of enzymic binding sites (n) and consequently of v_{max}.

There are several examples described in literature where a drug readily stimulated the metabolism of another drug in vitro and apparently failed to do so in man or in the animal. Such discrepancies may be explained by the following kinetic facts:

(1) When a drug is eliminated by two different pathways, I and II, characterized by the rate constants k_{I} and k_{II}, respectively, and only one of them – say pathway I – is stimulated, the overall elimination rate will hardly increase when $k_{I} \ll k_{II}$ (see the discussion of eq. 11).

(2) Let c_{in} and c_{out} be the concentrations of a drug in the blood entering and leaving a metabolizing organ respectively. When $\dot{F}$ is the blood flow, the amount of drug metabolized in one passage through the organ will be $-dm/dt = \dot{F} \times (c_{in} - c_{out})$. According to eq. 6b this is equivalent to $\dot{V} \times c_{in}$ when $\dot{V}$ is the metabolic clearance of the drug:

$$\dot{F} \times (c_{in} - c_{out}) = \dot{V} \times c_{in}. \tag{20}$$

It follows from eq. 20 that

$$\dot{F} \times \frac{c_{in} - c_{out}}{c_{in}} = \dot{F} \times z = \dot{V}. \tag{21}$$

The expression $(c_{in} - c_{out})/c_{in} = z$ is called '*extraction ratio*' because it describes the fraction of drug which is removed in one passage from the blood flowing through the metabolizing organ. It follows:

$$z = \frac{\dot{V}}{\dot{F}}. \tag{22}$$

When a drug is completely metabolized during one passage (i.e. when $\dot{V} = \dot{F}$) it follows $c_{out} = 0$ and $z = 1.0$. Consequently, 1.0 is the highest possible value of z. When a drug such as propranolol (Shand et al., 1971), has a high extraction ratio ($z \to 1.0$), the rate of its metabolism becomes flow-limited. As a result, even a marked increase of v_{max} caused by enzyme stimulation will not appreciably increase the metabolic rate as long as liver blood flow is not simultaneously increased. So far only one paper has been published in the literature (Ohnhaus et al., 1971) reporting an increase in liver blood flow concomitantly with enzyme induction.

These considerations are not valid in the case of *inhibition* of drug metabolism, because it follows from eq. 21 that the metabolic clearance will decrease in proportion to the degree of inhibition, irrespective of the value of z.

(3) When the rate-limiting step in a metabolic transformation is not the limited amount of enzyme but rather the availability of a conjugation substrate, enzyme induction will not result in an increased metabolic transformation rate unless the conjugation substrate is concomitantly administered. The transformation of benzoic acid to hippuric acid by conjugation with glycine mentioned above is an example.

1.2 DRUG DISTRIBUTION

The problem of drug distribution cannot be discussed without taking into consideration that most drugs are partly bound to the plasma proteins. (In this section all symbols relating to the total drug concentration will be denoted by a prime (c', V'). In contrast, c signifies the concentration of unbound drug in the plasma water and c'' the concentration of protein bound drug in the plasma.)

The term 'distribution' has two different meanings in medical literature. The word is used in the sense of a kinetic *process (distribution rate)* and in the sense of a state, i.e. of a spatial distribution *pattern (distribution equili-*

brium). The second connotation which is the subject of the following discussion led to numerous misinterpretations in medical literature because it is often not sufficiently realized that the kinetic term 'distribution volume' (V') is no more than a mathematical capacity constant (Dettli and Spring, 1970) relating the drug concentration in the plasma, c', to the drug amount in the organism, m:$V' = m/c'$. As a consequence, V' does not correspond to a physiological fluid space and tells little on the 'real' distribution of a drug in the organism and on the factors influencing the distribution equilibrium. When the problem is analyzed in the light of present knowledge, at least the following 'real' spaces should be considered: the plasma space, V_p, the interstitial space, V_i, the intracellular space, V_c, and the lipid space, V_f. Under conditions of equilibrium the concentrations of freely dissolved molecules in the interstitial water (c_i) and in the plasma water ($c = c_p$) are equal. However, c_p is only a fraction, $f = c_p/c'_p$, of the total concentration because the drug is partly protein-bound.
From this it follows that $c'_p = c_p/f_p$ and $c'_i = c_i/f_i$. Moreover, in order to account for the possible binding of drug molecules to enzymes and other macromolecules in the intracellular space, one has to write $c'_c = c_c/f_c$. In the case of acidic or basic drugs, pH differences between the intracellular and the interstitial spaces must be taken into consideration because the theory of non ionic partitioning predicts that only unionized molecules will equilibrate through the call walls until $c_i \times \varphi_i = c_c \times \varphi_c$. From this it follows that:

$$c_c = c_i \times \frac{\varphi_i}{\varphi_c} = c_p \times \frac{\varphi_i}{\varphi_c}. \tag{23}$$

Since many experimental findings indicate that the intracellular pH is lower than the pH of the interstitial fluid eqs. 9, 12 and 23 predict that a basic drug will reach a higher intracellular concentration of unbound molecules than an acidic drug, all other conditions being equal. Finally, the neutral molecules will penetrate into the lipid space according to their oil–water partition coefficient, γ. When we consider that $c_p = c_i = c$, the 'real' distribution of the drug amount, m, is described by the following expression:

$$m = c' \times V' = \left[c \times \left(\frac{V_p}{f_p} + \frac{V_i}{f_i}\right)\right] + \left[c \times \frac{\varphi_i}{\varphi_c} \times \left(\frac{V_c}{f_c} + V_f \times \gamma\right)\right] = [m_{ec}] + [m_{ic}] \tag{24}$$

The square brackets separate the amount of drug in the extracellular space, m_{ec}, from the intracellular amount of drug, m_{ic}.

Although the model described by eq. 24 is, of course, still far from reality it demonstrates the factors which could potentially influence the distribution equilibrium of a drug:

(1) It is evident that any agent influencing the volume of one of the fluid spaces (e.g. a diuretic) may influence the distribution equilibrium of a drug.

(2) Most disturbances of the acid–base equilibrium are more pronounced in the extracellular than in the intracellular space. The resulting abnormal value of the quotient φ_i/φ_c in eq. 24 will lead to an abnormal distribution of acidic and basic drugs between these compartments. This has been experimentally verified by the simultaneous administration of sodium bicarbonate and sulphonamides (Dettli and Spring, 1968a); as predicted by eq. 24, V' was found smaller than normal. In contrast, V' was shown to be greater than normal during sleep (Krauer, 1970). Thus, acidifying and alkalinizing agents and hypnotics may not only influence the renal excretion but also the distribution of cationic and anionic drugs.

(3) Eq. 24 predicts that any factor influencing the macromolecular binding of a drug will influence its distribution equilibrium. Since the binding is reversible and the number of the macromolecular binding sites (r_{max}) is limited, it is reasonable to assume that the binding equilibrium can be described by the law of mass-action (Klotz, 1953; Spring, 1966; Goldstein et al., 1969). In analogy to eq. 15 one can write:

$$r = r_{max} \times \frac{c}{c + K''} \qquad (25)$$

where r denotes the number of mols of drug bound per mol of macromolecules and K'' is the dissociation constant of the complex. It has been demonstrated experimentally that the binding of many drugs to the plasma proteins can be adequately described by eq. 25 and that the values of r_{max} and K'' vary within wide limits. For example, the values $r_{max} = 1$–2 and $K'' = 10^{-5}$–10^{-3} mol/l were found with sulphonamides (Spring, 1966); the corresponding values for digoxin are $r_{max} \rightarrow \infty$ and $K'' = 1.5 \times 10^5$ mol/l (Ohnhaus et al., 1972). Eq. 25 is the kinetic basis for possible drug interactions because a drug I characterized by the concentration c_{I} and the dissociation constant K''_{I} may be displaced by a concomitantly administered second drug II characterized by the concentration c_{II} and the dissociation constant K'_{II}. Arguing along the same lines as in the case of eq. 17 one obtains a very similar equation:

$$r_{\text{I}} = r_{\max} \times \frac{c_{\text{I}}}{c_{\text{I}} + K''_{\text{I}}(1 + c_{\text{II}}/K''_{\text{II}})} \qquad (26)$$

In the case of competitive displacement, drug II acts by increasing the denominator of eq. 26 by a factor $1+(c_{\text{II}}/K''_{\text{II}})$. The number of mols of the displaced drug I bound per mol of protein decreases to the same proportion. Consequently, the extent of displacement depends solely on the relationships between the concentrations (c_{I} and c_{II}) and between the affinities (K''_{I} and K''_{II}) of the displaced drug I and the displacing drug II. The probability that a drug displaces another drug from its protein binding sites increases with its concentration ($c_{\text{II}} > c_{\text{I}}$) and with its affinity to the serum proteins ($K''_{\text{II}} < K''_{\text{I}}$). Contrary to promotional arguments, the potency of a drug, i.e. the dose range within which it exerts its therapeutic action, is usually of minor therapeutic significance. Eq. 26 describes an exception to this rule: a drug acting in a lower concentration range has a lower tendency to displace, and a higher tendency to be displaced by a drug acting in a higher concentration range. (Similarly, a prerequisite of enzyme induction is usually a high molar concentration of the stimulating drug.)

Although eqs. 17 and 26 are almost identical, it should be emphasized that the pharmacotherapeutic consequences of these two equations are different in the following important respects:

(a) According to eqs. 15–17 the rate of drug elimination is directly proportional to the fraction, b, of molecules bound to the transporting macromolecules. In contrast, it is generally accepted (Anton, 1960; Krueger-Thiemer, 1960; Dettli, 1961) that the pharmacological activity of a drug is proportional to the concentration of unbound molecules $c = c' \times f$. The fraction f is found in the following way: multiplying both sides of eq. 25 by the molar concentration of the binding plasma protein, P, yields the concentration of bound drug molecules: $P \times r = c'' = c' - c$. It follows:

$$f = c/c' = \frac{c}{c + r \times P} \qquad (27a)$$

Substituting r by eq. 25 results in:

$$f = c/c' = \frac{1}{1 + \dfrac{r_{\max} \times P}{c + K''}} \qquad (27b)$$

As can be seen from eq. 27b, f is a function of the concentration of unbound drug in the plasma water, c, and increases with increasing values of c.

Furthermore, f decreases with decreasing values of K'', i.e. with the increasing affinity of the drugs to the plasma proteins (see Fig. 4). The effect of the displacing drug II on the unbound fraction f_{I} of drug I can be described when r in eq. 27a is substituted by eq. 26 (competitive displacement):

$$f_{\mathrm{I}} = c_{\mathrm{I}}/c'_{\mathrm{I}} = \frac{1}{1 + \dfrac{r_{\max} \times P}{c_{\mathrm{I}} + K''_{\mathrm{I}}\,(1 + c_{\mathrm{II}}/K''_{\mathrm{II}})}} \tag{28}$$

According to eq. 28, the displacing effect of drug II will be more pronounced the higher its concentration ($c_{\mathrm{II}} > c_{\mathrm{I}}$) and the smaller its dissociation constant ($K''_{\mathrm{II}} < K''_{\mathrm{I}}$) and vice versa.

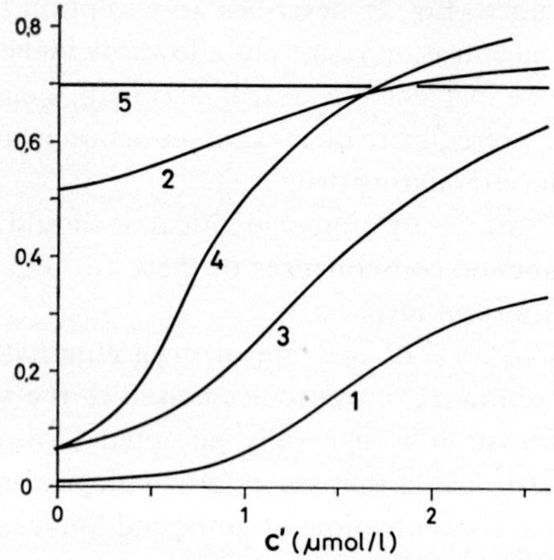

Fig. 4. Binding of drugs to the serum albumin: The unbound fraction, f, as a function of the total drug concentration, c', in the serum (equilibrium-dialysis experiments analysed according to eq. 27b). *Curve 1* represents a sulphonamide (sulphadimethoxine) with a very high binding affinity and *curve 2* a sulphonamide (sulphadiazine) with a relatively low binding affinity (Spring, 1966). *Curves 3 and 4* demonstrate the displacing effect of the metabolite acetyl-sulphamethoxypyridazine (ASMP) on its parent drug sulphamethoxypyridazine (SMP). *Curve 3* describes the binding of SMP alone and *curve 4* the binding of SMP after the addition of equimolar amounts of SAMP (Dettli and Spring, 1973). The kinetic analysis of these results according to the law of mass action is depicted in Fig. 6. Note that f increases with increasing values of c'. *Curve 5:* the maximum binding capacity for digoxin is extremely high and the affinity to the serum albumin extremely low resulting in a high value of f which is practically independent of c' (Ohnhaus et al., 1972). For further explanations see text.

(b) In principle, $v_{\max}$ in eqs. 15–17 and $r_{\max}$ in eq. 25 may have any value between zero and infinity. In contrast, the maximum value of the unbound fraction is $f = c/c' = 1.0$. It follows from this that a pronounced competitive

displacement of a drug from its plasma protein binding is impossible unless f is much smaller than 1.0.
(c) Eq. 28 describes the influence of a concomitantly administered interacting drug II on the concentration–time curve of a drug I in the plasma of the living organism. In contrast, when the displacing drug II is added to a protein-bound drug I in an in vitro experiment and an increased value of f_I and a correspondingly increased value of c_I is found as predicted by eq. 28, this result is only valid for the in vitro system where c increases in proportion to f according to the relation $c = c' \times f$. In the organism however, the increase in c is always less than the increase in f because, when c increases, redistribution of unbound drug molecules into the different fluid compartments will immediately take place until a new distribution equilibrium is established. As a consequence, c will decrease accordingly. Consequently, the results of displacement experiments in vitro should be interpreted in the light of eq. 24. The salient point is the fact that plasma proteins are only present in the extracellular space ($V_p + V_i$). Consequently, the interacting drug will displace drug molecules only there and c will not increase appreciably when most of the displaced molecules are trapped in the intracellular space. As indicated by eq. 26, this is the case when $\varphi_i/\varphi_c > 1$, when the drug molecules are bound by intracellular macromolecules ($f_c < 1$) or when the drug is markedly lipid soluble ($\gamma > 1$). In summarizing these pharmacokinetic predictions (Dettli and Spring, 1973), it may be stated for practical purposes that drug displacement from plasma protein binding will only be of practical significance when the displaced drug is highly protein bound ($f_p < 0.1$) and when its distribution volume does not exceed markedly the volume of the extracellular water. On the other hand, the displacing drug must have a high binding affinity to the plasma proteins ($K_{II} < K_I$) and/or be present in a high concentration ($c_{II} > c_I$). So far, practical experience appears to be in accordance with these predictions. For more details the reader is referred to the literature (Anton, 1968; Gillette, 1968; Dettli and Spring, 1973).

1.3 DRUG ABSORPTION

Numerous examples are described in the literature where a drug influences, on a kinetic basis, the rate or the extent of absorption of another drug. This is especially true in the case of gastrointestinal drug absorption (Wagner, 1971). The discussion of these biopharmaceutic interactions is beyond the scope of the present report. However, Rowland (1972) has recently emphasized the fact that drug molecules which have penetrated the gut wall, i.e. molecules which have been absorbed, do not necessarily reach the general circulation because they may be metabolized in the intestinal wall or during their first passage through the liver. When D is a perorally administered and completely absorbed dose of a drug and $z = \dot{V}/\dot{F}$ is the metabolic extraction ratio in the gut wall and in the liver (eq. 22), the amount of drug reaching the general circulation (m_{in}) will be

$$m_{in} = D - D \times z = D(1 - z) \tag{29}$$

According to Rowland (1972), the gastrointestinal bioavailability of a drug, θ, may be defined as follows:

$$\theta = \frac{m_{in}}{D} = 1 - z \tag{30}$$

If the hepatic clearance of the drug, $\dot{V}$, approaches the liver blood flow, $\dot{F}$, i.e. when the extraction ratio is high ($z \rightarrow 1.0$) then even a moderate stimulation of the metabolizing enzymes will markedly decrease the intestinal availability of a drug. On the other hand, when $z \ll 1.0$ an increase in enzyme activity will hardly influence, to a detectable extent, the intestinal availability of the drug.

2 Pharmacokinetic consequences of drug interactions

2.1 ONE-DOSE KINETICS

2.1.1 *Elimination*

When the metabolic transformation or the 'active' secretion of a drug is inhibited or stimulated by a second drug one expects a corresponding change in the slope of the descending limb of its concentration–time curve. In addition, one would expect that the area below the concentration–time curve will be greater or smaller than normal, accordingly. It should be realized however, that the pharmacokinetic effects of such drug interactions may be much more complex:

In the simplest case the interacting drug is administered by continuous infusion and will consequently reach a constant steady-state concentration in the different compartments of the organism. When the drug exerts an inhibitory effect on the elimination of another drug and when its concentration and its affinity to the macromolecules are not very high ($c_{II} < c_I$ and $K_{II} > K_I$), the possible consequence is a decreased slope of the elimination curve according to eq. 18. However, when $c_{II} > c_I$ and/or $K'_{II} < K'_I$ the elimination curve of the influenced drug will no longer be linear but will exhibit saturation phenomena (see eq. 17 and Fig. 1). As an extreme, zero order kinetics according to eq. 19 may be observed.

It should be mentioned in this connection that the analysis of the plasma concentration curve of a drug is not always the best way to detect kinetic drug interactions. When the inhibited pathway of elimination is of minor quantitative importance (see eq. 11), the influence of its inhibition on the plasma concentration curve may be so small that the interaction escapes detection (Sjöqvist et al., 1969). Similarly, in the case of capacity-limited kinetics, the deviation of the plasma concentration curve from linearity is often restricted to the highest concentration range and may be so small that it cannot be proven statistically. In such cases the effect of the interaction may be detected by analysing the pattern of metabolites in the urine because the relative amounts of metabolites excreted in the urine are usually proportional to the rate constants of their formation (Wagner, 1971).

When the interacting drug is administered as a single dose, its concentration in the organism will change with time. It is evident that this may result in a highly complex interaction pattern, because drug interactions depend on the concentrations of the interacting drugs.

In the case of enzyme induction, eq. 16 predicts that v_{max} increases, i.e. that the elimination process still follows first order kinetics and that the negative slope of the plasma concentration curve will increase, provided the stimulated process is of sufficient quantitative importance (eq. 11). When the drug is administered orally, a decreased area below the concentration–time curve is not sufficient proof for its increased elimination rate because its absorption could have been influenced by the interacting drug. Such an effect is unlikely when the time of the maximum concentration of the drug is reached earlier than normal. Furthermore, as discussed in connection with eq. 30, when the hepatic extraction ratio of a drug is high, a decrease in intestinal availability may be a much more sensitive indicator of enzyme induction than is an increased elimination rate.

2.1.2 *Distribution*

Although the fact is firmly established on theoretical and experimental grounds that it is not the total concentration (c') of a drug in the plasma but rather the concentration of unbound drug molecules in the plasma water (c) that is most closely related to the pharmacological effects, it is general practice in clinical research to predict therapeutic and toxic effects of a drug from its total plasma concentration because it is tacitly assumed that the fraction of unbound drug molecules (f_p) is nearly identical in all patients. It is evident that this assumption is no longer valid when a drug has been partly displaced from its protein binding sites. When f_p is abnormally high, therapeutic and toxic effects should occur at lower than normal total plasma concentrations.

When a drug is eliminated by glomerular filtration, its displacement from plasma protein-binding results in an increased renal clearance, $\dot{V}'$. However, as can be seen from eq. 24, an abnormally high value of f_p will at the same time increase the distribution volume of the drug, V'. When both, $\dot{V}'$ and V' increase to the same extent, eq. 6 predicts that the elimination rate constant (k') will remain unchanged. Expressing this in a more general way, it follows from eq. 6 that any change in the distribution equilibrium of a drug will influence its elimination rate. This is also true for drugs eliminated by tubular or biliary excretion or by metabolism although these mechanisms themselves apparently do not depend on the protein binding of the drug.

Finally, the possibility should be taken into consideration that a drug displaces another drug from intracellular macromolecular binding sites. In fact, Levy (1970) has shown that a much greater fraction of a dose may be bound by intracellular macromolecules than by plasma proteins even when the drug (e.g. dicumarol) is extremely bound to plasma albumin.

2.2 MULTIPLE-DOSE KINETICS

Many drugs (chemotherapeutic agents, cardiac glycosides etc.) are administered over a prolonged period of time in such a way that a constant dose, D, is repeatedly given at regular dosage intervals, τ. When the dose is not eliminated completely during the first dosage interval (i.e. before the second dose is administered) the drug concentration in the plasma, c', will increase from dose to dose. However, when c' increases, eq. 6b predicts that the rate of drug elimination will also increase until the amount of drug eliminated during one dosage interval is equal to the administered dose, D/τ. As a consequence, c' will no longer increase but approach a constant steady-state, c'_∞. This self-limiting process of utmost clinical importance is called *drug accumulation*. The principles of drug accumulation outlined above apply to both continuous and intermittent administration of drugs. For the sake of simplicity the influence of drug interactions on the process of drug accumulation will be discussed here using continuous drug administration as an example. It is evident that the drug concentration eventually reached in the plasma, c'_∞, is proportional to the dose administered during one dosage interval, D/τ, and inversely proportional to the rate constant of elimination, k', and to the distribution volume, V', of the drug:

$$c'_\infty = \frac{D/\tau}{k' \times V'} \tag{29}$$

When a drug is eliminated by enzymatic transformation, enzyme induction may increase the value of k'. It follows from eq. 29 that an identical dose, D/τ, will result in a lower value of c'_∞. On the other hand, when the metabolism or the tubular secretion of a drug I is inhibited by a second drug II, it follows from eq. 18 that k' decreases by a factor $(1+c_{II}/K'_{II})$ and c'_∞ will increase in proportion (see Fig. 5):

$$c'_{I\infty} = \frac{D_I/\tau}{k' \times V'/(1+c_{II}/K'_{II})} \tag{30}$$

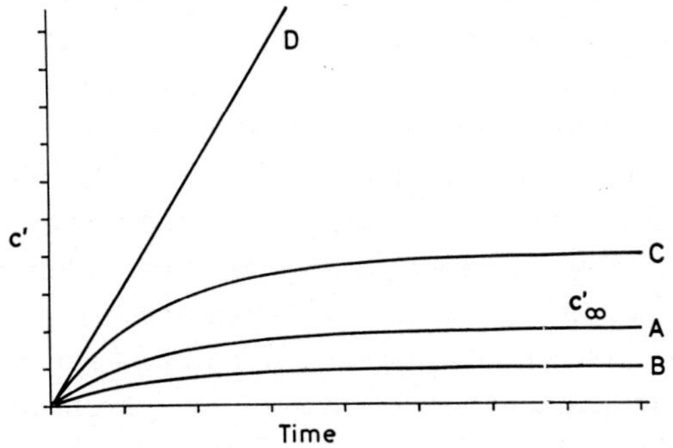

Fig. 5. Drug accumulation in the plasma during continuous infusion. The drug concentration in the plasma increases with time until the steady-state level (c'_∞) predicted by eq. 29 is eventually reached (*curve A*). After enzyme induction, the elimination rate constant will increase resulting in an accordingly lower value of c_∞ (*curve B*). In contrast, enzymatic inhibition will result in a higher than normal value of c_∞ (*curve C*). The difference will be still more pronounced when the drug interaction results in saturation phenomena. In the extreme case of complete saturation of the elimination process (zero-order kinetics), the drug concentration in the serum will increase indefinitely with time when the dose administered per unit of time exceeds the maximum rate of drug metabolism (*curve D*).

Eq. 30 is however only valid when the enzyme is far from being saturated. When saturation phenomena appear to a considerable extent, the elimination process will no longer follow first order kinetics but will become more and more capacity-limited and will therefore depend on c'_I and c'_{II}, i.e. on the doses administered per unit of time, D/τ. This results in a further abnormal increase in $c'_{I\infty}$. The corresponding mathematical relationships are too complex to be discussed here. The interested reader is referred to the work of Tsuchiya and Levy (1972). Finally, when the metabolizing enzyme is completely saturated, the elimination of the drug will follow apparent zero-order kinetics according to eq. 19. This means that c'_I will no longer approach a finite steady-state value when the administered doses surpass an upper critical limit. Instead c'_I will without limit increase linearly with time (see Fig. 5).

However, this will rarely occur because most drugs are eliminated by several different pathways and it is very unlikely that all of them are inhibited to such an extent by another drug that they are saturated. When one elimination process obeying first order kinetics exists besides a saturated mechanism, the first order process tends to mask the saturation phenomena, because the amount of drug eliminated per unit of time by the first-order process increases with increasing values of c'_{I}. As a consequence, c'_{I} will not increase indefinitely but eventually approach a constant, though abnormally high, steady-state value with all its potential toxicological consequences. These considerations may have therapeutic consequences. For example, the renal elimination of salicylic acid depends highly on the pH of the urine. Nevertheless, the concomitant administration of alkali will not influence profoundly the plasma concentration curve of the drug under normal circumstances because the renal pathway is of minor quantitative importance in the elimination of salicylic acid (see the discussion of eq. 11). However, when the metabolic transformation of the drug is greatly reduced by saturation kinetics after administering an overdose, or by competitive inhibition by the concomitant administration of a second inhibiting drug, then the administration of alkali may be a life-saving procedure (Levy and Leonards, 1971).

When two interacting drugs are administered chronically, the drug interactions may follow extremely complex patterns because, on the one hand, the extent and the nature of drug interactions depend on the concentrations of the drugs involved, and on the other hand, the concentrations of the drugs will increase during the accumulation process. It can be shown (Dost, 1968) that the time period necessary for reaching c'_{∞} increases with decreasing values of the elimination rate of the drug. Thus, when a fixed dose of a slowly eliminated interacting drug II (i.e. digitoxin, phenobarbital) is administered at constant dosage intervals, c'_{II}, may increase during several weeks until the steady-state, $c'_{\mathrm{II}\infty}$, is reached. It is therefore conceivable that drug II may inhibit the metabolism of another drug I during the first period of administration. In a later period, the concentration of drug II has increased and the main interaction may now be the displacement of drug I from protein binding sites, or enzyme induction may overshadow the inhibitory effects.

A very interesting fact of possible toxicological significance in multiple-dose therapy is the displacement of a drug from its plasma-protein binding sites by its own metabolites. As a rule, metabolites are structurally closely related to the parent drug. The assumption appears therefore reasonable that the drug and its metabolites will be bound by the same binding sites. Mutual displacement is therefore likely to occur. However, since metabolites are usually more polar than the parent drug, their renal elimination rates are higher. As a result, the plasma concentration is often so low that they will

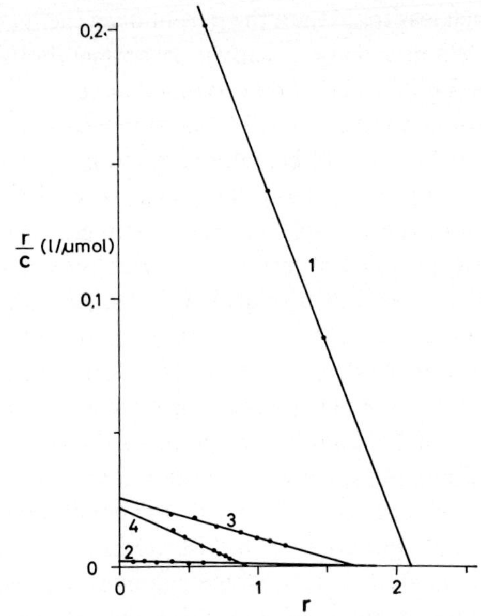

Fig. 6. Binding oi sulphonamides to the serum albumin: The results of the dialysis experiments with the three sulphonamides depicted in Fig. 4 were analysed based on a linearized equation of the law of mass-action. The resulting 'Scatchard-plots' allow the calculation of the dissociation constant of the drug–albumin complex (K'') and of the apparent maximum binding capacity (r_{max}). *Curve 1* represents sulphadimethoxine ($K''=7.3\times10^{-6}$ mol/1). *Curve 2* corresponds to sulphadiazine ($K''=8.6\times10^{-4}$ mol/1). *Curve 3* describes the binding of sulphamethoxypyridazine (SMP) to the serum albumin ($K''=6.6\times10^{-5}$ mol/1). The apparent maximum binding capacity is about $r_{max}=2$ binding sites for these sulphonamides (Spring, 1966). *Curve 4* demonstrates the displacing effect of a metabolite of SMP, acetyl-sulphamethoxypyridazine (ASMP) on its parent drug. After addition of equimolar amounts of ASMP the following values of the binding constants of SMP were found: $K''=3.9\times10^{-5}$ mol/1 and $r_{max}=0.9$ binding sites (Dettli and Spring, 1973). For further explanations see text.

hardly displace the parent drug to a significant degree. However, when a drug which is partly metabolized and partly excreted by the kidneys, is administered to patients with renal disease, its dosage regimen can be adapted in such a way to the functional capacity of the kidneys that the drug concentration in the plasma remains in the 'usual' range (Dettli et al., 1971). For example, in an anuric patient, when only a fraction of the normal dose corresponding to the fraction which is normally metabolized, is administered the plasma drug concentration will be in the 'usual' range as long as the drug is metabolized at a normal rate. However, the metabolites of the drug are not eliminated by the kidneys in such patients. They may therefore accumulate tremendously (Kunin et al. 1959) and may reach concentrations ten times higher or even more than the parent drug (Rieder, 1974). Although most metabolites are much less toxic than the parent drug the increased risk of side effects is evident. When a drug is known to be metabolized to pharmacologically active metabolites it should be avoided in patients with renal failure.

Using sulphamethoxypyridazine (SMP) and its acetyl metabolite (ASMP) in equal concentrations, it could be demonstrated in our laboratory that the parent drug, SMP, is displaced from the plasma proteins by its metabolite, ASMP. The results of these displacement experiments are shown in Fig. 6. As can be seen, the experimental results are perfectly described by the law of mass action. In principle, the displacement is of a non-competitive type because the number of binding sites decreases. In addition however, the dissociation constant of the drug decreases also considerably indicating that the affinity of the drug to the plasma proteins increases under the influence of the displacing action of the metabolite. None of the equations presented in this report can explain this phenomenon either on a competitive or on a non-competitive basis. Therefore, the following concluding remarks may be appropriate: our simple equations demonstrate in a quantitative way many mportant factors contributing to kinetic drug interactions. They constitute therefore a useful tool of predictive pharmacology. However, a much more sophisticated mathematical and physico-chemical language would be needed in order to approximate all the complexities of biological reality (Goldstein et al., 1969; Wagner, 1971).

Acknowledgement

The experiments performed in the author's laboratory have been supported by Schweizerischer Nationalfonds zur Förderung der wissenschaftlichen Forschung.

References

Accocella, G., Nicolis, F. and Tencohi, L.T. (1965): The effect of an intravenous infusion of Rifamycin SV on the excretion of Bilirubin, Bromsulfalein, and Indocyan Green in man. *Gastroenterology*, **49**, 521.

Anton, A. H. (1960): The relation between the binding of sulfonamides to albumin and their antibacterial efficacy. *J. Pharmacol. exp. Therap.*, **129**, 282.

Anton, A. H. (1968): The effect of disease, drugs and dilution on the binding of sulfonamides in human plasma. *Clin. Pharmacol. Therap.* **9**, 561.

Conney, A. H. (1967): Pharmacological implications of microsomal enzyme induction. *Pharmacol. Rev.*, **19**, 317.

Dettli, L. (1961): Der Konzentrationsbegriff in der Chemotherapie mit Sulfanilamiden. *Arzneimittelforsch.*, **11**, 861.

Dettli, L. and Spring, P. (1966): Diurnal variations in the elimination rate of a sulfonamide in man. *Helv. med. Acta*, **33**, 291.

Dettli, L. and Spring, P. (1968a): Pharmacokinetics as a basic medical Problem. *Proc. 3rd Int. Congr. Pharmacol.* Vol. 7, p. 5. Pergamon Press, Oxford and New York.

Dettli, L. and Spring, P. (1968b): Factors influencing drug elimination in man. *Farmaco* (Ed. sci.), **23**, 795.

Dettli, L. and Spring, P. (1970): A hydrokinetic simulator as a teaching aid in pharmacokinetics. *Proc. 4th Int. Congr. Pharmacol.* Vol. 1, p. 227. Verlag Benno Schwabe, Basel.

Dettli, L. and Spring P. (1973): The modifying effects of physiological variables and diseases upon pharmacokinetics. *Proc. 5th Int. Congr. Pharmacol.* Vol. 3, p. 165. Verlag Karger, Basel–New York.

Dettli, L., Spring, P. and Ryter, S. (1971): Multiple dose kinetics and drug dosage in patients with kidney disease. *Acta Pharmacol.*, **29**, Suppl. 3, 211.

Dost, F. H. (1968): *Grundlagen der Pharmakokinetik.* Georg Thieme-Verlag, Stuttgart.

Gillette, J. R. (1968): Problems associated with problems of the extrapolation of data from in vitro experiments to experiments in intact animals. In: *Importance of Fundamental Principles in Drug Evaluation.* Editors: D. H. Tedeschi and R. E. Tedeschi. Raven Press, New York.

Goldstein, A., Aronow, L. and Kalman, S. M. (1969): *Principles of drug action.* Harper & Row, New York.

Klotz, I. M. (1953): Protein Interactions. In: *The proteins.* Editors: H. v. Neurath & K. Bailey. Academic Press, New York.

Krauer, B. (1970): unpublished observations.

Krüger-Thiemer, E. (1960): Dosage schedule and pharmacokinetics in chemotherapy. *J. Amer. pharm. Ass.* (Sci. Ed.), **49**, 311.

Kunin, C. M., Glatzko, A. J. and Finland, M. (1959): Persistence of antibiotics in blood of patients with acute renal failure. II. Chloramphenicol and its metabolic products in the blood of patients with severe renal disease or hepatic cirrhosis. *J. clin. Invest.*, **38**, 1498.

Levy, G. (1968): Dose dependent effects in pharmacokinetics. In: *Importance of fundamental Principles in Drug Evaluation.* Editors: D. H. Tedeschi and R. E. Tedeschi. Raven Press, New York.

Levy, G. (1970): Effect of protein binding on the distribution and metabolism of a highly plasma protein bound drug (bishydroxycoumarin). *Proc. 4th Int. Congr. Pharmacol.* Verlag Benno Schwabe, Basel.

Levy, G. and Amsel, L. P. (1966): Kinetics of competitive inhibition of salicylic acid conjugation with glycine in man. *Biochem. Pharmacol.*, **15**, 1033.

Levy, G. and Leonards, J. R. (1971): Urine pH and salicylate therapy. *J. Amer. med. Soc.*, **217**, 81.

Levy, G. and Matsuzawa, R. (1967): Pharmacokinetics of Salicylamide elimination in man. *J. Pharmacol. exp. Therap.*, **156**, 285.

Milne, M. D., Scribner, B. H. and Crawford, M. A. (1958): Non-ionic diffusion and the excretion of weak acids and bases. *Amer. J. Med.*, **24**, 709.

Ohnhaus, E. E., Spring, P. and Dettli, L. (1972): Protein binding of digoxin in human serum. *Europ. J. clin. Pharmacol.* **5**, 34.

Ohnhaus, E. E., Thorgeirsson, S. A., Davies, D. S. and Breckenridge, A. (1971): Changes in liver blood flow during enzyme induction. *Biochem. Pharmacol.*, **26**, 2561.

Rieder, J. (1974): Pharmacokinetics of the antibacterial combination sulfamethoxazole plus trimethoprim in patients with normal or impaired kidney function. *Antibiot. Chemother.*, **18**, 148.

Rowland, M. (1972): Influence of route of administration on drug availability. *J. pharm. Sci.*, **61**, 70.

Rowland, M., Beckett, A. H. and Turner, P. (1965): Influence of urinary pH on excretion of amphetamine. *Lancet*, *1*, 303.

Shand, D. G., Evans, G. H. and Nies, A. S. (1971): The almost complete hepatic extraction of propranolol during intravenous administration in the dog. *Life Sci.*, **10**, I, 1417.

Sjöqvist, F., Berglund, F., Berga, O., Hammer, W., Andersson S. and Thorstrand, C. (1969): The pH-dependent excretion of monomethylathed tricyclic antidepressants. *Clin. Pharmacol. Therap.*, **10**, 826.

Spring, P. (1966): Die Bindung einiger Sulfonamide an die Bluteiweisskörper der Menschen. *Arzneimittelforsch.*, **16**, 346.
Tsuchiya, T. and Levy, G. (1972): Relationship between dose and plateau levels of drugs eliminated by first-order and capacity-limited kinetics. *J. pharm. Sci.*, **61**, 541.
Wacker, E. C., Haynes, H., Druyan, R., Fisher, W. and Coleman, J. E. (1965): Treatment of ethylene glycol poisoning with ethyl alcohol. *J. Amer. med. Assoc.*, **194**, 1231.
Wagner, J. G. (1971): Biopharmaceutics and relevant pharmacokinetics. Hamilton Press, Hamilton.
Weiner, I. M. and Mudge, G. H. (1964): Renal tubular mechanisms for excretion of organic acids and bases. *Amer. J. Med.*, **36**, 743.

CHAPTER 5

Drug interactions resulting in loss of action

E. J. ARIËNS AND A. M. SIMONIS

1 Introduction

Complications of drug therapy due to drug interactions have a high incidence as is demonstrated by various recent monographs (Hartshorn, 1970; Hansten, 1971; Garb, 1971; Martin, 1971; Swidler, 1971; Viars and Seebacher, 1971). Up to now emphasis has almost exclusively been on drug-induced side-effects. With regard to medical health care in certain highly advanced countries about 15% of the hospital beds appeared to be occupied by patients requiring treatment because of unwanted drug effects, probably partly due to drug interactions. The terms drug-induced diseases and iatrogenic diseases are used.

Drug interaction may also be involved in resistance to therapy – iatrogenic therapy resistance – often shown by the failure of the patient or eventually of the infectious agent to respond, or as a failure of the drug to act, but in fact it is often the prescribing physician who has failed. Drug interactions resulting in a loss of therapeutic response are undoubtedly another contribution to unnecessarily occupied hospital beds or, what is worse, patients unnecessarily hospitalized.

2 The main phases in drug action

For a systematic discussion of drug interactions and their possible consequences for drug action, consideration of the three main phases in drug action and their essential aspects with regard to therapeutic efficacy is required (see Scheme 1) (Ariëns 1974, Ariëns and Simonis, 1972).

The pharmaceutical phase is the first phase. It is determinant for the quantity of the drug available for absorption. In this phase the disintegration of the application form (tablets, capsules, etc.) and the dissolution of the active compound take place. It is followed by the pharmacokinetic phase

Scheme 1

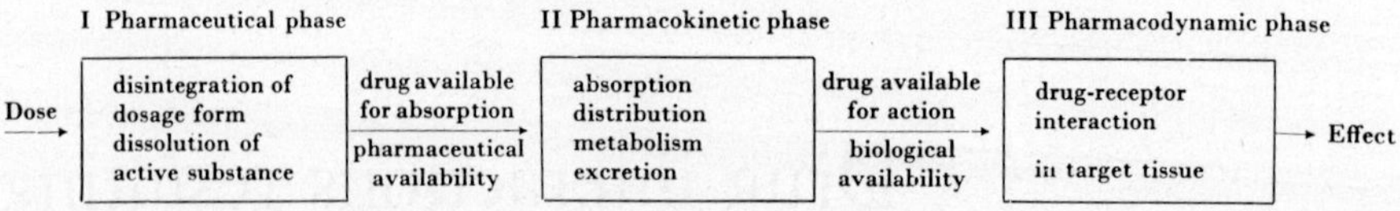

which comprises absorption, distribution, excretion and metabolic conversion of the drug, and is determinant for the concentration of the active compound in the plasma and therewith in the target tissues and at the sites of action – the specific receptors. The final phase, the pharmacodynamic phase, concerns the interaction between the drug and its specific receptors and therewith the induction of a stimulus and the generation of the effect.

3 Drug parameters

3.1 PHARMACEUTICAL AVAILABILITY, BIOLOGICAL AVAILABILITY, SYSTEMIC AVAILABILITY, AND AVAILABILITY PROFILE

The pharmaceutical availability of a drug is the fraction of the dose of the active compound available for absorption. It is comparable to that fraction of the dose of the drug that goes into solution under standardized in vitro conditions. These should simulate as much as possible the conditions operant in the case of application of the drug, for instance, by the use of test media simulant of the intestinal fluids. There is confusion around the term bioavailability. It is sometimes used for the fraction of the active compound that is dissolved after disintegration of the application form, sometimes for the fraction of the dose absorbed, sometimes for the fraction of the dose that reaches general circulation, sometimes for the surface under the plasma concentration curve, and sometimes for the plasma concentration at a certain time. For reasons of clearness it may be advisable to differentiate between biological availability and systemic availability. The latter then represents the fraction of the dose of the compound which reaches general circulation in its active form (Ritschel, 1972). It can be calculated from the time–plasma concentration curve, taking into account the rate of absorption and the elimination at first liver passage. The latter is the elimination which takes place after intestinal absorption, as a result of the metabolic inactivation due to liver passage before the drug reaches the general circulation. In case of a chronic application aimed at a continuous plasma level (a steady-state level) of the drug, the systemic availability as such may give a suitable indication of the therapeutic efficacy of the drug preparation. Then the quantity of the drug absorbed in the dosage interval should match the quantity eliminated in that period.

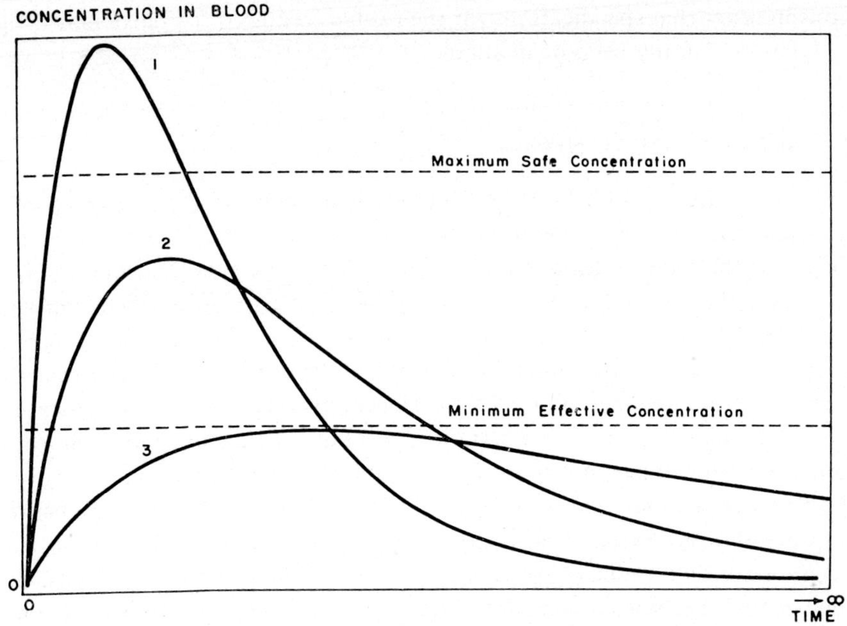

Fig. 1. Time–blood concentration relationships – biological availability profiles – for three drug preparations which differ in the rate of uptake, while the values of the rate of elimination, the size of the dose, and the biological availability – the surface under the curve – are equal. Minimum effective and maximum safe concentrations are indicated. *Note*: The 3 preparations, although of equal biological availability, are essentially different in their availability profiles and therewith in their therapeutic efficacy (modified after Notari, 1971).

In other situations two preparations with an equal biological or systemic availability may, however, essentially differ in their therapeutic efficacy which often depends on the availability profile, the profile of the time–plasma concentration curve. Depending on the type of preparation, for instance, high plasma levels for a short period or low plasma levels for a longer period may be obtained with preparations with an equal biological or systemic availability (see Fig. 1) (Notari, 1971). The systemic availability does not give information relevant to the therapeutic efficacy of the preparation and the availability profile gives more useful information (Ariëns, 1974). Drug preparations should be compared for their availability profiles and the comparisons should take place under standardized conditions (before, with, after the meals, time of the day, etc.).

The availability profile of a drug should fit that required for optimal therapeutic efficacy of that drug. Clinicians should study and compare the therapeutic efficacy and the availability profiles of different drug preparations in order that specifications for the profiles required for particular drugs or types of therapy become available.

3.2 HALF-LIFE AND STEADY-STATE LEVEL

The availability profile of a drug is greatly dependent on the rate of absorption and the rate of elimination of the drug. A useful parameter in this respect is the half-life time ($t_{\frac{1}{2}}$) of the drug. The time $t_{\frac{1}{2}}$ is the time required to reduce the concentration of the drug in plasma or in another compartment to 50% of its original value. For most elimination processes, such as drug metabolism, active excretion and ultrafiltration, it holds true that the quantity processed per unit of time is proportional to the concentration available. This implies that a certain percentage of the concentration available is eliminated per unit of time. As a consequence the elimination curves have an exponential character (Fig. 2). Only if the eliminating systems, for instance enzyme systems, are saturated with the drug – which as a rule occurs only at extremely high concentrations – the quantity processed per unit of time becomes a constant. This is the case for instance with alcohol in the usual dosages.

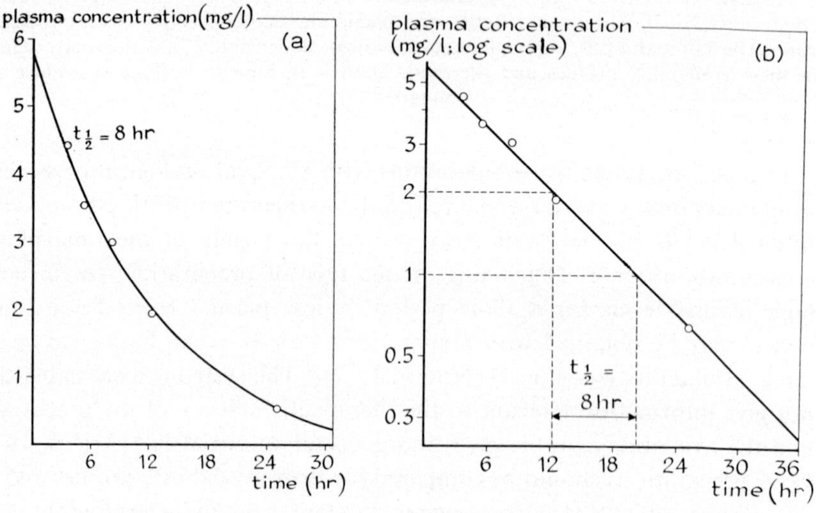

Fig. 2. Time–plasma concentration relationship for the elimination of a drug from plasma on a linear (a) and semilogarithmic (b) scale for the case that per unit of time a certain fraction of the compound available is eliminated – a first-order process. The half-life time of the compound is indicated. *Note*: On a semi-logarithmic scale the time–concentration curve is a straight line. The half-life time is independent of the concentration.

For a drug chronically applied with dosage intervals equal to or smaller than $t_{\frac{1}{2}}$, the plasma level will increase with subsequent dosages; thus accumulation will occur. With the increase of the plasma level, the quantity eliminated per unit of time increases, until at a certain plasma level the quantity eliminated in the dosage interval will match the dose given – the steady-state level. Given a certain dose and dosage interval, the steady-state level reached depends on the half-life time of the compound (Fig. 3) (Van Rossum, 1968). Consequently, if drug interactions influence the eliminating processes, the half-life time of a drug is changed, and the steady-state level obtained on a certain dosage regimen will change. Enhancement of the elimination will shorten the half-life time and lower the steady-state plasma level, possibly below the effective level.

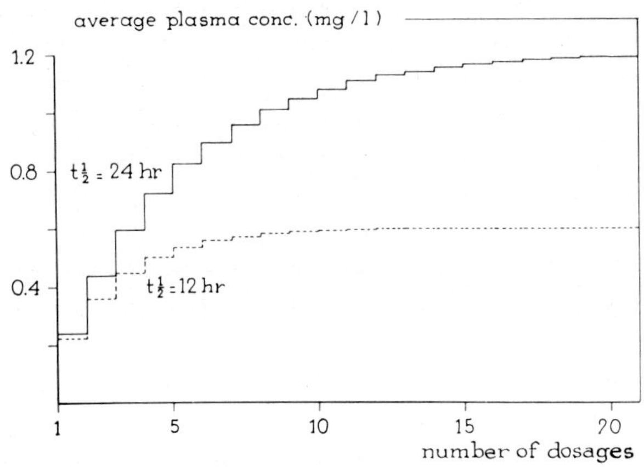

Fig. 3. Cumulation curves based on average plasma concentrations for the dosage intervals for 2 drugs given in equal dosages 3 times a day, but with half-life times of 24 and 12 hr, respectively. *Note*: The steady-state level of accumulation finally reached after chronic application of a drug strongly depends on the half-life time. Doubling of the half-life time results in almost doubling of the steady-state concentration in the plasma. (After Van Rossum, 1968.)

3.3 THERAPEUTIC EFFICACY

The therapeutic efficacy of a drug is dependent on the availability profile of that drug in its active form in the target tissue (biophase, target compartment) where the sites of action or specific receptors for the bioactive compound are located. Usually a simple relationship is assumed between the systemic availability and the availability in the target compartment, the latter also indicated as physiological availability.

For therapeutic efficacy, besides the availability profile of the drug, the condition of the patient and the indication for which a drug is prescribed are determinant factors. A drug will have the character of a therapeutic agent only in the hands of a skilled physician. If applied to a healthy individual or on a wrong indication, the drug may still be 'effective' but instead of acting as a therapeutic agent it will become a nuisance or even a poison to the 'patient'.

4 Drug interactions

In 1923 the Dutch clinician Storm van Leeuwen wrote in his *Fundamentals of Pharmacology*: "In the use of combinations of two or more drugs, the intensity of action of the combination will be strongly dependent on the dose–response curves of the compounds combined", and "it frequently occurs that one compound changes the action of the other one in a quantitative or qualitative sense". In 1924 in an article on antagonism of drugs he wrote: "It may be assumed that every drug before acting must be absorbed by dominant receptors present at the site of action of the drug". He further postulated secondary receptors as indifferent binding sites for the drug. With regard to combinations of drugs he continued: "... replacement of one drug by another one on the dominant receptors or on the secondary receptors will per se be an important feature in drug action, as it will certainly influence the general action of both drugs". He thus emphasized the significance of an interaction between drugs in the pharmacokinetic phase – displacement from the secondary receptors – and interaction between drugs in the pharmacodynamic phase – displacement from 'dominant receptors'. The significance of drug interactions, recognized and clearly formulated by Storm van Leeuwen, 50 years ago, has in recent years become well established. He also was a great advocate of an integration of pharmacology in the clinical approach to the patient. In this respect he was bitterly disappointed by the declinatory attitude of the clinicians of his time (Beumer, 1968).

5 Drug combinations

Drug combinations may be incidental or intentional (Ariëns, 1973, 1974). If intentional, they are based on a rationale. One should well distinguish here between a rationale and 'wishful thinking'. Incidental drug combinations may be involved in complicated diseases, e.g., the use of antibiotics to deal with infections in diabetic patients treated with antidiabetic agents. Self-medication next to professional medication or medication by different mutually non-informed physicians is a less acceptable cause for incidental drug combination. The drugs combined may be applied simultaneously, possibly as fixed-ratio combinations, or in a regular or irregular sequence. The dosages of the drugs to be combined as a rule have to be adapted to the individual needs of the patient on the basis of the therapeutic response. The pharmacokinetics of the compounds combined should also be adapted to the particular requirements. Therefore, fixed-ratio combinations, mostly industrial products, are often inadequate. The same holds true for standard fixed-ratio combinations prescribed by a particular clinician to his patients and sometimes misleadingly represented as a form of 'individualized' therapy.

5.1 RATIONAL DRUG COMBINATIONS

Rationales for drug combination and therefore rational drug combinations undoubtedly exist. The rationale may involve any of the three main phases of drug action (Scheme 1). Examples of rational drug combinations based on drug interactions in the various phases of drug actions will be given with an elucidation of the objectives of the combinations.

With regard to the pharmaceutical phase the aim of the combination may be to increase the pharmaceutical availability, and thus the bioavailability and to achieve an optimal availability profile and thus improved therapeutic efficacy. The following may serve as examples: the combination of ferrous salts with ascorbic acid to maintain the iron in the well absorbed reduced ferrous form; the combination of anthelmintics with saline laxatives to prevent or reduce the absorption of the relatively toxic anthelmintic and the use of carbo adsorbens to reduce intestinal absorption of overdosed drugs or toxins in general, can be mentioned as rational combinations.

With regard to the pharmacokinetic phase an increase in the biological availability and adaptation of the availability profile to the therapeutic requirements are the main aims. In this respect there can be mentioned the combination of penicillins with probenecid to delay excretion (Gibaldi et al., 1970; Riggs, 1972), the combination of penicillinase-resistant penicillins – which also act as inhibitors of penicillinase – with penicillinase-sensitive penicillins which thus become more effective (Nishida et al., 1969; Sabath et al., 1967), the combination of L-DOPA with a peripherally acting dopa-decarboxylase inhibitor to obtain higher concentrations of the compound in the CNS (Ferel, 1972; Siegfried et al., 1969), and the alkalinization of the urine to enhance renal reabsorption of CNS stimulants such as amphetamine to make them more effective and reduce the concentration of the drugs in the urine (Beckett and Rowland, 1965) – a procedure practised by drug addicts and soigneurs in cycling sports. The combination of penicillin G with procaine–penicillin and of insulin with protamine–insulin are aimed at complementarity in the bioavailability profiles. Other examples are the combination of local anaesthetics with vasoconstrictor agents to localize the action of the anaesthetic, and the use of hyaluronidase with subcutaneously applied drugs to enhance tissue penetration. The use of combinations of sulfonamides to avoid crystalluria may also be mentioned. The alkalinization of the urine decreases the bioavailability in the case of barbiturate poisoning since the excretion of the barbiturates is enhanced.

With regard to the pharmacodynamic phase the objective of the combination is to increase the therapeutic efficacy by potentiation, complementarity or reduction of the side-effects without an interference with the therapeutic effect. Examples of a complementarity in action are combinations of diuretics with antihypertensive agents, of estrogens with progestogens in oral contraceptives, of expectorants with antitussives, of general anaesthetics with muscle relaxants, and of contact amoebicides with agents which are effective against the tissue forms in the treatment of amoebic dysentery. Suppression of side-effects without affecting the therapeutic response has been aimed at in the combination of mercurial diuretics causing alkalosis with ammonium chloride; the combination of diuretics causing a loss of potassium with diuretics which bring about potassium retention; the combination of broad-spectrum antibiotics with antimycotics (e.g. nystatin); the combination of corticoids for local use with antimycotics or antibiotics to counteract the increased risk for infections, e.g. in ophthalmology; the combination of immunosuppressives or cytostatics with antibiotics in order to protect against the increased infectious risk, and the combination of p-aminosalicylic acid with isonicotinic acid hydrazide to avoid development of resistance in tuberculostatic therapy. Combinations of cycloguanil and sulfones serve the same purpose in antimalarial therapy. The combination is more effective than the single compounds in the case of development of resistance to one of them (Elslager and Worth, 1965). Enhancement of the therapeutic effect is aimed at with the combination of dihydrofolic acid reductase inhibitors with sulfonamides, known to be highly synergistic with regard to the antibacterial action (Bushby and Hitchings, 1968; Editorial, 1969) and with the combination of neuroleptic agents as pre-medication with general anaesthetics.

Although combinations of drugs may be rational, they can be accepted for therapy only after clinical confirmation of the advantages of the combination over one of the drugs given alone, and in many commonly used combinations such confirmation is not available.

6 Complications with drug combinations

As a rule unwanted complications of drug combinations are indicated as side-effects. They may occur in both incidental and intentional drug combinations. Detection of unwanted enhanced drug responses and thus toxic side-effects is apparently more easy than detection of reduction or loss of therapeutic response. Side-effects of drugs are emphasized in the literature while a lack of therapeutic response is accepted as a more or less normal phenomenon. One should be aware of the fact that in those cases that drugs are prescribed on correct indication, the deprivation of the patient from the drug effect – the therapeutic effect – may be more detrimental to him than many of the side-effects extensively discussed in literature. In this Chapter special attention will be paid to the complications of drug combinations in the sense of a loss of therapeutic action and therewith a deprivation of the patient of the therapeutic benefit due to drug interactions: the iatrogenic therapy resistance (Ariëns, 1969a, 1971, 1974; Ariëns and Simonis, 1972). The various types of interaction will be discussed against the background of Scheme 1. The reduction in drug action by the use of antidotes will not be discussed.

6.1 LOSS OF DRUG ACTION DUE TO INTERACTIONS IN THE PHARMACEUTICAL PHASE

In the pharmaceutical phase the active substance is released from the pharmaceutical preparation and becomes available for absorption. Drug interactions in this phase may decrease the pharmaceutical availability – the fraction of the dose of the drug available for absorption. Unwanted interactions between the components in a pharmaceutical preparation are known as pharmaceutical incompatibilities. There is an extensive literature on this topic (Dale, 1966; Ariëns and Simonis, 1972; Thompson, 1969).

Not only interactions between the components in a drug preparation, but also between the pharmaceutical preparation and the package (container) may take place (Neuwald, 1969). Repacking of nitroglycerine tablets by a pharmacist into plastic packages resulted in a loss of action due to migration of the strongly fat-soluble and volatile nitro-compound from the tablets to the plastic (Shangraw, 1972). The same may happen if such tablets are kept in one pill box together with other tablets. The disinfectant chlorhexidine, which is effective in low concentrations, may be inactivated by the tannin present in cork stoppers (Informatorium Medicamentorum, 1972). Additives used in the pharmaceutical preparations may also be involved. Phenylephrine is inactivated if combined with formaldehyde caseine used as a disintegrating agent in tablets (Cordes and Göbbeler, 1971). In addition combination of drugs in injections especially in intravenous infusions, may cause a loss of action (Kramer et al., 1971).

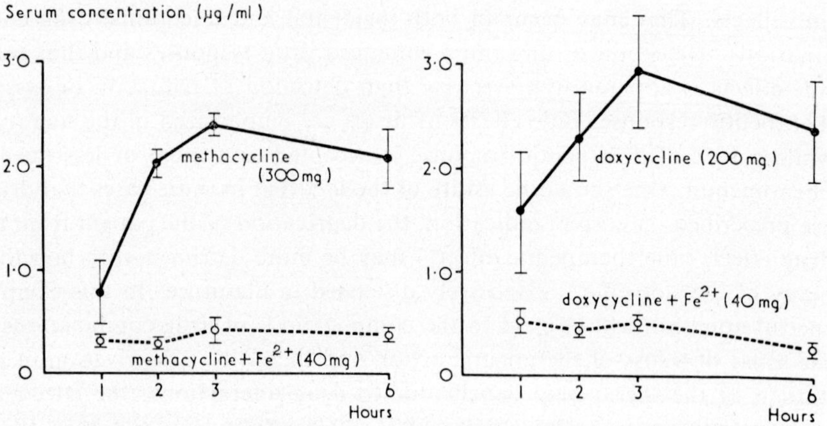

Fig. 4. Mean serum levels (±S.E.) after single doses of methacycline and deoxycycline, administered either alone or simultaneously with 200 mg ferrous sulfate (40 mg Fe^{2+}). The number of subjects in each group is 5. *Note*: If combined with ferrous sulfate, these antiinfective drugs hardly reach the circulation due to the formation of insoluble complexes in the gut. (After Neuvonen et al., 1970).

Unwanted interactions between drugs, if applied separately in two application forms, may occur even with self-medication by the patient. Examples of a loss of therapeutic action due to such interactions in the pharmaceutical phase are the combination of anionic detergent cleaners (soaps) with cationic disinfectants (disinfectant onium compounds) which are inactivated because of a complex salt formation of the agents combined. Further, combination of tetracyclines with preparations containing polyvalent metals such as iron, magnesium and aluminium, may form poorly soluble complexes which are not absorbed (Neuvonen et al., 1970; Greenberger, 1971; Tatro, 1972) (see Fig. 4). Often in the past the conclusion will have been: "... the patient does not respond to the therapy" or "... the infection is not sensitive to the antibiotic". However, measurement of the plasma level of the drug would have indicated an adverse pharmaceutical interaction. A reduction in the drug available for absorption if combined with gastric antacidic aluminium oxide or magnesium oxide preparations and other adsorbents also occurs (Wagner, 1966; Hall and Davis, 1969; Hurwitz, 1971; Tsuchiya and Levy, 1972) (see Fig. 5). In case of dicumarol, simultaneous administration of magnesium oxide or hydroxide increases the plasma level of anticoagulant up to 75% (Akers et al., 1973; Ambre and Fischer, 1973). This phenomenon is not general, since it is not observed with Warfarin. One also has to take into account that magnesium, part of many stomach preparations, is converted in the intestinal tract to a laxative magnesium salt. The resulting enhanced gastrointestinal passage and dilution due to water retention in the intestinal tract may reduce the absorption of other drug. This is true for laxatives and for drugs that cause diarrhoea, such as sympatholytic agents (reserpine and guanethidine) and broad-spectrum antibiotics.

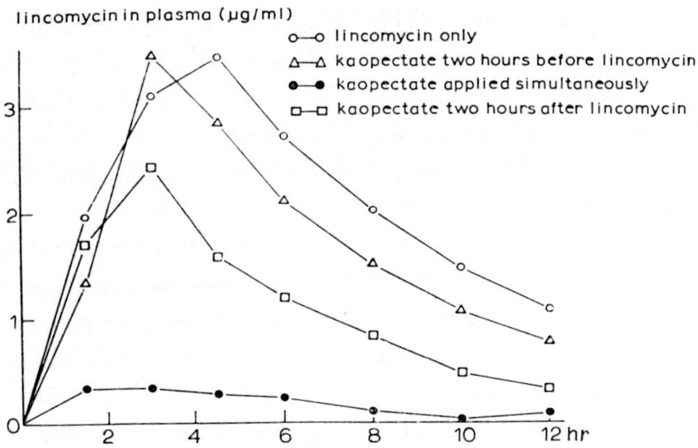

Fig. 5. The influence of kaopectate (kaolin and pectinic acid) on the absorption of lincomycin in man after oral application. *Note:* The decrease in plasma levels caused by the simultaneous application of the adsorbent. (After Wagner, 1966.)

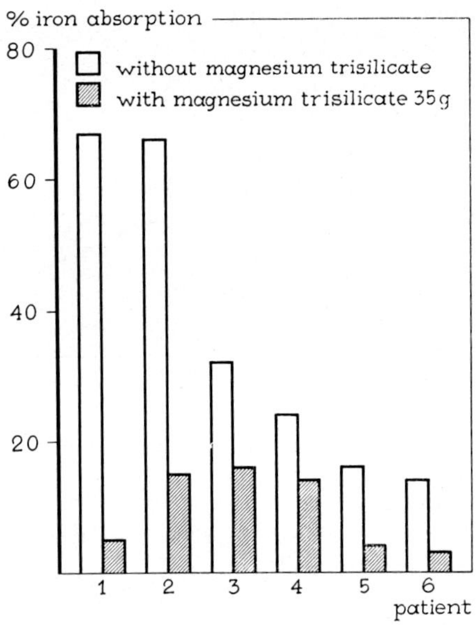

Fig. 6. The influence of magnesium trisilicate (35 g p.o.) on the absorption of iron (5 mg ferrous sulphate in 20 ml water p.o.) in 6 various patients suffering from: (1) hiatal hernia; (2) haemochromatosis; (3) cirrhosis; (4) gastric ulcer; (5) jejunitis; (6) duodenal ulcer. *Note:* The use of magnesium trisilicate strongly decreases the absorption of iron. (After data of Hall and Davis, 1969.)

Acid-neutralizing preparations may also interfere with drug absorption. At a higher pH in the stomach, iron from iron preparations will precipitate and become converted to the poorly absorbed ferric form (Hall and Davis, 1969) (Fig. 6), and acidic drugs may become strongly ionized and thus poorly absorbed (Crouthamel et al., 1971). Drug absorption may also be delayed and reduced by anticholinergics and ganglionic blocking agents which reduce peristalsis of the gastrointestinal tract and secretion of fluids therein (Orrego-Matte et al., 1971; Manninen et al., 1973; Nimmo et al., 1973) (see Fig. 7). If this happens to a patient treated with anticoagulants, the reduced anti-coagulant response may lead to increase of the dosage of the anticoagulant. Once the anticholinergic therapy is stopped, then the anticoagulant accumulated in the gastrointestinal tract will be absorbed and overdose may result. Not only well-known anticholinergics, but also various antihistamines, drugs used in Parkinson's disease, and antidepressive compounds, such as imipramine, have a relatively strong anticholinergic action and thus may bring about this type of complication (Consolo and Garattini, 1969; Kato et al., 1972). The interactions in which gastrointestinal peristalsis is involved are on the verge of the pharmaceutical and the pharmacokinetic phase.

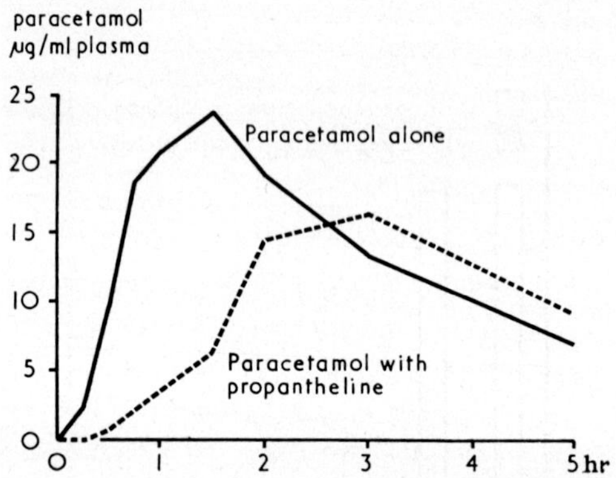

Fig. 7. The delay in the absorption of the analgesic paracetamol (1.5 g in 400 ml water p.o.) by administration of the anticholinergic propantheline (30 mg i.v. 15 min before). Average values obtained with 6 patients are given. *Note:* The spasmolytic strongly influences the plasma concentration and therewith the effect of the analgesic. (After Nimmo et al., 1973.)

6.2 LOSS OF DRUG ACTION DUE TO INTERACTIONS IN THE PHARMACOKINETIC PHASE

In the pharmacokinetic phase of drug action, there are various processes in which drugs can interact. As such may be mentioned binding to plasma proteins, active excretion in the liver and the kidney, passive reabsorption in the renal tubules, and metabolism of drugs.

In many cases the objectives of drug combination are simultaneous actions of the combined drugs. This necessitates a synchronisation of the availability profile, i.e. the plasma and/or tissue concentrations of the compounds. These requirements may be easily fulfilled if both drugs are applied intravenously or locally (if locally active), but the situation is rather problematic especially in the case of oral application. A combination therefore may fail in its therapeutic effect because of lack of concordance in the availability profiles of the compounds combined. Therapeutic failure may also be the result of an interaction between the drugs in the combination at the level of the binding sites, transport systems, metabolizing enzyme systems, etc. In these cases the interactions result in changes in the availability profiles and thus in the action of the drugs.

In the following sections examples will be given of a loss of action due to drug interactions on the level of drug metabolism, plasma protein binding, active transport processes, and the pH-dependent passive transport.

6.2.1 *Interactions in drug metabolism*

In drug metabolism two phases can be distinguished (Fig. 8). In the first phase the drugs are degraded by hydrolytic enzymes, esterases, amidases and glucosidases, by reductions, and expecially by oxidative processes, such as: oxidative deamination, N-dealkylation and O-dealkylation, oxidative breakdown of longer alkyl chains and introduction of hydroxyl groups into aromatic rings. With the exception of some plasma esterases, drug-metabolizing enzymes are located intracellularly, mainly in the endoplasmic reticulum, especially in the liver cells. This implies that in order to be metabolized the drugs must have a certain degree of lipid solubility to penetrate the cells and to reach the enzymes. Strongly hydrophilic drugs, such as the highly ionized quaternary onium compounds and strongly acidic compounds, are therefore not involved in this type of conversion. The ester-type quaternary onium compounds such as suxamethonium can be hydrolyzed by plasma esterases. The hydrolysis of esters and amides as well as the oxidative degradation of drugs results in the formation of products containing –OH, –COOH, and other relatively polar groups.

The introduction of such groups makes the drug metabolite accessible for the conjugation reactions which form the second phase of drug metabolism. The products of the first phase are coupled with molecules, such as glucuronic acid, glycine and sulphate, bound to the polar groups mentioned before. The conjugation products are strongly ionized acids, highly water-soluble

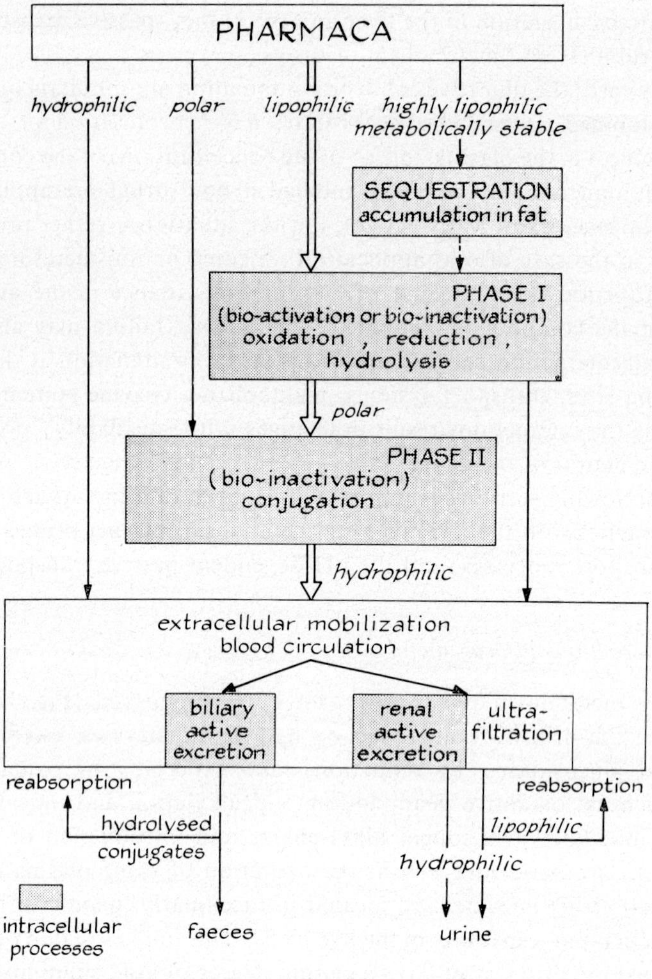

Fig. 8. Schematic representation of the main steps in drug metabolism.

and therefore mobilized in the extracellular fluid compartments. Since they show little or no plasma protein binding, they are fully available for excretion by ultrafiltration in the kidneys.

Considering the extreme variety of exogenous chemicals, including therapeutic agents, that have to be metabolized and eliminated from the body it is quite understandable that nature did not provide for enzyme systems specific for each particular compound. A rather small number of enzyme systems mainly in the endoplasmic reticulum of the liver and a small number of active excretion systems in the kidney and liver take care of the processing of the unlimited variety of foreign compounds. The enzymes are not substrate-specific, as in the case of the general metabolic processes, but they can perform specific types of chemical changes in a very large variety of chemical compounds as long as these compounds are suitable for the particular conversion. Certain esterases split a large variety of esters; a few monoamine oxidases take care of the oxidative deamination of nearly all compounds which contain a suitable amino group; there are enzymes for general N-dealkylation, and O-dealkylation, and for ring hydroxylation, etc. In a similar way the systems involved in active excretion process large groups of compounds with one common characteristic.

An important phenomenon in relation to drug interactions in drug metabolism is enzyme induction, i.e. an increased drug-metabolizing capacity induced by drugs. This induction phenomenon is especially observed after administration of relatively lipid-soluble and slowly metabolized drugs. The phenomenon is not restricted to the enzymes involved in the metabolism of the inducing agent, but comprises nearly the whole spectrum of drug-metabolizing enzymes. Even drugs which are not metabolized themselves can act as inducing agents (Ariëns, 1964; Conney, 1967; Remmer, 1967; Conney, 1969; Sher, 1971).

A consequence of the induction is a shortening of the half-life time of the inducing drug itself – if metabolized – and of other drugs. The resulting reduction in the bioavailability will as a rule cause a reduction in the response. Since a variety of drugs are metabolized by one enzyme system, and the induction phenomenon is extended to a variety of enzyme systems, induction

TABLE I

Shortening of half-life time by drug combination in man

Half-life time Warfarin (min)	Warfarin after pretreatment with	Half-life time reduced to (min)	References
52.0 ±6.7	Glutethimide 1 g 21 days	28.5 ±2.9	MacDonald et al., 1969
54.3 ±5.8	Phenobarbital 120 mg 21 days	29.1 ±3.1	MacDonald et al., 1969
Half-life time phenylbutazone (min)	Phenylbutazone after pretreatment with	Half-life time reduced to (min)	References
78 ±5	Phenobarbital 90 mg	57 ±8	Levi et al., 1968
Half-life time ethylbiscoumacetate (min)	Ethylbiscoumacetate after pretreatment with	Half-life time reduced to (min)	References
60	Phenobarbital 150 mg 10 days	25	Van Dam and Gribnau-Overkamp, 1967
65	Glutethimide 50 mg 10 days	40	Van Dam and Gribnau-Overkamp, 1967

of drug-metabolizing enzymes is a common cause of the loss of drug action based on drug interaction. Also as a matter of fact, drugs which inhibit certain drug-metabolizing enzyme systems will influence the rate of metabolism of other drugs processed by the enzyme system. Only in the case that the metabolic conversion implies a bioactivation will the inhibition result in a decreased bioavailability of the active product formed and thus a reduction of the response.

A variety of cases have been reported in which enzyme-inducing drugs are reported to shorten the half-life time and thus to lower the plasma levels and decrease the response of other drugs with which they are combined (see

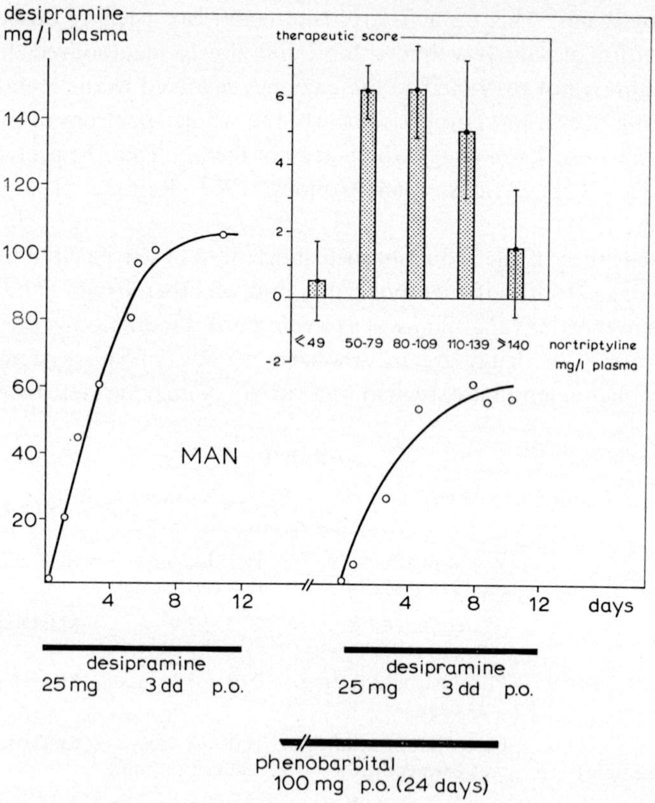

Fig. 9. The effect of phenobarbital on the steady-state plasma levels obtained with chronic application of desipramine. *Note:* The steady-state levels reached with desipramine in combination with phenobarbital medication are about 60% of those reached with desipramine alone. (After data of Sjöqvist et al., 1968.) In the inset: the dependency of the therapeutic score on the plasma concentration of nortriptyline. (After Åsberg et al., 1971.) *Note:* The therapeutic score greatly depends on the plasma levels reached. Plasma levels below 50 mg/l are ineffective while high plasma levels have a low therapeutic score due to the predominant side-effects.

Table I). Fig. 9 (Sjöqvist et al., 1968) gives an example how the steady-state level obtained by chronic treatment with desipramine decreases if phenobarbital is added to the medication. Similar observations are described for combinations of phenobarbital with anticoagulants, corticosteroid hormones and phenytoin (Fig. 10) (MacDonald et al., 1969; Brooks et al., 1972; Cucinell, 1972; Reynolds, 1972). In case of anticoagulants the decrease in the efficacy of the anticoagulant may lead the physician to increase the dose of the anticoagulant in order to restore the prothrombin time to the therapeutic level. If the patient now stops using the enzyme-inducing drug, for instance phenobarbital, with return to normal in the metabolic capacity, an overdosage of the anticoagulant will occur with the risk of haemorrhage. The lowering of the phenytoin concentration below the therapeutically required level by enzyme-inducing agents may have serious consequences (Morselli et al., 1971; Cucinell, 1972).

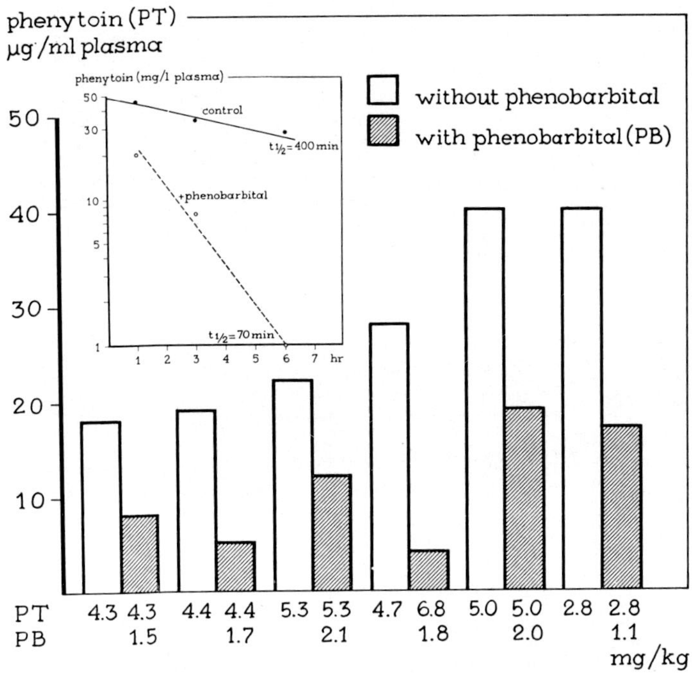

Fig. 10. Plasma levels of phenytoin in epileptic patients treated for 21 days with phenytoin alone and for 21 days with phenytoin in combination with phenobarbital. (After Morselli et al., 1971.) *Note:* In combination with phenobarbital the plasma levels of phenytoin are significantly reduced. In the inset: the influence of phenobarbital on the rate of elimination of phenytoin from plasma (dog). (After Burns and Conney, 1965.) *Note:* Phenobarbital strongly enhances the rate of elimination of phenytoin and thus reduces the half-life time of this drug from 400 to 70 min.

Although a metabolic conversion of the compound to an active metabolite has been reported for a number of drugs, a loss of action due to combination with inhibitors of the enzymes involved in this conversion has only been achieved experimentally. Under certain circumstances, however, it may be of clinical significance.

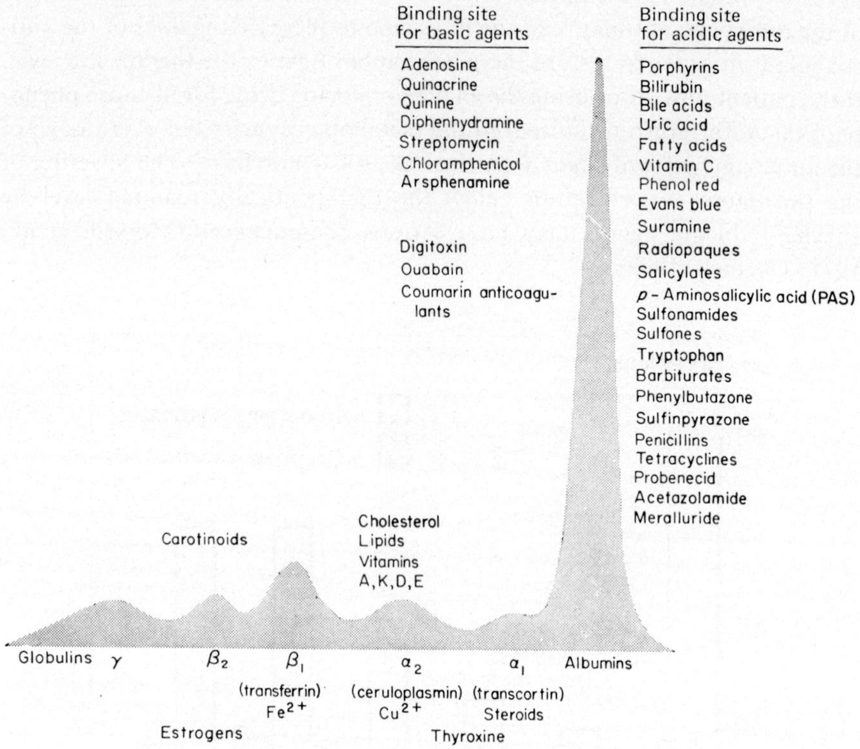

Fig. 11. Schematic representation of the binding of a variety of drugs to various plasma proteins. (Modified after Bennhold, 1966.) *Note:* The prevalence of drug binding to albumins, the great variability of the drugs involved, and the binding to only a few types of binding sites.

6.2.2 *Loss of action due to displacement from plasma proteins*

With regard to a drug circulating in plasma, the drug free in solution and therefore freely exchangeable with the extravascular compartments via the vascular wall must be differentiated from the protein-bound drug which is restricted to the vascular compartment. Strongly hydrophilic compounds, such as the highly water-soluble conjugates formed in the second phase of drug metabolism, are slightly or not bound to plasma proteins. Many drugs, especially those which are rather lipophilic, have a usually strong tendency to bind to plasma proteins. Again a large variety of compounds are bound on only a few types of binding sites. On plasma albumin, for instance, there are binding sites for lipophilic (hydrophobic) acidic compounds and binding sites for lipophilic (hydrophobic) bases (Bennhold, 1966) (see Fig. 11). Mutual displacement of compounds bound to common binding sites will therefore not be uncommon. Besides binding to plasma albumin, binding of drugs to other tissue components should be taken into account. Certain strongly basic compounds such as various bisquaternary onium compounds are found bound to tissues rich in acid mucopolysaccharides such as cartilaginous tissue (Hespe and Wieriks, 1971; Wassermann, 1972). Displacement can also take place in these tissues.

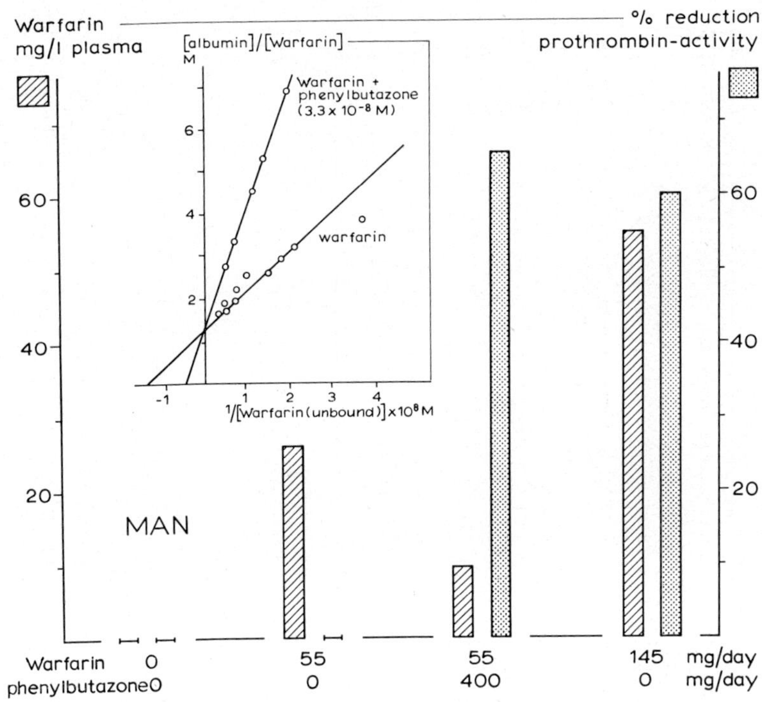

Fig. 12. The paradoxical relationship between plasma concentration and effect of the anticoagulant Warfarin if combined with phenylbutazone. (After data of Aggeler et al., 1967.) *Note:* If combined with phenylbutazone a dose of Warfarin 55 mg/day reaches a much lower plasma concentration; nevertheless its effect (reduction of prothrombin activity) is much stronger, and more or less equal to that of a much higher dose given alone (145 mg/day). – In the inset: the displacement of Warfarin from albumin in the presence of phenylbutazone. (After Solomon and Schrogie, 1967.) *Note:* The relationship observed indicates a competitive displacement of Warfarin from its binding sites on albumin by phenylbutazone.

The consequence of a displacement of drugs from plasma proteins will be an increase in the concentration of the drug in its unbound form which, due to the fact that the compound liberated from the plasma proteins can pass the vascular wall and thus distribute over a much larger volume, remains restricted as compared to the relatively strong decrease in the total plasma concentration of the drug concerned. Therefore, if a drug bound 99% to

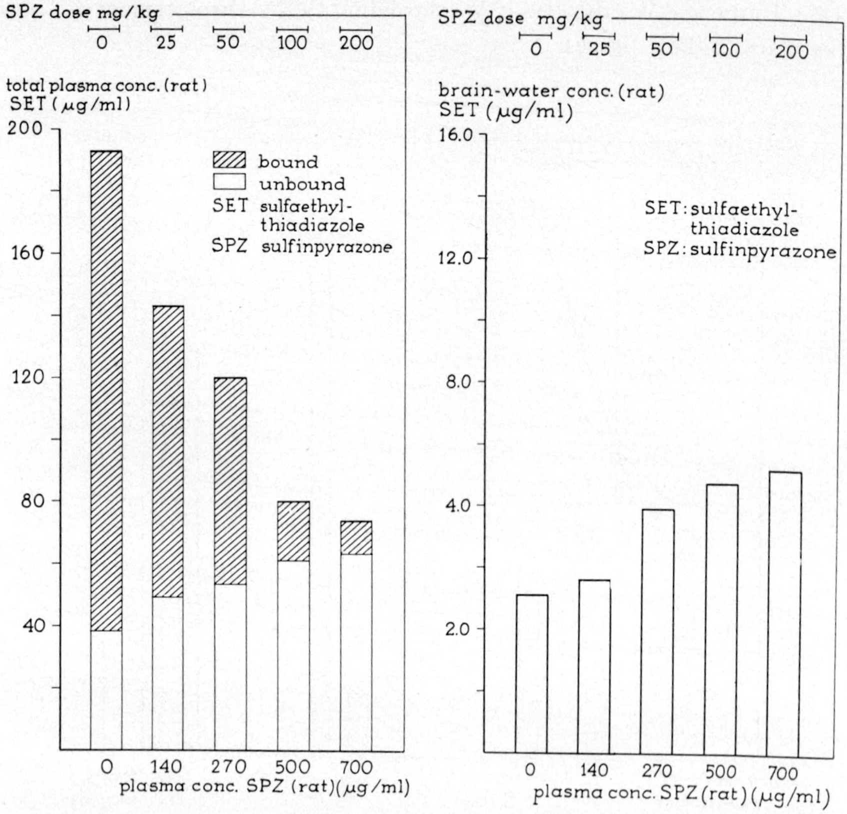

Fig. 13. The displacement of sulphaethylthiadiazole (SET), a strongly plasma albumin-bound drug, from the plasma compartment to the tissues under the influence of sulfinpyrazone (SPZ), an also strongly plasma protein-bound drug. (a) The decrease in total plasma concentration of SET with a concomitant increase in the concentration of SET in the unbound form under the influence of SPZ. (b) The increase in the concentration of SET in brain tissue fluid under the influence of SPZ. (After data of Anton, 1961.) *Note:* The displacement on the level of the plasma proteins results in a decrease in the total plasma concentration and an increase in the concentration of SET in its unbound form in plasma and a corresponding increase in the concentration of SET in tissue fluids

plasma proteins is displaced so that only 50% remains bound, this does not imply that the free concentration then rises to the 50-fold of the original one. The rise in this concentration and in the concentration of the drug in the interstitial fluid remains restricted but a doubling or more of the free plasma concentration may easily be reached. This then implies an increase in the availability of the compound also in the target compartment and thus an increase in the response. A decrease in plasma concentration therefore does not necessarily imply a loss of action (Gillette, 1967; Ariëns, 1969b; 1973; Ariëns and Simonis, 1972). Fig .12 shows this paradox for a combination of the anticoagulant Warfarin and phenylbutazone (Solomon and Schrogie, 1967; Aggeler et al., 1967).

Differences observed between the concentrations of a drug in plasma and cerebrospinal fluid may be due to the so-called blood–brain barrier. Highly ionized onium compounds, for instance, do not pass this barrier, therefore do not reach the CNS and thus are devoid of CNS actions. Often, however, a difference in the plasma and liquor concentration is due to a high binding of the agent involved to proteins in plasma while such proteins are nearly absent in the cerebrospinal fluid. The concentration in the cerebrospinal fluid then will be practically equal to the concentration of the drug in its unbound form in plasma. For drugs able to penetrate the blood–brain barrier, a displacement from the plasma proteins thus may result in a rise in the levels of the drug in the CNS (Fig. 13) (Anton, 1961) and thus in an increased central response.

The rise in the concentration of the drug in its unbound form in the circulation implies an increase in the concentration available for excretion by ultrafiltration in the kidney. On the other hand, a substantial decrease in the total plasma concentration due to displacement and redistribution will imply a decrease in the load of the drug offered to the eliminating systems, such as drug-metabolizing enzymes in the liver and active excretion systems in the kidney. If the rate of dissociation of the drug–protein complex is sufficiently high, and the clearance of the drug approaches that of the blood flow through the liver or the kidney such that the blood is cleared of drug to a greater degree, the displacement and the inherent decrease in the total plasma load will result in a decrease in the quantity of drug eliminated per unit of time by drug metabolism and active excretion, and thus in a prolonged action (Fig. 14) (Ariëns, 1969b; Ariëns and Simonis, 1972).

Not only for body-foreign, but also for body-own compounds bound to plasma proteins, such as bilirubin, displacement by drugs may take place. Again a shift of the compound to the tissues will be the result. In the case of bilirubin such a shift may result in a damage to the CNS in the sense of a 'kern'-icterus (see Fig. 15) (Silverman et al., 1956; Watson, 1962).

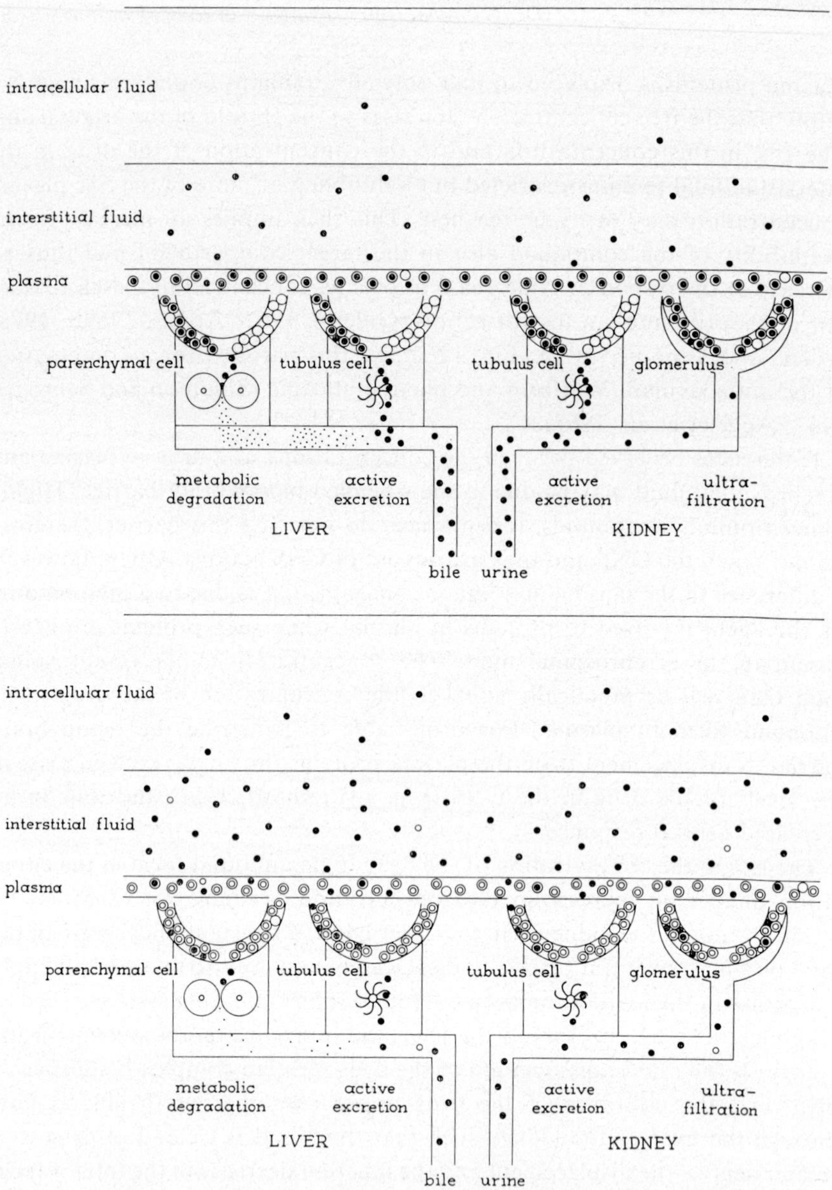

Fig. 14. Schematic representation of the excretion by the kidney and the liver of a drug (•) with a strong plasma protein binding but a high rate of dissociation of the drug–protein complex (a), and the influence thereon of a second drug (o) displacing the first one from the plasma proteins (b). *Note:* Glomerular filtration is restricted to the unbound drug, while active excretion and metabolic degradation extend themselves to the total plasma concentration of the drug. The displacing drug enhances the concentration of the first drug in its unbound form, and therefore its excretion by ultrafiltration. Due to the decrease in the total plasma concentration as a result of the redistribution after displacement the rate of active excretion and metabolic degradation will be decreased. This will especially be the case if the clearance approximates the plasma flow through the organ systems concerned.

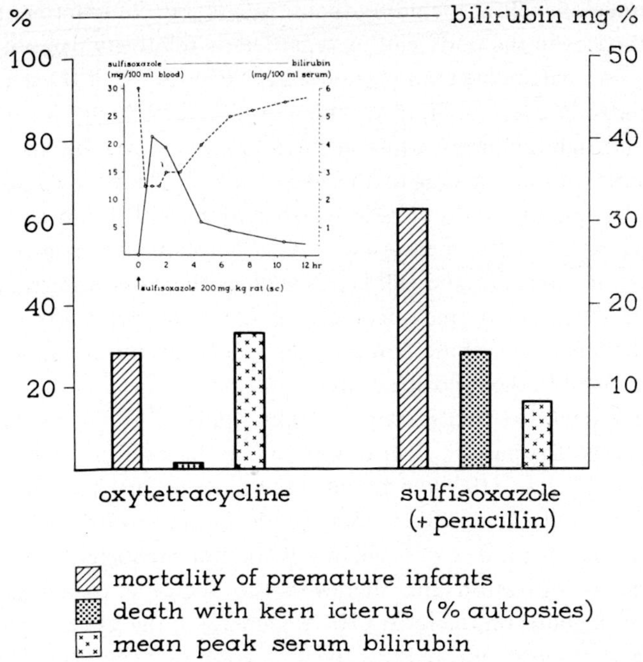

Fig. 15. The influence of prophylactic treatment of premature children with oxytetracycline and with a combination of sulphisoxazole and penicillin. (After Silverman et al., 1956.) *Note* the relatively high mortality in the sulphisoxazole-treated group, and the concomitant large frequence of 'kern' icterus and relatively low plasma bilirubin level. This is in contrast with the oxytetracycline treated group where the frequency of 'kern' icterus is very low although the bilirubin levels are significantly higher. The inset gives the relation between the plasma levels of sulphisoxazole and bilirubin studied in the rat. (After Watson, 1962.) *Note:* The decrease in bilirubin serum level in the presence of high sulphisoxazole blood levels due to the displacement of bilirubin by sulphisoxazole from plasma albumin.

6.2.3 *Loss of action due to interactions in excretion processes*

The drug products of conjugation reactions as a rule are substrates for the systems in kidney and liver involved in the active excretion of body-foreign compounds with the urine and the bile. After active excretion with the urine because of the high water-solubility there will be little or no passive reabsorption; in this way efficient elimination is guaranteed. As a rule the conjugation products as such are already inactive such that detoxification has taken place. Conjugation products excreted with the bile into the intestine may be hydrolyzed there and the drugs or drug metabolites originally conjugated may become available again for absorption and possibly action.

As already mentioned, the strongly hydrophilic and highly ionized conjugation products are mobilized and restricted in their distribution mainly to the extracellular fluid including the intravascular compartment. The various membranes in the body can be regarded as relatively lipophilic barriers separating compartments containing water. Penetration of these membranes will be relatively easy for lipid-soluble compounds which can pass by free diffusion through the lipids, while the membranes are real barriers for highly water-soluble compounds, with the exception of the very small inorganic ions, such as sodium and chloride which may pass through the very small water-filled pores in the membranes. As a consequence, passive transport through cell membranes and cell layers such as the gastrointestinal wall and the wall of the renal tubules depends on the water-solubility of the compound. Extremely lipophilic compounds may be accumulated and more or less sequestrated in the lipid structures of the organism. Compounds with an intermediate position, that is with a certain lipid- as well as water-solubility are most suited for passive distribution. Weak bases and weak acids, comprising the majority of the compounds used as drugs, are partially ionized at the pH of the body fluids. Such compounds will penetrate the lipid barriers in the unionized form and pass the water compartments in the ionized form. The degree of ionization and therewith the degree of penetration of the membranes depends on the local pH. A decrease in the pH promotes ionization of the weak bases and reduces the ionization of weak acids. An increase in the pH has the opposite effect. In the extramural fluid compartments such as the fluid in the intestinal lumen and the urine, the pH, which can strongly deviate from that in the extracellular and intracellular compartments, strongly influences the degree of ionization of drugs. A high degree of ionization

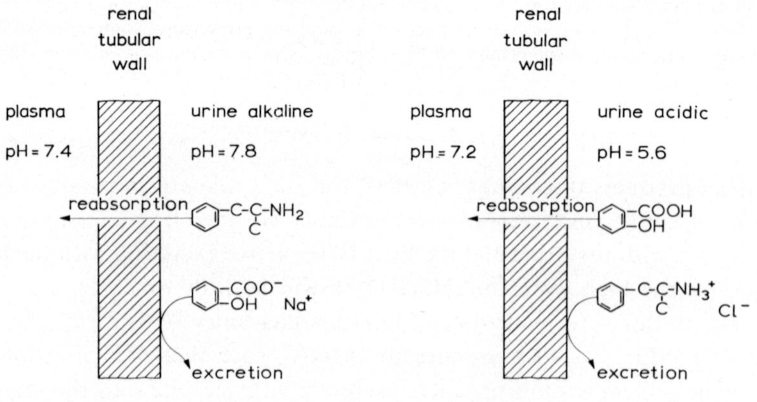

Fig. 16. Schematic representation of the influences of the urinary pH on the passive reabsorption of a weak acid and a weak base from the urine in the renal tubules. *Note:* At a high pH the passive reabsorption of the weak base and the excretion of the weak acid are enhanced while at a low pH value the reabsorption of the weak acid and the excretion of the weak base are enhanced.

in the extramural compartment will limit absorption and reabsorption of the compound, while a low degree of ionization will facilitate absorption and reabsorption (Hogben et al., 1959; Ariëns, 1964) (see Fig. 16). Thus drugs which bring about changes in the pH in the intestinal fluid or in the urine may greatly change the absorption from the gut or reabsorption from the renal tubules of other drugs.

As mentioned, the pH of the urine is an important factor in renal reabsorption of weakly acidic and weakly basic drugs. The consequence is that, for instance, systemically alkalinizing substances, e.g. sodium bicarbonate used in tablets to neutralize acid production in the stomach, will enhance the excretion of weakly acidic compounds such as salicylic acid. If chronic treatment with salicylic acid preparations, e.g. aspirin, is combined with sodium bicarbonate, such that the pH of the urine which normally is around 5.8 rises to about 6.5., the steady-state plasma level of salicylate is only about 50% of that obtained under normal circumstances (Levy and Leonards, 1971) (see Fig. 17). Similar phenomena will occur with other weak acid-type organic agents, especially those with a high lipid-solubility in the unionized form such as many of the sulphonamides. This especially holds true for the long-acting sulphonamides since their prolonged action greatly depends on their passive renal reabsorption. For various urinary antiinfectious agents, e.g. nalidixic acid and amygdalic acid, which require a low pH to be effective, alkalinization also results in a loss of action, but this is not based on changes

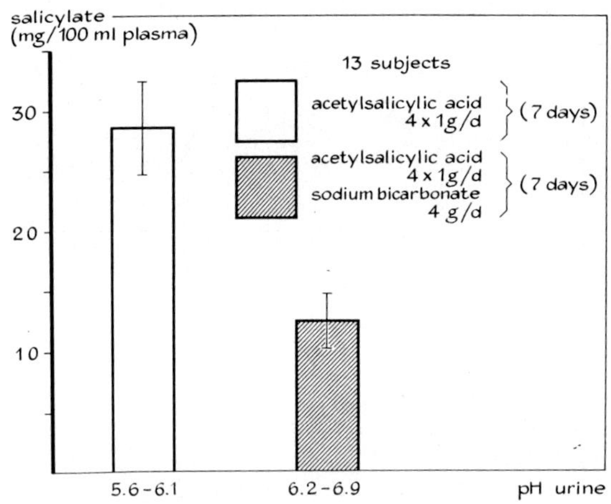

Fig. 17. The influence of the systemically alkalinizing agent sodium bicarbonate on the plasma levels obtained with acetylsalicylic acid after chronic treatment. (After Levy and Leonards, 1971.) *Note:* Due to the increased urinary pH and the consequential increased degree of ionization passive reabsorption of salicylic acid is decreased, excretion is enhanced, thus plasma level is lowered. (See Fig. 16.)

in the reabsorption. Since combination of stomach preparations with other drugs is not uncommon, taking into account the fact that many drugs cause gastrointestinal side-effects, there is no doubt, that such combinations in many cases will result in a loss of therapeutic efficacy. Fig. 18 shows that for basic drugs like quinidine the plasma levels and the therapeutic response are dependent on the pH of the urine (Gerhardt et al., 1969). The use of systemically alkalinizing or acidifying drugs may easily upset the dosage regimens for patients treated with basic drugs to which, by the way, belong most psychopharmacological drugs, antihistamines, adrenergic blocking agents, narcotic analgesics, etc.

The complications observed with combinations of drugs are not always easy to interpret as far as the mechanisms involved. Often the changes in the plasma concentration, in the half-life time of the drug, and in the rate of excretion of the drug or its metabolites in the urine, may give sufficient

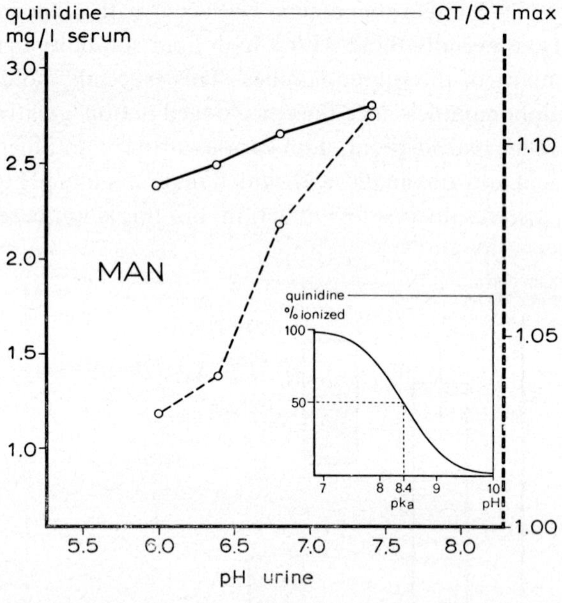

Fig. 18. Serum quinidine levels (——) and the change in the response (the ratio of the measured Q–T interval to the maximum normal Q–T interval) (.......) plotted as a function of the pH of the urine. (After Gerhardt et al., 1969.) *Note:* Increase in the urinary pH results in an increase in the degree of ionization of quinidine and therewith its passive reabsorption increases and consequently plasma levels and response increase. A decrease in urinary pH has the opposite effect. The inset gives the dependence of the degree of ionization of quinidine on the local pH. *Note* the decrease in the amount of ionized and therewith charged drug at low pH values and the increase in the unionized and therewith uncharged fraction at high pH values. At the pH value equal to pK_a value 50% of the drug is present in the ionized and 50% in the unionized form.

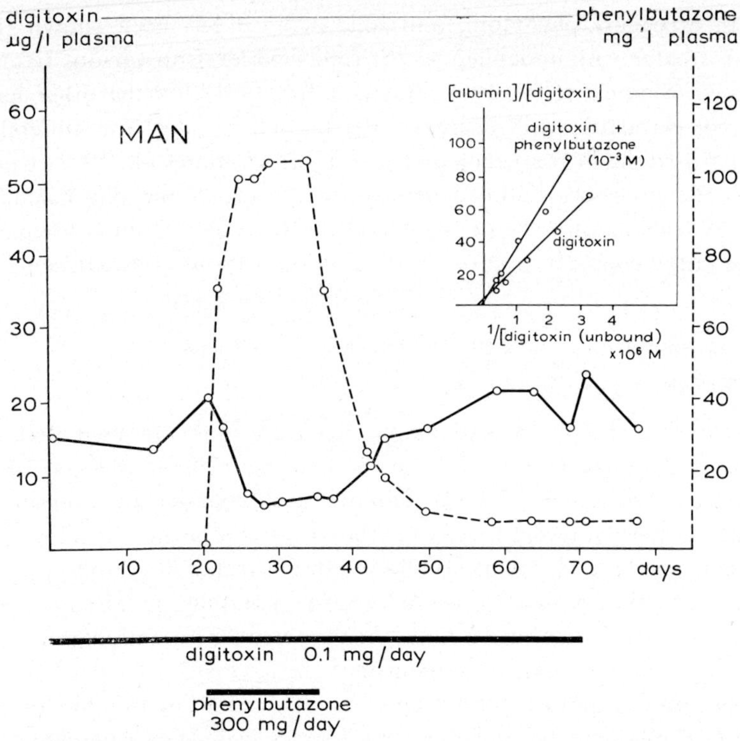

Fig. 19. The plasma concentration of digitoxin (——) after chronic application and the change therein by application of phenylbutazone, the plasma concentration of which is also given (- - - -) (Solomon et al., 1971.) *Note:* These phenomena suggest a redistribution of digitoxin due to displacement of this drug from plasma albumin by phenylbutazone. The inset gives the displacement of digitoxin by phenylbutazone from plasma albumin. (After Solomon et al., 1971). *Note:* The relationship observed indicates a competitive displacement of digitoxin by phenylbutazone. For further comment see text.

information to draw conclusions; frequently, however, the situation may be rather complex. Fig. 19 shows a patient on chronic treatment with digitoxin and a temporary additional therapy with phenylbutazone (Solomon et al., 1971). During phenylbutazone treatment there is a clear decrease in the digitoxin concentration in plasma. Although phenylbutazone can displace digitoxin from plasma albumin, this is not the main cause of the decrease in glycoside concentration. This may be concluded from the latency time in this decrease and from the enhanced excretion of digitoxin metabolites in the urine observed after application of phenylbutazone (Solomon et al., 1971). It is probable that, besides displacement from plasma proteins, phenylbutazone also induces an increase in drug-metabolizing capacity.

Similarly puzzling is the interaction between various antiepileptic compounds, especially phenytoin, and folic acid. It has been shown that in patients treated with antiepileptics the folic acid levels in various tissues are decreased (Sjöqvist et al., 1968; Baylis et al., 1971); on the other hand, a supply of extra folic acid decreases the plasma levels of the antiepileptics and increases the fit frequency and severity (Morselli et al., 1971; Cucinell, 1972). The processes outlined before are aspects of the pharmacokinetic phase of drug action. The drug interactions have as a main consequence a change in the concentration of the drug in the various compartments.

6.3 LOSS OF DRUG ACTION DUE TO INTERACTIONS IN THE PHARMACODYNAMIC PHASE

Interactions in the pharmacodynamic phase are more frequent than interactions in the pharmaceutical or in the pharmacokinetic phase (Cohen of Birkenhead, 1965). One of the possibilities is competitive antagonism at the level of the specific receptor sites for the drugs combined. Since the consequence of combination of metabolites with antimetabolites and of agonists with competitive antagonists is well known, non-intentional combinations of this type are an exception. Only the treatments with antidotes are sometimes based on this type of antagonism.

An example of an incidental drug combination leading to a loss of action is that of sulphonamides and local anaesthetics such as procainamide which rapidly hydrolyze in plasma under liberation of *p*-aminobenzoic acid, a highly effective antagonist of sulphonamides.

The various other types of antagonisms such as *functional antagonism*, which in fact is an antagonism between two agonists, and *non-competitive antagonism*, where the antagonists block the effector system for the agonist will not be discussed here.

In many cases of drug antagonism in the pharmacodynamic phase there is not sufficient understanding of the exact mechanism behind it to come to a clear-cut classification (Ariëns and Simonis, 1972; Ariëns, 1974).

Interesting is the loss of action of the guanethidine-type antihypertensive agents in the presence of tricyclic antidepressants (e.g. imipramine), certain of the chlorpromazine-type neuroleptic agents, and CNS-stimulant drugs such as amphetamine (Day and Rand, 1962; Skinner et al., 1969; Meyer et al., 1970; Medical News, 1972; Ober and Wang, 1973). The antihypertensive agents mentioned are known to act as depletors of the norepinephrine stores at the sympathetic nerve terminals. Imipramine, chlorpromazine in higher doses, and amphetamine block the uptake of the guanethidine-type compound into the storage sites of norepinephrine at the nerve endings, and counteract in this way the norepinephrine-depleting and the hypotensive action of the guanethidines. The blockade of the central effects of amphetamine by amantadine has also been described (Menon et al., 1973).

An intriguing interaction is the inhibition of the analgesic effect of morphine by β-adrenergic blocking agents observed in mice (Heller et al., 1968) and recently confirmed with regard to the induction of an abstinence syndrome by β-adrenergic blocking agents in heroin addicts (Grosz, 1972; Lowenstein, 1973). The full significance of these observations with regard to clinical implications for combinations of β-adrenergic blocking agents and narcotic analgesics and with regard to our understanding of the mode of action of these compounds cannot be estimated yet.

Of particular importance is the loss of the bactericidal action of a number of antibiotics if combined with bacteriostatic agents (see Chapter 9, p. 184). Bactericidal agents, such as the penicillins, the cephalosporins, vancomycin and cycloserine, act by inhibiting the synthesis of the constituents of the bacterial wall and thus interfere with the multiplication of bacteria which require the synthesis of new bacterial wall material. If bacterial growth is stopped, these agents lose their action. Consequentially combinations of these antibiotics with tetracyclines, chloramphenicol, sulphonamides, streptomycins, etc., result in a loss of the action of the bactericidal compound, at least if the bacteriostatic agents reached effective concentration before or simultaneously with the second agent (see Tables II and III) (Jawetz and Gunnison, 1953; Hartshorn, 1969). This also holds true for combinations of the bactericidal compound nalidixic acid with bacteriostatic agents such as the tetracyclines and chloramphenicol, and with nitrofurantoin. Such an

TABLE II

Classification of antiinfectious agents

I. Bactericidal inhibitors of mucopeptide synthesis	III. Bacteriostatic inhibitors of protein synthesis
Penicillins	Tetracyclines
Cephalosporins	Chloramphenicol
D-Cycloserine	Sulphonamides
Vancomycin	Erythromycin
Ristocetin	Lincomycin
II. Attacking membranes	IV. Bactericidal inhibitors of protein synthesis
Polymyxin	Streptomycins
Bacitracin	Kanamycin
Colistin	Neomycin

Combinations of type I with type III are of questionable value since these bacteriostatic agents tend to antagonize these bactericidal agents.

TABLE III

Antibiotics interfering with penicillin activity

Drugs inhibiting effect of penicillin	Drugs not inhibiting effect of penicillin
Tetracyclines	Bacitracin
Chloramphenicol	Vancomycin
Erythromycin	Cephalothin
Oleandomycin	Polymyxin
Kanamycin	Colistin
Neomycin	Cycloserine
Paromomycin	
Streptomycin	

antagonism is not observed if the bactericidal compounds mentioned are combined with bactericidal agents such as polymyxin and bacitracin which act by attacking the bacterial membranes (Hartshorn, 1969).

Awareness of the complications of drug combinations and the far-reaching consequences which they may have is based on the many reports of such complications especially in treatment with anticoagulant drugs and oral antidiabetic agents. This does not mean that such complications are characteristic especially for these groups of drugs, but arises because monitoring the response of the patient under treatment with these groups of drugs is a common procedure. In the meantime a massive body of evidence for complications for the antiepileptic drugs due to drug combinations has been built up (Woodbury et al., 1972). No doubt, once the medical profession pays as much attention to therapy as to diagnosis, which from the point of view of the patient is highly desirable, still more evidence for undesirable consequences of drug combinations will be found. This will then supply us with solid evidence about the possibilities and especially the limitations of drug combinations.

The various examples given are only a selection out of the wide variety of drug combinations leading to iatrogenic therapy resistance. They may be sufficient, however, to make the physician aware of the fact that unintentional and incidental drug combinations will often appear to be deleterious combinations, not only due to overdosage effects and toxic reactions in general, but also because of deprivation of the patient of therapeutic benefit.

References

Aggeler, P. M., O'Reilly, R. A., Leong, L. and Kowitz, P. E. (1967): Potentiation of anticoagulant effect of warfarin by phenylbutazone. *New. Engl. J. Med.*, **276**, 496.

Akers, M. J., Lach, J. L. and Fischer, L. J. (1973): Alterations in absorption of dicumarol by various excipient materials. *J. Pharm. Sci.*, **62**, 391.

Ambre, J. J. and Fischer, L. J. (1973): Effect of coadministration of aluminum and magnesium hydroxides on absorption of anticoagulants in man. *Clin. Pharmacol. Therap.*, **14**, 231.

Anton, A. H. (1961): A drug-induced change in the distribution and renal excretion of sulfonamides. *J. Pharmacol. exp. Therap.*, **134**, 291.

Ariëns, E. J. (1964): Molecular Pharmacology. Vol. 1. Academic Press, New York.

Ariëns, E. J. (1969a): Reduction of drug action by drug combination. *J. Mond. Pharm.*, **12**, 263.

Ariëns, E. J. (1969b): Modulation of pharmacokinetics by modification of the various factors involved. *Il Farmaco*, **24**,3.

Ariëns, E. J. (1971): Adverse drug interactions. Interaction of drugs on the pharmacodynamic level. Proc. XIII Meeting Europ. Soc. for the Study of Drug Toxicity, Berlin. Excerpta Medica Int. Congr. Series no. 254, p. 137.

Ariëns, E. J. (1973): Combinatie van geneesmiddelen; mogelijkheden en beperkingen. *Ned. T. Geneesk.*, **117**, 434.

Ariëns, E. J. (1974): Drug action; Target tissue, dose–response relationships, receptors. Proc. Conf. Pharmacol. Pharmacokin.: Problems and Perspectives 1972. Editors: P. G. Condliffe, Fogarty Intern. Center.

Ariëns, E. J. and Simonis, A. M. (1972): The mechanisms of adverse drug reactions. In: *Drug-Induced Diseases*. Vol. 4, p. 110. Editors: L. Meyler and H. M. Peck. Excerpta Medica, Amsterdam.

Åsberg, M., Crönholm, B., Sjöqvist, F. and Tuck, D. (1971): Relationship between plasma level and therapeutic effect of nortriptyline. *Brit. med. J.*, **3**, 331.

Baylis, E. M., Crowley, J. M., Preece, J. M., Sylvester, P. E. and Marks, V. (1971): Influence of folic acid on blood-phenytoin levels, *Lancet*, **1**, 62.

Beckett, A. H. and Rowland, M. (1965): Urinary excretion kinetics of amphetamine in man. *J. Pharm. Pharmacol.*, **17**, 628.

Bennhold, H. (1966): Transport function of the serum proteins: Historical review and report on recent investigations on the transport of dyestuffs and of iron. In: *Transport Function of Plasma Proteins*. West European Symposium on Clinical Chemistry. Vol. 5, p. 1. Editors: P. Desgrez and P. M. de Traverse. Elsevier, Amsterdam.

Beumer, H. M. (1968): Willem Storm van Leeuwen und seine Bedeutung für die Asthmaforschung. Triltsch, Düsseldorf.

Brooks, S. M., Werk, E. E., Ackerman, S. J., Sullivan, I. and Thrasher, K. (1972): Adverse effects of phenobarbital on corticosteroid metabolism in patients with bronchial asthma. *New Engl. J. Med.*, **286**, 1125.

Burns, J. J. and Conney, A. H. (1965): Enzyme stimulation and inhibition in the metabolism of drugs, Symposium No. 7, Section I, Clinical effects of interaction between drugs. *Proc. roy. Soc. Med.*, **58**, 955.

Bushby, S. R. M. and Hitchings, G. H. (1968): Trimethoprim, a sulphonamide potentiator. *Brit. J. Pharmacol. Chemother.*, **33**, 72.

Cohen of Birkenhead, Rt. Hon. Lord (1965): Panel discussion: drug interaction in relation to acute poisoning. *Proc. roy. Soc. Med.*, **58**, 995.

Conney, A. H. (1967): Pharmacological implications of microsomal enzyme induction. *Pharmacol. Rev.*, **19**, 317.

Conney, A. H. (1969): Drug metabolism and therapeutics. *New Engl. J. Med.*, **280**, 653.

Consolo, S. and Garattini, S. (1969): Effect of desipramine on intestinal absorption of phenylbutazone and other drugs. *Europ. J. Pharmacol.*, **6**, 322.

Cordes, G. and Göbbeler, K. H. (1971): Onverenigbaarheid van fenylefrinehydrochloride met formaldehyde-caseïne. *Pharm. Ind.*, **33**, 299.

Crouthamel, W. G., Tan, G. H., Dittert, L. W. and Doluisio, J. T. (1971): Drug absorption, IV. Influence of pH on absorption kinetics of weakly acidic drugs. *J. Pharm. Sci.*, **60**, 1160.

Cucinell, S. A. (1972): Phenobarbital, interactions with other drugs. In: Antiepileptic Drugs, p. 319. Editors: D. M. Woodbury, J. K. Penry and R. P. Schmidt. Raven Press. New York.

Dale, J. K. (1966): Pharmaceutical incompatibilities and adverse drug reactions. In: Pharmaceutical dispensing, 6th ed. p. 496. Editors: E. W. Martin and J. E. Hoover. Mack Easton, Pa.

Day, M. D. and Rand, M. J. (1962): Antagonism of guanethidine by dexamphetamine and other related sympathomimetic amines. *J. Pharm. Pharmacol.*, **14**, 541.

Editorial (1969): Synergy of trimethoprim and sulphonamides. *Brit. med. J.*, **2**, 507.

Elslager, E. F. and Worth, D. F. (1965): Repository antimalarial drugs: n,n-diacetyl-4,4-diaminodiphenylsulphone and related 4-acylaminodiphenylsulphones. *Nature*, **206**, 630.

Ferel, D. (1972): Die Behandlung des Parkinson-Syndroms mit L-Dopa und einem Dekarboxylasehemmer (Ro 4-4602). *Schweiz. med. Wschr.*, **102**, 88.

Garb, S. (1971): Clinical Guide to Undesirable Drug Interactions and Interferences. Springer, New York.

Gerhardt, R. E., Knouss, R. F., Thyrum, P. T., Luchi R. J. and Morris, J. J. (1969): Quinidine excretion in aciduria and alkaluria. *Ann. intern. Med.*, **71**, 927.

Gibaldi, M., Davidson, D., Plaut, M. E. and Schwartz, M. A. (1970): Modification of penicillin distribution and elimination by probenecid. *Intern J. clin. Pharmacol.*, **3**, 182.

Gillette, J. R. (1967): In: Animal and Clinical Pharmacologic Techniques in Drug Evaluation, Vol. 2, p. 48. Editors: P. E. Siegler and J. H. Moyer. Year Book Med. Publ. Inc., Chicago.

Greenberger, N. J. (1971): Absorption of tetracyclines: interference by iron. *Ann. intern. Med.*, **74**, 792.

Grosz, H. J. (1972): Narcotic withdrawal symptoms in heroin users treated with propranolol. *Lancet*, **2**, 564.

Hall, G. J. L. and Davis, A. E. (1969): Inhibition of iron absorption by magnesium trisilicate. *Med. J. Aust.*, **2**, 95.

Hansten, P. D. (1971): Drug interactions. Lea and Febiger, Philadelphia.

Hartshorn, E. A. (1969): Drug interactions. III. Classes of drugs and their interactions; anti-infective agents. Drug Intell., **3**, 70.

Hartshorn, E. A. (1970): Handbook of Drug interactions. Francke, Cincinnati.

Heller, B., Saavedra, J. M. and Fischer, E. (1968): Influence of adrenergic blocking agents upon morphine and catecholamine analgesic effect. Experientia, **24**, 804.

Hespe, W. and Wieriks, J. (1971): Metabolic fate of the short-acting peripheral neuromuscular blocking agent Stercuronium in the rat, as related to its action. *Biochem. Pharmacol.*, **20**, 1213.

Hogben, C. A. M., Tocco, D. J., Brodie, B. B. and Schanker, L. S. (1959): On the mechanism of intestinal absorption of drugs. *J. Pharmacol. exp. Therap.*, **125**, 275.

Hurwitz, A. (1971): The effects of antacids on gastrointestinal drug absorption. II. Effect on sulfadiazine and quinine. *J. Pharmacol. exp. Therap.*, **179**, 485.

Informatorium Medicamentorum (1972): Vol. 1, p. 97. Koninklijke Nederlandse Maatschappij ter bevordering der Pharmacie, 's-Gravenhage, The Netherlands.

Jawetz, E. and Gunnison, J. B. (1953): Antibiotic synergism and antagonism: an assessment of the problem. *Pharmacol. Rev.*, **5**, 175.

Kato, R., Takanaka, A., Onoda, K. and Omori, Y. (1972): Drug affecting the gastric emptying rate and drug absorption. *Jap. J. Pharmacol.*, **22**, 434.

Kramer, W., Inglott, A. and Cluxton, R. (1971): Some physical and chemical incompatibilities of drugs for i.v. administration. *Drug Intell. Clin. Pharm.*, **5**, 211.

Levi, A. J., Sherlock, S. and Walker, D. (1968): Phenylbutazone and isoniazid metabolism in patients with liver disease in relation to previous drug therapy. *Lancet*, **2**, 1275.

Levy, G. and Leonards, J. R. (1971): Urine pH and salicylate therapy. *J. Amer. med. Assoc.*, **217**, 81.

Lowenstein, H. (1973): Propranolol as a psychotropic agent. *Lancet*, **1**, 559.

MacDonald, M. G., Robinson, D. S., Sylwester, D. and Jaffe, J. J. (1969): The effects of phenobarbital, chloral betaine, and glutethimide administration on warfarin plasma levels and hypoprothrombinemic responses in man. *Clin. Pharmacol. Therap.*, **10**, 80.

Manninen, V., Melin, J., Apajalahti, A. and Karesoja, M. (1973): Altered absorption of digoxin in patients given propantheline and metoclopramide. *Lancet*, **1**, 398.

Martin, E. W. (1971): Hazards of medication. Editors: S. F. Alexander, D. J. Farage and W. E. Hassan. Lippincott, Philadelphia.

Medical News (1972), Chlorpromazine, another guanethidine antagonist, *J. Amer. Med. Assoc.*, **220**, 1288.

Menon, M. K., Clark, W. G. and Fleming, R. M. (1973): Blockade of the central effects of D-amphetamine sulfate by amantadine hydrochloride. *Europ. J. Pharmacol.*, **21**, 311.

Meyer, J. F., McAllister, C. K. and Goldberg, L. I. (1970): Insidious and prolonged antagonism of guanethidine by amitriptyline. *J. Amer. med. Assoc.*, **213**, 1487.

Morselli, P. L., Rizzo, M. and Garattini, S. (1971): Interaction between phenobarbital and diphenylhydantoin in animals and in epileptic patients. *Ann. N.Y. Acad. Sci.*, **179**, 88.

Neuvonen, P. J., Gothoni, G., Hackman, R. and Björksten, K. af (1970): Interference of iron with the absorption of tetracyclines in man. *Brit. med. J.*, **4**, 532.

Neuwald, F. (1969): Problems of packaging drugs in plastic containers. *W. African Pharmacist*, **11**, 60.

Nimmo, J., Heading, R. C., Tothill, P. and Prescott, L. F. (1973): Pharmacological modification of gastric emptying: effects of propantheline and metoclopromide on paracetamol absorption. *Brit. med. J.*, **1**, 587.

Nishida, M., Mine, Y. and Kuwahara, S. (1969): Synergistic activity of ampicillin and cloxacillin. *J. Antibiot.*, **22**, 144.

Notari, R. E. (1971): *Biopharmaceutics and Pharmacokinetics – an introduction.* Marcel Dekker, Inc., New York.

Ober, K. F. and Wang, R. I. H. (1973): Drug interactions with guanethidine. *Clin. Pharmacol. Therap.*, **14**, 190.

Orrego-Matte, H., Fernandez, O. and Mena, I. (1971): Effect of anticholinergic agents on the intestinal absorption of Fe 59 ferrous citrate. *Amer. J. Dig. Dis.*, **16**, 789.

Remmer, H. (1967): Die Induktion arzneimittelabbauender Enzyme im endoplasmatischen Retikulum der Leberzelle durch Pharmaka. *Dtsch. med. Wschr.*, **92**, 2001.

Reynolds, E. H. (1972): Diphenylhydantoin, hematologic aspects of toxicity. In: *Antiepileptic Drugs*, p. 247. Editors: D. M. Woodbury, J. K. Penry and R. P. Schmidt. Raven Press, New York.

Riggs, M. (1972): Ampicillin-probenecid treatment of gonorrhea. *J. Amer. med. Assoc.*, **220**, 420.

Ritschel, W. A. (1972): Bioavailability in the clinical evaluation of drugs. *Drug Intell. Clin. Pharm.*, **6**, 246.

Sabath, L. D., Elder, H. A., McCall, C. E. and Finland, M. (1967): Synergistic combinations of penicillins in the treatment of bacteriuria. *New Engl. J. Med.*, **277**, 232.

Shangraw, R. F. (1972): Instable nitroglycerin tablets: *New Engl. J. Med.*, **286**, 950.

Sher, S. P. (1971): Drug enzyme induction and drug interactions: literature tabulation. *Toxicol. appl. Pharmacol.*, **18**, 780.

Siegfried, J., Klaiber, R., Perret, E. and Ziegler, W. H. (1969): Behandlung des Morbus Parkinson mit L-dopa in Kombination mit einem Decarboxylasehemmer. *Dtsch. med. Wschr.*, **94**, 2678.

Silverman, W. A., Andersen, D. H., Blanc, W. A. and Crozier, D. N. (1956): A difference in mortality rate and incidence of kernicterus among premature infants allotted to two prophylactic antibacterial regimens. *Pediatrics*, **18**, 614.

Sjöqvist, F., Hammer, W., Ideström, C. M., Lind, M., Tuck, D. and Åsberg, M. (1968): Plasma levels of monomethylated tricyclic antidepressants and side effects in man. In: Toxicity and Side Effects of Psychotropic Drugs. Proc. Europ. Soc. for the Study of Drug Toxicity. Vol. 9, p. 246. Congr. Series No. 145. Editors: S. B. de C. Baker, J. R. Boissier and W. Koll. Excerpta Medica Intern.

Skinner, C., Coull, D. C. and Johnston, A. W. (1969): Antagonism of the hypotensive action of bethanidine and debrisoquine by tricyclic antidepressants. *Lancet*, **2**, 564.

Solomon, H. M. and Schrogie, J. J. (1967): The effect of various drugs on the binding of Warfarin-^{14}C to human albumin. *Biochem. Pharmacol.*, **16**, 1219.

Solomon, H. M., M. J. Barakat and C. J. Ashley (1971): Mechanisms of drug interaction. *J. Amer. med. Assoc.*, **216**, 1997.

Storm van Leeuwen, W. (1923): Grondbeginselen der algemeene pharmacologie. Wolters, Groningen.

Storm van Leeuwen, W. (1924): On antagonism of drugs. *J. Pharmacol. exp. Therap.*, **24**, 21.

Swidler, G. (1971): *Handbook of Drug Interactions.* Wiley–Interscience, New York.

Tatro, D. S. (1972): Tetracycline–antacid interactions. *J. Amer. Med. Assoc.*, **220**, 586.

Thompson, J. H. (1969): Drug interactions and incompatibility. In: *Essentials of Pharmacology*, p. 628. Editor: J. A. Bevan. Hoeber, New York.

Tsuchiya, T. and Levy, G. (1972): Relationship between effect of activated charcoal on drug absorption in man and its drug adsorption characteristics in vitro. *J. Pharm. Sci.*, **61**, 586.

Van Dam, F. E. and Gribnau-Overkamp, M. J. H. (1967): The effect of some sedatives (phenobarbital, glutethimide, chlordiazepoxide, chloral hydrate) on the rate of disappearance of ethyl biscoumacetate from the plasma. *Folia med. Neerl.*, **10**, 141.

Van Rossum, J. M. (1968): Pharmacokinetics of accumulation. *J. Pharm. Sci.*, **57**, 2162.

Viars, P. and Seebacher, J. (1971): Les Interférences Médicamenteuses. Librairie Arnette, Paris.

Wagner, J. G. (1966): Design and data analysis of biopharmaceutical studies in man. *Can. J. Pharm.*, **1**, 55.

Wassermann, O. (1972): Studies on the pharmacokinetics of bis-quaternary ammonium compounds, *Naunyn-Schmied. Arch. Pharmacol.*, **275**, 251.

Watson, D. (1962): The transport of bile pigments: the binding of sodium bilirubinate to plasma protein. *Clin. Sci.*, **22**, 435.

Woodbury, D. M., Penry, J. K. and Schmidt, R. P. (1972): Antiepileptic Drugs. Raven Press, New York.

CHAPTER 6

Clinical drug interactions in the gastrointestinal tract in man

A. BARTELINK

1 Introduction

There is much concern about drug interaction because in many diseases the concomitant prescription of several drugs is the rule. Patients also commonly consume drugs that are available without prescription. In addition there can be interaction between an administered drug and a known or unknown bioactive material in the form of food, food additives, insecticides and cleaning agents.

The following mechanisms have been suggested as possible causes for interactions between drugs: alteration of gastrointestinal absorption, stimulation or inhibition of enzyme systems, displacement of drugs from binding sites on proteins or receptor sites and alteration of urinary excretion. These mechanisms have been reviewed by Macgregor (1965). Diseases which primarily affect the organs of drug absorption, metabolism or excretion may also alter the pharmacological response to drugs. Finally, nutrients may enhance or impair the intestinal absorption of drugs and vice versa.

In this chapter clinical drug interaction in the gastrointestinal tract, the influence of gastrointestinal disease on drug interaction and the interaction of drugs and foods during absorption will be discussed. The pathogenesis of the side effects of drugs in the gastrointestinal tract has been reviewed elsewhere (Bartelink, 1972).

2 Alteration of gastrointestinal absorption

2.1 ALTERATION OF PH

The pH in the gastrointestinal tract varies widely from one region to another, e.g. in the stomach it is about 1.0 and in the duodenum 6.6. The absorption of drugs is governed by the pH of the medium, by the rate of dissociation (characterized by the pK_a of the drug), by its lipid solubility, by its particle size and by its physical form. The pK_a of a drug affects the rate of absorption because the non ionized form of a molecule is less polar and therefore more lipid soluble and so more readily transported across the cell membrane of gastric and/or intestinal mucosal cells. Weak acids (high pK_a) are well absorbed from the stomach because ionization is suppressed, and less well absorbed from the duodenum. The converse is true of weak bases (low pK_a). Neutral substances do not display definite preference for a particular site of absorption.

The antiinflammatory agents acetylsalicylic acid (Aspirin), phenylbutazone, oxyphenbutazone, and indomethacin are weak organic acids and are bound to plasma albumin. At pH 3.5 or lower these drugs are in the non-ionized form, as such readily lipid soluble and able to penetrate the lipoprotein membrane of the gastric epithelial cells. At the same time increased mucosa-to-lumen fluxes of sodium, potassium and chloride take place. This increase in gastric mucosal permeability has also been demonstrated after instillation of fatty acids, bile salts, urea and ethanol. Increased mucosal permeability induced by acetylsalicylic acid is a function of diffusion of its undissociated, lipid soluble moiety through the mucosa in the presence of acid. The magnitude of permeability change is directly proportional to the concentrations of hydrochloric acid and acetylsalicylic acid. The increased gastric mucosal permeability to H^+ ions may be a basic feature in the pathogenesis of ulceration and bleeding from the stomach (Hingson and Ito, 1971; Cooke, 1973). Vane (1971) showed that aspirin and indomethacin are able to block the production of the prostaglandins E_2 and $F_{2\alpha}$ locally in the tissues. It has been suggested that inhibition of prostaglandin synthesis could explain the antiinflammatory, antipyretic and other effects of non-steroidal antiinflammatory drugs. Prostaglandins are known to participate in various defensive reactions (Collier, 1971). The increased mucosal permeability after administration of aspirin may be caused by lack of prostaglandins locally. Changes in mucosal permeability caused by ethanol are dependent upon the concentration of ethanol and also upon the concentration of hydrogen ions in the lumen. Ethanol is known to stimulate fluid and acid production by the stomach and ethanol in combination with acetylsalicylic acid is especially harmful by producing mucosal bleeding (Needham et al., 1971; Smith et al., 1971). The combination of the non-steroidal antiinflammatory drugs with corticosteroids enhances also the risk of ulcer formation.

Aspirin interferes with platelet aggregation and platelet adenosine diphosphate release and causes a mild prolongation of bleeding time. The mechanism of aspirin-induced bleeding seems to be variable (Cooke, 1973) but the local mechanism is probably the most important (Smith et al., 1971).

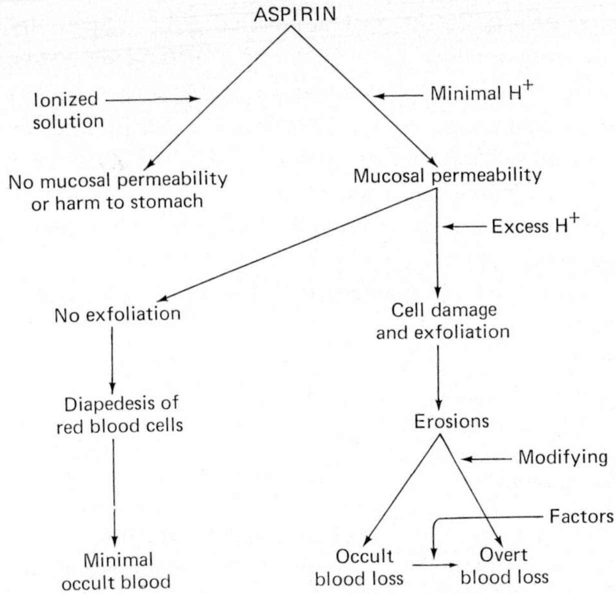

Fig. 1. A schematic diagram to represent the effect of hydrogen-ion and other factors on aspirin-induced gastrointestinal damage.

The gastric mucosa in patients with pernicious anemia, gastritis and chronic ulcers and in patients hospitalized in intensive treatment units, in whom uremia, hypotension, respiratory failure and jaundice are common complications, has an increased permeability to hydrogen ions. Spontaneous or drug-induced gastric ulceration or bleeding or both are frequent complications in these patients.

Stimulants of gastric secretion include many bitter substances which form the basis of appetizers or aperitifs. Many amino acids and meat extracts initiate acid secretion, probably through the release of gastrin, and in combination with e.g. aspirin may cause gastric bleeding or ulceration. Drugs which reduce or neutralize stomach secretion (anticholinergic drugs and antacids) may have a beneficial action in this respect.

Barr et al. (1971) have reported a decrease of about 50% in tetracycline absorption in man by sodium bicarbonate, but only when tetracycline was given as a capsule, not when it was given as a solution. The rate of dissolution and thus the fraction of tetracycline absorbed seems markedly reduced at the higher pH values. Any substance (antacids) or condition (achlorhydria) which significantly increases gastric pH may decrease dissolution and, hence, absorption of tetracycline. After administration of antacids containing polyvalent cations such as Ca^{2+}, Mg^{2+} or Al^{3+} the absorption of tetracyclines is decreased by yet another mechanism, namely chelation.

The presence of food in the gastrointestinal tract induces changes in pH, osmolality, motility and secretion. The effect of food on absorption of the antibiotic erythromycin may depend on gastric acidity. In achlorhydria due to pernicious anemia prior ingestion of breakfast did not affect adversely the blood concentrations of erythromycin. An adverse effect of food on the absorption of lincomycin has been observed (McCall et al., 1967), on the absorption of cloxacillin (Garrod and O'Grady, 1971) and also on the absorption of minocycline.

The influence of pH on the activity of pancreatic enzymes, especially ilpase, will be mentioned below.

2.2 CHELATION

2.2.1 *Cholestyramine*

Cholestyramine, a basic anion exchange resin, which contains quaternary ammonium groups attached to a polymer, forms unabsorbable complexes with bile salts, thus interrupting their enterohepatic circulation. Bile acids are formed from cholesterol and, although hepatic cholesterol synthesis rises in response to the stimulus of bile acid depletion, utilization of preformed plasma and tissue cholesterol for bile acid synthesis is an important factor in lowering plasma cholesterol levels in man by cholestyramine. Bile salts perform several functions, but their most important property is their key role in micelle formation. In addition, they also help to provide monoglycerides and fatty acids by enhancing the activity of pancreatic lipase and they are essential for intraluminary hydrolysis of ingested cholesterol esters. At a mucosal level bile salts probably activate cellular esterification of cholesterol and might play an important role in the transfer of cholesterol from the intestinal wall to the lymph. After administration of cholestyramine bile salt deficiency may cause steatorrhoea and malabsorption of the vitamins A, D, E and K. Cholestyramine also impairs absorption of calcium and of the anticoagulant Warfarin (Koch-Weser and Sellers, 1971) and of digoxin and digitoxin (Caldwell et al., 1971). On the other hand, in the malabsorption and diarrhoeal states associated with a high colonic concentration of bile acids as occurs following resection or bypass of the ileum, cholestyramine treatment may be beneficial (Hofmann and Poley, 1969). In patients with acquired hypogammaglobulinaemia a watery diarrhoea without steatorrhoea might occur due to increased concentrations of uncommon secondary bile acids derived from bacterial conversion of primary bile acids. The diarrhoea of such patients may also respond to the administration of cholestyramine (Gleich and Hofmann, 1971).

Neomycin precipitates sodium salts of taurocholic, glycocholic and deoxycholic acids at a pH slightly less than 6.0 and so exerts the same effect as cholestyramine.

p-Aminosalicylic acid (PAS), also lowers the plasma cholesterol level and may cause steatorrhoea. The intestinal epithelium remains histologically unchanged, even after oral administration of 12 g PAS daily for 4 weeks (Levine, 1968). The mechanism is still unclear, perhaps chelation of bile acids may be involved.

PAS impedes the gastrointestinal absorption of rifampicin. The mechanism remains to be elucidated, but the clinical implication is that PAS and rifampicin should be given with an interval of about 12 hrs (Boman and Borgå, 1971).

2.2.2 *Tetracyclines*

Tetracyclines (oxytetracycline, chlortetracycline, methacycline, doxycycline) are all close derivatives of a single polycyclic compound. These compounds act as bacteriostatic agents, so their plasma levels should never be allowed to fall below the minimum inhibitory concentration. Milk, antacids, bivalent and trivalent cations (e.g. calcium, magnesium and aluminium-ions) are known to reduce the absorption of tetracyclines by formation of chelates. Ferrous sulphate administered together with tetracyclines seriously impairs the absorption of these antibiotics (Neuvonen et al., 1970). Because the binding of Fe^{2+} to tetracyclines takes place in equimolar ratios, methacycline and doxycycline when given with iron suffer the greatest reduction in serum concentration, owing to their use in smaller doses.

Some tonics contain so much iron that the serum levels of concurrently administered tetracyclines dropped below the usually accepted minimum level of 0.6 μg/ml. Not only does iron inhibit the absorption of tetracyclines, but the reverse also occurs. Ferric salts were found to have the same inhibitory action on the absorption of tetracyclines as ferrous salts.

After absorption tetracyclines form complexes with calcium-ions especially in growing bones and teeth. In children, hypoplasia of dental enamel occurs and yellow discoloration of the teeth may be permanent if the drug has been given during pregnancy particularly after the first four months, or administered to children under seven years of age.

2.2.3 *Foods*

Foods, especially milk products, interfere significantly with the absorption of erythromycin, oleandomycin, tetracyclines and most of the oral penicillins (penicillin K, benzylpenicillin G, oxacillin and 2-biphenylpenicillin). However, the closely related drugs phenoxymethyl penicillin (V) and α-aminobenzylpenicillin are not affected by food. Whole milk and cottage cheese contain calcium caseinate which may chelate e.g. tetracyclines, thus rendering these antibiotics no longer available for absorption. The effect of food on the absorption of antibiotics also may depend on the lipid solubility of the drug. Griseofulvin is only lipid soluble and the dietary fat load governs its absorption. If no fat is included in the meal, no rise in blood level of griseofulvin is observed. Several other possible chelating agents are present in foods, e.g. starch (Krondl, 1970).

2.3 ALTERED MOTILITY OF THE GASTROINTESTINAL TRACT

The cathartics oxyphenisatin, bisacodyl and phenolphthalein have been shown to decrease the absorption of glucose. Anthraquinone derivatives have no such effect. Oxyphenisatin is partially absorbed from the intestine, taken up by the liver and excreted in the bile in a peristalsis-stimulating form. Recently jaundice has been reported after taking oxyphenisatin-containing laxatives (Reynolds et al., 1971). The changes in the liver function tests and the histological appearances of the liver tissue resembled those of acute viral hepatitis or of active chronic hepatitis due to an autoimmune reaction. Several of the oxyphenisatin-containing laxatives also contain dioctyl sodium sulphosuccinate, a surface-active agent which might enhance absorption and hence the hepatotoxicity of oxyphenisatin. Challenge experiments with pure oxyphenisatin have proved that the substance itself is hepatotoxic.

A deficiency of the lipid soluble vitamins A, D, E and K may occur after long term administration of liquid paraffin which acts as a cathartic because it is poorly absorbable. The same mechanism may lead to malabsorption of concurrently administered lipid soluble drugs. Any cathartic when used in excess may produce steatorrhoea, protein loss and hypokalaemia. Hypokalaemia causes paralysis of the intestinal musculature with resulting megacolon. On the other hand hypokalaemia in a digitalized patient will increase the risk of digitalis-induced cardiac arrhythmias. The ganglion-blocking drugs such as methantheline bromide may inhibit absorption of some nutrients by their action on the autonomic system of the gut (Fordtran and Dietschy, 1966).

2.4 ALTERED CELLULAR STRUCTURE OF THE GUT WALL

Neomycin impairs fat absorption by precipitation of bile salts in the lumen of the small gut, by changing the bacterial flora in the gut in favor of bacteroides, clostridia and certain anaerobic lactobacilli. These possess an amidase capable of removing taurine and glycine from bile acids (deconjugation of bile salts) and in addition have a direct toxic effect on the intestinal mucosal cell. This toxic effect is exerted chiefly on crypt cells, causing reversible changes in the villi with increased cellularity of the lamina propria and the occurrence of pigment-loaded macrophages. The villous height is reduced and on electron-microscopic examination the crypt cells show mitotic arrest with marked dilatation of the endoplasmic reticulum.

The activity of the mucosal enzymes (e.g. disaccharidases and peptidases) is decreased and may cause malabsorption of acrbohydrates and proteins. Malabsorption of carotene, hexoses, iron and vitamin B12 have also been reported (Dobbins et al., 1968).

Polymyxin, kanamycin and bacitracin may cause malabsorption of fat, carbohydrate and protein and an increased loss of bile acids but less than neomycin. These drugs act by interfering with the protein synthesis of bacteria. Their toxic effect on the mucosal cell may occur on the same basis.

Cytostatics (colchicine, aminopterin, methotrexate) cause injury of the intestinal absorptive surface including villous atrophy, cellular invasion of the lamina propria and arrest of mitosis. Simultaneously mucosal enzyme

TABLE I

Alteration of gastrointestinal absorption of drugs by interactions with other drugs, foods, bioactive materials or the mucosal cell of the gastrointestinal tract

Interfering compounds A	Interfering compounds B	Mechanism	Promoting pathological conditions	Unwanted effects
Gastric hydrochloric acid stimulants – ethanol, appetizers, meat extracts, amino acids	Weak acidic drugs: aspirin®, phenylbutazone, oxyphenbutazone, indomethacin	Lowering gastric pH	Gastritis, chronic ulcers, uremia, hypotension, respiratory failure, jaundice	Increased gastric absorption of these non-steroidal anti-inflammatory agents →increased gastric mucosal permeability to H^+-ions→ gastric ulceration and/or bleeding
	in combination with corticosteroids cytostatics	Decrease of gastric epithelial cell renewal		Aggravation of the tendency to gastric ulceration and/or bleeding
Food	Erythromycin Lincomycin Cloxacillin Minocycline Oleandomycin Oral penicillins	Lowering gastric pH? Chelation?		Decreased absorption of these antibiotics

Interfering compounds A	B	Mechanism	Promoting pathological conditions	Unwanted effects
Antacids (Na-bicarbonate) Anticholinergic drugs	Tetracyclines Capsules	Rise of gastric pH	Achlorhydria	Decreased absorption of tetracyclines given as capsules
Antacids (Ca, Mg and Al ions) Milk Cheese Tonics Ferrous sulphate	Tetracyclines	Chelation		Decreased absorption of tetracyclines unrelated to the form of administration. Precipitation of calcium–tetracycline complexes in growing bones and teeth→yellow discoloration of teeth
Tetracyclines	Ferrous sulphate	Chelation		Decreased absorption of ferrous sulphate
Cholestyramine	Bile salts Calcium Warfarin Digoxin Digitoxin	Chelation	Small bowel disease (Crohn's disease, resection etc.)	Bile salt deficiency→steatorrhoea→malabsorption of lipid soluble drugs and vitamins (A,D,E,K) Decreased absorption of calcium, Warfarin, digoxin and digitoxin
Neomycin Polymyxin Kanamycin Bacitracin Cytostatics Drug-induced folic acid deficiency and/or vitamin B_{12} deficiency	Bile salts Mucosal cell	Precipitation Villous atrophy	Small bowel disease (Sprue, Crohn's disease etc.)	Bile salt deficiency→steatorrhoea Malabsorption of fat, protein, carbohydrate, vitamins, drugs
p-Aminosalicylic acid (PAS)	Bile salts	Chelation?		Bile salt deficiency→steatorrhoea→malabsorption
	Rifampicin Vitamin B_{12}	Unknown		Decreased absorption of rifampicin Decreased absorption of vitamin B_{12}
Griseofulvin	Dietary fat restriction	Lipid-solubility of the drugs	Malabsorption syndrome	Malabsorption of griseofulvin
Lipid soluble drugs and vitamins	Liquid paraffin			Malabsorption of these drugs and vitamins

activity is inhibited and the absorption of nutrients, vitamins and water is blocked. Drugs given concurrently are malabsorbed.

Anticonvulsant drugs (phenobarbitone and phenytoin) may interfere with folic acid absorption. Folic acid deficiency may give rise to cellular damage and cause malabsorption (Bartelink, 1972). In patients with a malabsorption syndrome, e.g. gluten-induced enteropathy or Crohn's disease, drug absorption is impaired to a greater or lesser extent.

3 Stimulation or inhibition of enzyme systems

3.1 GENERAL

The normal digestive and absorptive action of the intestinal enzymes upon the dietary constituents have been studied intensively but until recently very little has been known about the effect of dietary constituents, hormones and drugs on the enzyme activities in the normal and diseased human intestine.

The three common dietary disaccharides are lactose, sucrose and maltose and to be absorbed they must be hydrolysed into their component monosaccharides (glucose, galactose and fructose) by the disaccharidases lactase, sucrase and maltase. These enzymes are located in the brush border of the epithelial cells of the small intestine, especially of the jejunum. Patients suffering from lactose intolerance with or without lactase deficiency are well on a lactose-free diet. Lactose however, is used as a convenient vehicle of various pharmacologically active chemicals thus present in many tablets or powders. Lactose-intolerant patients relapse if they take lactose-containing drugs.

Rosensweig et al. (1971) point out that the intestine might be used to reflect changes occurring elsewhere in the body by drugs. Since it is relatively easy and safe to obtain human jejunal mucosal tissue by peroral intestinal biopsy this tissue could be a convenient tool to study regulation of enzyme activities in both normal and diseased states and after administration of drugs.

3.2 FOLIC ACID METABOLISM

Folic acid antagonists (aminopterin), iron deficiency, alcohol ingestion, anticonvulsant drug therapy (phenytoin), tuberculostatic agents, vitamin B12 deficiency and oral contraceptives all may interfere with folic acid metabolism.

Folic polyglutamates, the principal dietary forms of folate, consist of folic acid bound to 1–6 glutamic acid residues in a gamma-peptide linkage. The small intestinal enzyme conjugase is necessary for hydrolysis and absorption of the polyglutamates (Rosenberg and Godwin, 1971). Conjugase inhibition is suggested as the cause of low serum folate levels after administration of phenytoin. This has not been confirmed in recent studies and neither has the suggestion that phenytoin displaces folate from its carrier protein. Recently Maxwell et al. (1972) reported a significant association between the extent of hepatic microsomal enzyme induction, as measured by the urinary excretion of D-glucaric acid, and the levels of both serum and red cell folate. This finding is consistent with their hypothesis that folate deficiency results from accelerated metabolism of folate after the induction of hepatic drug metabolizing enzymes caused by anticonvulsant drug therapy. Folic acid antagonists such as aminopterin exert an inhibitory action on folate reductase which converts folic acid into the co-enzyme tetrahydrofolic acid. Inhibition of this enzyme affects primarily the production of thymidylic acid, inosinic acid and some precursors of RNA and DNA.

Oral contraceptive drugs have been associated with folate deficiency as a result of a reduction in absorption of folate polyglutamate, not of the monoglutamate form. It has been suggested that conjugase inhibition in the intestinal mucosa could be the cause (Streiff, 1970). Oestrogens however also have the property of inducing the activity of hepatic microsomal enzymes and this effect may explain the development of folate deficiency in women on oral contraceptives. The same mechanism may occur in chronic ethanol ingestion (Maxwell et al., 1972).

The mechanisms of interaction between tuberculostatic agents (isoniazid, cycloserine) and folic acid upon folate metabolism are still obscure.

A great deal of additional work is still needed to clarify the influence of various drugs on the folate metabolism. The recent introduction of a new technological tool, namely the synthetic folate polyglutamates, may soon lead to some clear answers.

3.3 VITAMIN B12 METABOLISM

Neomycin and colchicine may cause malabsorption of vitamin B12 by altering the intestinal morphology. PAS may produce vitamin B12 malabsorption either selectively or as a manifestation of a more extended malabsorption syndrome including malabsorption of D-xylose and of folic acid.

Profuse overgrowth of intestinal microorganisms secondary to stasis or to alteration of the normal flora by antibiotics may lead to malabsorption, and also malabsorption of vitamin B12. The mechanism is not clear, perhaps intestinal bacteria compete for dietary vitamin B12. Although intrinsic factor may protect vitamin B12 from being utilized by intestinal bacteria in normal subjects, it affords only partial protection in patients with an abnormal flora.

3.4 DIGESTIVES ENZYMES OF THE PANCREAS

Pancreatic enzymes are generally not involved in the absorption of drugs. There is no convincing evidence of interaction between drugs and gastrointestinal enzymes in the various drug-induced gastrointestinal diseases. In neomycin-induced steatorrhoea inhibition of lipase activity does not occur, even enhanced lipase activity has been reported.

The consequences of pancreatic insufficiency can be controlled with success by oral administration during the meals of 6–12 g of a potent pancreatic extract three-times daily. Gastric acidity however should be low or absent because pancreatic extract is inactive at low pH. In case of considerable gastric acid secretion bicarbonate has to be given concurrently with the pancreatic extract, in a dose of 5 g three times daily (Veeger et al., 1962).

3.5 THE LIVER

Many of the interactions between drugs are due to alterations in the activity of drug-metabolizing enzymes, particularly in the liver. Also insecticides have been shown in animals to stimulate drug metabolizing enzymes in the liver (D'Arcy and Griffin, 1972). In man the significance of this phenomenon is unknown but it presents a potential hazard to everyone.

Stimulation or inhibition of drug-metabolizing enzymes in the liver are discussed elsewhere in this volume.

3.6 MONOAMINE OXIDASE INHIBITORS (MAOI)

Monoamine oxidase inhibitors (MAOI) are compounds which block the synthesis of certain sympathomimetic amines. Monoamine oxidase destroys dopamine, tyramine, serotonin, noradrenaline and adrenaline by oxidative deamination. MAOI also affect other enzyme systems, for example those concerned with the detoxification of drugs in the liver. MAOI interact with many other drugs, e.g. pargyline, amphetamines, antiparkinsonism drugs, tricyclic antidepressants and they potentiate the hypoglycaemic effect of insulin and sulphonylureas.

MAOI also interact with various foodstuffs, especially those which contain tyramine. Tyramine is a sympathomimetic agent normally inactivated in the liver after oral ingestion. In the presence of MAOI tyramine reaches the general circulation and produces hypertension, attacks of forceful heart beats and severe headache. Death from intracranial haemorrhage has been reported. Tyramine-containing foods include: cheese, wines (Chiantis), beer and yeast extracts (Marmite). Also pickled herrings, fruits and caffeïne-containing drinks may interact with MAOI due to their dopamine, tyramine or serotonin content.

3.7 METOCLOPRAMIDE

Metoclopramide is an antiemetic drug also used as an adjunct to X-ray examinations of the upper alimentary tract. It accelerates emptying of the stomach possibly by an action on autonomic centres. In combination with phenothiazines symptoms of dystonia were reported, but recently Casteels-van Daele et al., (1970) reported serious extrapyramidal reactions in children receiving a normal dosage of metoclopramide. The symptoms included neck pain, torticollis, retrocollis, oculogyric crises, trismus, dysarthria, dysphagia and involuntary movements. These symptoms are very similar to the extrapyramidal reactions caused by the chemically unrelated phenothiazines. Possibly the syndrome may be due to interaction of metoclopramide with central catecholamines, particularly dopamine, or to interference with central histamine.

4 Displacement of one drug by another from carrier proteins or from receptor sites

Almost all drugs are reversibly bound to proteins in plasma and tissues. The unbound fraction is biologically active; the bound fraction acts as a reservoir and prevents the occurrence of toxic levels of the unbound fraction. Many acidic drugs are highly bound to albumin molecules and may displace other drugs.

The non-steroidal antiinflammatory drugs, phenylbutazone, indomethacin and salicylates, may displace coumarin anticoagulants from plasma proteins and thus promote bleeding tendencies (Koch-Weser, 1971); they also displace in animal experiments corticosterone from plasma proteins.

Gastric bleeding may occur if long acting sulphonamides are administered to patients on tolbutamide due to release of tolbutamide with resulting hypoglycaemia and thus increased hydrogen-ion secretion in the stomach (D'Arcy and Griffin, 1972). When patients on salicylates receive sulphonamides concurrently the toxicity and ulcerogenic action of the salicylates is increased.

The sulphonylurea drugs may act by displacing insulin from proteins (D'Arcy and Griffin, 1972). Alcohol ingestion potentiates the hypoglycaemic effect of the sulphonylurea drugs.

Many diseases of the gastrointestinal tract may lead to protein-loss and hypoalbuminaemia may develop in the absence of liver disease. Toxic levels of free drugs may readily occur in patients with hypoalbuminaemia (Lewis et al., 1971).

Competitive inhibition, e.g. atropine–acetylcholine or histamine–antihistamine, will not be discussed in detail.

5 Alteration of urinary excretion

The elimination of many drugs occurs predominantly by renal excretion. The factors involved are discussed in detail in Chapter 10.

6 Final remarks

Four types of mechanisms by which drugs may interact are described but many others are as yet undiscovered. Interactions between drugs are not only determined by each separate drug, but also by each individual patient. Patients with a serious illness, who receive many drugs, patients of old age, patients with abnormal renal function or disturbed liver function, with fever and hypothermia or with gastrointestinal disease are all in different ways predisposed to adverse or allergic drug reactions (Smith et al., 1966). However drug interactions are not always dangerous to the patient: synergistic actions of drugs may also be therapeutically important and may contribute to the benefit of the patient.

Drugs should be used for definite indications, with a predefined therapeutic end point. The clinician must be alert to the possibility of drug interactions. Caution is necessary when a drug is added or deleted from a therapeutic regimen.

References

Barr, W. H., Adir, J. and Garrettson, L. (1971): Decrease of tetracycline absorption in man by sodium bicarbonate. *Clin. Pharmacol. Therap.*, **12**, 779.

Bartelink, A. (1972): Diseases of the gastrointestinal tract due to drugs. In: *Drug-Induced Diseases*, Vol. IV, p. 403. Editors: L. Meyler and H. Peck. Excerpta Medica Foundation, Amsterdam.

Boman, G. and Borgå, O. (1971): Drug interaction: decreased serum concentrations of rifampicin when given with PAS. Lancet, **1**, 800.

Caldwell, J. H., Bush, C. A. and Greenberger, N. J. (1971): Interruption of the enterohepatic circulation of digitoxin by cholestyramine. *J. clin. Invest.*, **50**, 2626.

Casteels van Daele, M., Jaeken, J., Van der Schueren, P., Zimmerman, A., Van der Ben, P. (1970): Dystonic reactions in children caused by metoclopramide. *Arch. Dis. Childhood*, **45**, 130.

Collier, H. C. J. (1971): Prostaglandins and aspirin. *Nature*, **232**, 17.

Cooke, A. R. (1973): The role of acid in the pathogenesis of aspirin-induced gastro-intestinal erosions and hemorrhage. *Digestive Dis.*, **18**, 225.

D'Arcy, P. F. and Griffin, J. P. (1972): Iatrogenic Diseases, p. 10. Oxford University Press, London.

Dobbins, W. O., Herrero, B. A. and Mansbach, C. M. (1968): Morphologic alterations associated with neomycin-induced malabsorption. *Amer. J. med. Sci.*, **255**, 63.

Fordtran, J. S. and Dietschy, J. M. (1966): Water and electrolyte movement in the intestine. *Gastroenterology*, **50**, 263.

Garrod, L. P. and O'Grady, L. (1971): *Antibiotics and Chemotherapy*, p. 77. E. & S. Livingstone, London.

Gleich, G. J. and Hofmann, A. F. (1971): Use of cholestyramine to control diarrhea associated with acquired hypogammaglobulinemia. *Amer. J. Med.*, **51**, 281.

Hingson, D. J. and Ito, S. (1971): Effect of aspirin and related compounds on the fine structure of mouse gastric mucosa. *Gastroenterology*, **61**, 156.

Hofmann, A. F. and Poley, J. R. (1969): Cholestyramine treatment of diarrhea associated with ileal resection. *New. Engl. J. Med.*, **281**, 397.

Koch-Weser, J. and Sellers, E. M. (1971): Drug interactions with coumarin anticoagulants. *New. Engl. J. Med.*, **285**, 487 and 547.

Krondl, A. (1970): Present understanding of the interaction of drugs and food during absorption. *C.M.A. J.*, **103**, 360.

Levine, R. A. (1968): Steatorrhoea induced by para-aminosalicylic acid. *Ann. intern. Med.*, **68**, 1265.

Lewis, G. P., Jusko, W. J., Burke, C. W. and Graves, L. (1971): Prednisone side-effects and serum-protein levels. *Lancet*, II, 778.

Macgregor, A. G. (1965): Review of points at which drugs can interact. *Proc. roy-Soc. Med.*, **58**, 943.

Maxwell, J. D., Hunter, J., Stewart, D. A., Ardeman, S. and Williams, R. (1972): Folate deficiency after anticonvulsant drugs: an effect of hepatic enzyme induction? *Brit. med. J.*, **1**, 297.

McCall, C. E., Steigbigel, N. H. and Finland, M. (1967): Lincomycin: activity in vitro and absorption and excretion in normal young men. *Amer. J. med. Sci.*, **254**, 144.

Needham, C. D., Kyle, J., Jones, P. F., Johnston, S. J. and Kerridge, D. F. (1971): Aspirin and alcohol in gastrointestinal haemorrhage. *Gut*, **12**, 819.

Neuvonen, P. J., Gothoni, G., Hackman, R. and Björksten, K. (1970): Interference of iron with the absorption of tetracyclines in man. *Brit. med. J.*, **4**, 532.

Reynolds, T. B., Peters, R. L., Yamada, S. (1971): Chronic active and lupoid hepatitis caused by a laxative, oxyphenisatin. *New. Engl. J. Med.*, **285**, 813.

Rosenberg, I. H. and Godwin, H. A. (1971): The digestion and absorption of dietary folate. *Gastroenterology*, **60**, 445.

Rosensweig, N. G., Herman, R. H. and Stifel, F. B. (1971): Dietary regulation of small intestinal enzyme activity in man. *Amer. J. clin. Nutr.*, **24**, 65.

Smith, B. M., Skillman, J. J., Edwards, B. G. and Silen, W. (1971): Permeability of human gastric mucosa, alteration by acetylsalicylic acid and ethanol. *New Engl. J. Med.*, **285**, 716.

Smith, J. B. and Willis, A. L. (1971): Aspirin selectively inhibits prostaglandin production in human platelets. *Nature New Biol.*, **231**, 235.

Smith, J. W., Seidl, L. G. and Cluff, L. E. (1966): Studies on the epidemiology of adverse drug reactions. *Ann. Intern. Med.*, **65**, 629.

Streiff, R. R. (1970): Folate deficiency and oral contraceptives. *JAMA*, **214**, 105.

Vane, J. R. (1971): Inhibition of prostaglandin synthesis as a mechanism of action for aspirin-like drugs. *Nature New Biol.*, **231**, 232.

Veeger, W., Abels, J., Hellemans, N. and Nieweg, H. O. (1962): Effect of sodium bicarbonate and pancreatin on the absorption of vitamin B12 and fat in pancreatic insufficiency. *New Engl. J. Med.*, **267**, 1341.

CHAPTER 7

Drug interactions affecting cardiovascular therapy

C. T. DOLLERY, C. F. GEORGE AND M. L'E. ORME

1 Introduction

Many patients are treated with 5 or more drugs at the same time (Lasagna, 1965; Smith et al., 1966); the number of possible combinations is very large indeed and it is beyond the grasp of a physician's memory to retain all the possible interactions that he may encounter. Interactions are most likely to have a substantial effect if one or more of the drugs being used has a steep dose response curve. Many interactions probably pass unnoticed because they do not cause a recognisable change in response. For example, an interaction that caused the plasma concentration of penicillin to be doubled would be most unlikely to be detected under ordinary circumstances, whereas a change of the same magnitude with an anticoagulant would be both noticeable and potentially hazardous. Many cardiovascular drugs, such as digitalis glycosides, potent antihypertensive agents and anticoagulants have a steep and progressive relationship between dose and response. It is not surprising that cardiovascular drugs figure disproportionately often in reports of drug interactions.

Many drug interactions are interesting but of little significance in therapy and only a few are hazardous. The importance of interactions should not be overstated. Inappropriate and unskilful use of drugs by physicians and failure to take medicines as prescribed are more important problems under most circumstances. However, interactions are important because they may lead to unexpected loss of therapeutic effect or occasionally to toxicity. Drug interactions should not be considered solely from the standpoint of unwanted actions and hazards. Most drugs have more than one pharmacological action. In some circumstances, this combination of properties may be useful but often one action is unwanted. The undesirable effect can sometimes be modified by use of a second drug, for example, a potassium-sparing diuretic combined with one that causes potassium loss. Sometimes, the desired combination of pharmacological properties cannot be achieved in a single chemical structure and it is appropriate to combine two different drugs to achieve it. The combined use of a vasodilator and a β-receptor blocking drug in the treatment of hypertension would be a case in point. Deliberate manipulation of drug interactions plays a large part in drug therapy.

2 Types of interaction

There are many different ways that drugs can interfere with one another's actions but a useful simplification can be made by considering these to be of only two types.

The first type are interactions where one drug causes a change in the steady state plasma concentration of another. The pharmacological action of drugs depends upon the concentration of free drug in plasma water because only this moiety is able to diffuse into cells and tissues. The concentration may be modified in several ways. Renal excretion may be altered by competition for a transport system; a familiar example is the interaction between penicillin and probenecid. Such interactions are not of great importance with cardiovascular drugs although the action of digoxin may be enhanced if excessive use of diuretics causes a severe fall in glomerular filtration rate. The free concentration may be increased if other drugs or disease displace from binding to plasma proteins a drug that is normally extensively bound. Examples of this type of interaction are often quoted with the anticoagulant Warfarin. Such effects may be expected to be short-lived for once the drug has been displaced the mechanisms normally controlling the free plasma concentration will bring the free concentration down to approximately its previous level.

The most important interactions which alter steady state plasma concentrations occur when a drug changes the rate of drug oxidation in the liver. Most lipid soluble drugs have their action terminated by oxidation or conjugation in the liver which renders them more water soluble and available for renal excretion. Drug oxidation for many different chemical structures is mediated by a single mixed function oxidase system in liver microsomes. The amount and activity of this enzyme system can be altered by administration of other drugs, or environmental contaminants such as dicophane (DDT). Increased activity of the drug-metabolising enzymes will lower the steady state plasma concentration of other drugs that are oxidised and decreased activity will cause the concentration of other drugs using this route to rise. The most important interactions of this kind concern coumarin anticoagulants,

The second main group of interactions concern pharmacological actions at receptors or upon control mechanisms such as those that regulate blood pressure. The concentration of drug in the plasma is not altered but the effect may be greatly changed. The loss of pressor response to tyramine after administration of reserpine is an example of this type of action. The main importance of this division into types of interactions lies in their predictability. Interactions due to pharmacological effects are in the main predictable from a knowledge of the pharmacological actions of the drugs being used. Those that change drug effects by changing the rate of drug oxidation in the liver cannot be predicted from a knowledge of pharmacology or are difficult to anticipate unless the prescriber knows the metabolic fate of the drugs he is using and their capacity to induce or inhibit drug-metabolising enzymes. Such knowledge is not widespread and in many cases the necessary information has not yet been obtained in man.

3 Oral anticoagulants

Since the oral anticoagulants were introduced into clinical practice some 30 years ago, they have been found to interact with many other drugs and at present they are the most frequently quoted example of drug interactions. In a recent survey by Starr and Petrie (1972) a potential source of drug interaction was noted in 33% of 254 patients on long term Warfarin. There are a number of reasons for this. Firstly, the oral anticoagulants are often given for long periods of time and because of the nature of the disease processes for which they are given many other drugs are often given concurrently. Secondly, the intensity of the pharmacological response must be carefully regulated when using these drugs and this response can be easily and accurately measured. Thirdly, the concentrations of the coumarin oral anticoagulants can be readily measured in body fluids and this fact enables the mechanism behind any drug interaction that may be detected to be analysed.

Oral anticoagulants are basically of two types. Firstly, the inandiones, of which phenindione is the best known example, and secondly, the coumarin group of which Warfarin is the most widely prescribed drug. Since Warfarin has fewer side effects than phenindione, it is more widely prescribed and so most reported interactions concern Warfarin. The oral anticoagulants work by inhibiting the vitamin K dependent synthesis of certain clotting factors in the liver. These factors are factor II (prothrombin), factor VII (proconvertin), factor IX (Christmas factor) and factor X (Stuart–Prower). The degree of depression of clotting factor synthesis at any time depends on the plasma concentration of the oral anticoagulant concerned (O'Reilly et al., 1963; Nagashima et al., 1969). Any drug which alters the plasma concentration of the oral anticoagulants will materially affect the degree of hypoprothrombinaemia.

3.1 INTERACTIONS IN THE GUT

Drugs may interact in the lumen of the gastrointestinal tract before absorption. A well-known example of this is the formation of insoluble chelates of tetracycline when cations such as aluminium, calcium or magnesium are administered at the same time (Kunin and Finland, 1961). Bishydroxycoumarin is the only coumarin anticoagulant that is not well absorbed (O'Reillyand Aggeler, 1969) and its absorption is further impaired by heptabarbital (Aggeler and O'Reilly, 1966, 1969; O'Reilly and Aggeler, 1969) and by allopurinol (Vessell et al., 1970). Warfarin which is more commonly used, is well absorbed (O'Reilly et al., 1963) and the only drug which has been shown to interfere with its absorption is cholestyramine (Council on drugs, 1966; Benjamin et al., 1970). The administration of cholestyramine in standard dosage has been shown to markedly reduce the absorption of Warfarin whether Warfarin is given with the cholestyramine or up to 3 hr after it (Robinson et al., 1971). Significant reductions in prothrombin time were also noted in these patients, with reductions of 4–5 sec in prothrombin time and 25% reductions in plasma Warfarin concentration. It is probably better to give the Warfarin 2 hr or so before cholestyramine by which time Warfarin absorption will be complete in most people.

3.2 INTERACTIONS IN THE PLASMA

Two drugs administered simultaneously can influence one another's binding to plasma proteins or at inactive tissue sites although this latter mechanism has not been demonstrated for the oral anticoagulants.

All the commonly used oral anticoagulants are highly bound to plasma albumin, Warfarin for example being 98% bound. Thus, only 2% of the drug in plasma is in free solution and able to exert its pharmacological effect (Brodie, 1965). The amount of drug bound to albumin is determined by the number of binding sites available, their affinity for the drug and the concentration of the drug present. Drugs or drug metabolites that displace oral anticoagulants from protein binding are generally highly protein-bound themselves, and are often given in large dosage and may accumulate to high levels in plasma (Sellers and Koch-Weser, 1970b). Most drugs that can displace Warfarin are acidic compounds (Solomon and Schrogie, 1967c; Solomon et al., 1968; Sellers and Koch-Weser, 1970b), although many basic drugs are also protein-bound (diphenylhydantoin, imipramine). Since basic drugs are bound to different sites on the albumin molecule, they do not compete for the same sites but the presence of a basic drug bound to the albumin may interfere with the binding of an acidic drug to an adjacent site.

Many studies have been performed on the displacement of oral anticoagulants from plasma albumin by a variety of drugs. These studies are often performed in vitro sometimes with unphysiological conditions of pH, temperature, drug concentration or artificial buffers and the conclusions that one can draw and transpose to the clinical situation are limited.

There are many clinical reports of haemorrhage or an increase in prothrombin time in patients on oral anticoagulants given phenylbutazone or oxyphenbutazone (Eisen, 1964; Hoffbrand and Kininmonth, 1967; Kotler et al., 1966; Nordoy, 1959; Seiler and Duckert, 1968). Udall (1969a) found a significant prolongation of the prothrombin time in all patients on Warfarin when given phenylbutazone. Phenylbutazone appears to have a higher affinity for plasma albumin than Warfarin (Solomon et al., 1968) and up to 40% of bound Warfarin may be displaced (O'Reilly and Aggeler, 1968). Oxyphenbutazone has a similar clinical effect (Fox, 1964; Hobbs et al., 1965). Recently, some doubt has been cast on this explanation and suggestions have been made that phenylbutazone inhibits the metabolism of oral anticoagulants such as Warfarin, leading to an increase in the plasma concentration (Weiner et al., 1965). This might explain why other highly protein-bound drugs do not appear to interfere with anticoagulant control. Indomethacin, for example, will displace Warfarin from protein binding in vitro (Hucker et al., 1966; Solomon et al., 1968) but has little effect in vivo (Hoffbrand and Kininmonth, 1967). Salicylates which are also protein-bound, have no effect on anticoagulant control in patients on Warfarin (Udall, 1969a) although they may affect coagulation by inhibiting platelet aggregation (O'Brien, 1968; Weis and Aledort, 1967).

If an oral anticoagulant is displaced from protein binding by another drug, the rise in free concentration will result in an increased pharmacological effect which will be only temporary. Theoretical calculations suggest that in a patient on Warfarin which will be 97–98% bound to plasma albumin, displacement of only 0.7% of this albumin-bound Warfarin can increase the prothrombin time from 20 to 26 sec (Sellers and Koch-Weser, 1971). The increase in the free concentration of Warfarin in the plasma means that more drug is available for metabolic transformation and this is reflected in practice by a shortened plasma half-life (Aggeler et al., 1967). The amount of oral anticoagulant eliminated from the body each day now exceeds the intake and the plasma concentration falls until a new steady state is achieved in which the total plasma concentration of oral anticoagulant is lower than before the interaction, but the free concentration and therefore the pharmacological effect is the same. An increase in prothrombin time should be expected within 24 hr of administration of a drug that may displace Warfarin. The effect will be maximal in 3–5 hr and the prothrombin time will return to its previous level in less than 2 weeks. Such an effect may be completely missed if the patient is seen only once a month.

Other drugs have been shown to displace Warfarin from protein binding. Chloral hydrate is metabolised to trichloroacetic acid which is strongly protein-bound and will displace Warfarin from its binding sites (Breckenridge and Orme, 1971; Sellers and Koch-Weser, 1970a; Koch-Weser, 1971). Some workers have found a small but significant effect of chloral hydrate on anticoagulant control (Griner et al., 1971; Boston Collaborate Drug Surveillance Program, 1972a) while other investigators have detected no change in anticoagulant control (Breckenridge and Orme, 1971; Sellers and Koch-Weser, 1970a, b; Koch-Weser, 1971).

TABLE I

Drugs potentiating the pharmacological response of oral anticoagulants by displacement from protein binding

Phenylbutazone	Sulphonamides
Oxyphenbutazone	Ethacrynic acid
Chloral hydrate	Nalidixic acid
Diazoxide	Mefenamic acid

A number of other drugs (Table I) have been shown to displace Warfarin from protein binding in vitro and while they pose a theoretical risk of interaction, there are no clinical reports of harmful hypoprothrombinaemia. If they must be given to a patient on oral anticoagulants, the prothrombin time should be carefully checked daily for the next 4 or 5 days. The use of phenylbutazone and oxyphenbutazone should be avoided in a patient on oral anticoagulants.

The effects of the lipid-lowering agent, atromid, on oral anticoagulants are particularly difficult to decipher. Atromid is a combination of ethyl chlorophenoxyisobutyrate (CPIB) and androsterone and soon after its introduction in 1962 reports began to appear of its potentiating effect on oral anticoagulants (Howard et al., 1963; Roberts and Pantridge, 1963). This effect was the same whether androsterone was present in the formulation or not and CPIB is now marketed alone.

CPIB is bound to plasma protein and, in vitro, it will displace Warfarin from protein binding (Solomon and Schrogie, 1967c; Solomon et al., 1968) but this does not explain its effects in vivo. CPIB produces a marked potentiation of the pharmacological effect of Warfarin in man that is maintained and necessitates a reduction in Warfarin dosage (Oliver et al., 1963). In dogs, a prolongation of the plasma half-life of Warfarin has been demonstrated (Hunningbake and Azarnoff, 1968) but studies in man both with Warfarin (Pyorola et al., 1968) and with bishydroxycoumarin (Schrogie and Solomon, 1967) have failed to show any change in plasma half-life. The current theory as yet unproven is that CPIB potentiates the effect of oral anticoagulants by 'increasing the affinity of the receptor site for the anticoagulant' (Schrogie and Solomon, 1967). An alternative hypothesis is that enzyme inhibition which has been demonstrated in dogs (Hunningbake and Azarnoff, 1968) contributes to the potentiation of hypoprothrombinaemia in man and prevents the fall in total plasma Warfarin and the reduction in the plasma Warfarin half-life that would occur due to displacement of Warfarin from protein binding. If a patient taking Warfarin is commenced on CPIB a reduction in Warfarin dosage of between 25 and 30% will be needed and the degree of hypoprothrombinaemia should be checked daily for the next few days.

3.3 DRUG METABOLISM

Many drugs are lipid soluble compounds that can only be eliminated slowly by the kidneys because they diffuse back across the renal tubules as the urine is concentrated. Metabolic transformation by a variety of chemical processes in the liver converts them to more water soluble compounds which can be excreted by the kidney. The oral anticoagulants are hydroxylated by mixed function oxidase enzymes located in the endoplasmic reticulum of the liver cell. Any drug that increases or decreases the activity of these enzymes will cause a change in the concentration of oral anticoagulant in the blood and hence a reduction or an increase in the resultant hypoprothrombinaemia. Warfarin in particular is not excreted unchanged, and the rate of its metabolism is the prime determinant of the pharmacological effect on a fixed dose regime.

Over the last ten years many compounds have been discovered that increase the activity of the hepatic drug-metabolising enzymes (Conney, 1967). The enhanced activity is primarily due to the increased synthesis of enzyme protein and is known as enzyme induction.

3.4 ENZYME INDUCTION

The barbiturates are the best known group of drugs that induce the hepatic drug-metabolising enzymes. It was known that barbiturates would reduce the pharmacological effect of oral anticoagulants for some years before the phenomenon of enzyme induction was discovered (Avellaneda, 1955; Grilli, 1959). Induction of the enzymes that metabolise the oral anticoagulants leads to a shortening of the plasma half-life, and therefore, to a lowering of the steady state plasma concentration and reduction of the hypoprothrombinaemic effect. Many drugs are now known to be inducers of the hepatic drug-metabolising enzymes in man, and these are listed in Table II. Other drugs have been shown to induce drug-metabolising enzymes in animals but information on their ability to do so in man is lacking.

TABLE II

Drugs that diminish the pharmacological effect of oral anticoagulants, by induction of the hepatic drug-metabolising enzymes

Barbiturates	Griseofulvin
Glutethimide	Dichloralphenazone
Ethchlorvynol	Haloperidol

There are many reports of the effect of the barbiturates on oral anticoagulants. Fig. 1 shows the effect of giving quinalbarbitone 100 mg at night to a patient on Warfarin 5 mg daily.

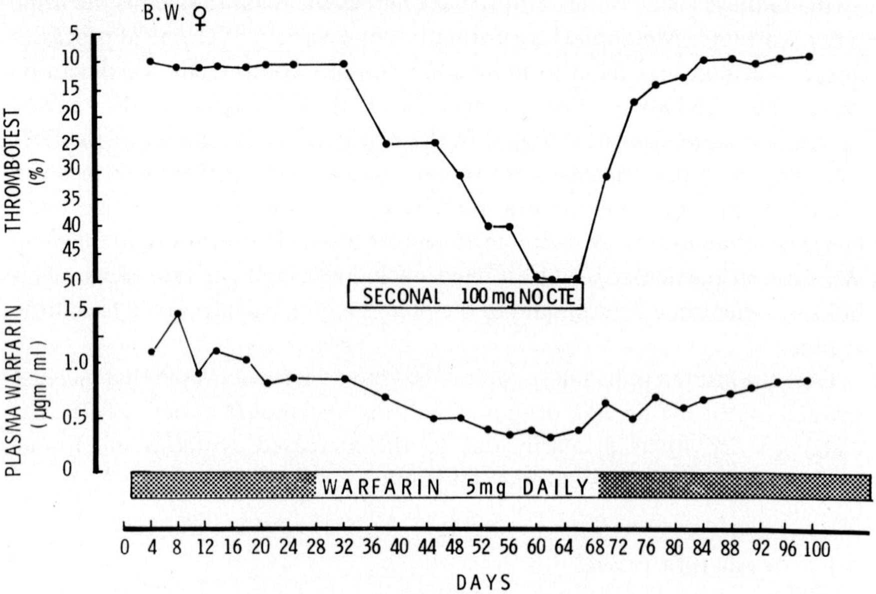

Fig. 1. The effect of a hypnotic (quinalbarbitone) on anticoagulant control and plasma Warfarin.

Most reports concern phenobarbitone (Corn, 1966; Corn and Rocket, 1965; Cucinell et al., 1965; Goss and Dickhouse, 1965; Levy et al., 1970; MacDonald et al., 1969; Reverchon and Sapir, 1961; Robinson and MacDonald, 1966; Van Dam and Gribnau-Overkamp, 1967; Van Dam et al., 1966) but butobarbitone (Antlitz et al., 1968a), amylobarbitone (Breckenridge and Orme, 1971; Robinson and Sylvester, 1970) and quinalbarbitone (Breckenridge and Orme, 1971) have all been shown to diminish the pharmacological effect of oral anticoagulants. Many studies have shown a shortening of the plasma half-life of the anticoagulant concerned and this would indicate that the effect is probably due to enzyme induction.

Glutethimide was originally reported not to affect the pharmacological effect of oral anticoagulants (Grilli, 1959) but this has been corrected by a number of studies with both Warfarin (Corn, 1966; Hunningbake and Azarnoff, 1968; MacDonald et al., 1969) and with ethyl biscoumacetate (Van Dam and Gribnau-Overkamp, 1967; Van Dam et al., 1966). Glutethimide appears to be a potent enzyme inducer. Chloral hydrate was at one time thought to be aninducer of hepatic drug metabolising enzymes (Cucinell et al., 1967) but further work has shown that its metabolite, trichloroacetic acid will displace Warfarin from protein binding (Sellers and Koch-Weser, 1970a) although in a clinical context this does not seem to have any significant effect on anticoagulant control. Dichloralphenazone, however, which is used widely in the United Kingdom as a hypnotic, causes a reduction in the pharmacological response to Warfarin due to the enzyme-inducing properties of phenazone. Chloral hydrate itself does not appear to induce hepatic drug metabolising enzymes (Breckenridge et al., 1971).

Ethchlorvynol (Placidyl) will also inhibit the hypoprothrombinaemic effect of Warfarin (Blank, 1967; Catalano and Cullen, 1966; Johansson, 1968) but in animals no evidence of enzyme induction has been seen (Martin, 1967). Griseofulvin will produce a fall in prothrombin time in patients on Warfarin (Catalano and Cullen, 1966; Cullen and Catalano, 1967) probably because of enzyme induction and haloperidol has been shown to increase the requirements of phenindione for anticoagulant control (Oakley and Lautch, 1963).

The degree of induction of the hepatic drug metabolising enzymes on exposure to a potential inducing agent varies widely from individual to individual. Some patients may show very little evidence of enzyme induction while other patients may have a profound change in the Warfarin requirements. Fig. 1 shows the response to 100 mg of quinalbarbitone taken at night. The effect of quinalbarbitone as an enzyme inducing agent is not seen at once even on the plasma Warfarin concentration. It takes 2 or 3 days to show any change after the quinalbarbitone is started and the effect is maximal by about two weeks. After stopping the enzyme-inducing agent the effect usually wears off slowly over the next 4–6 weeks although it can take longer. The degree of induction in this patient with a fall in plasma Warfarin concentration to 50% of its previous value would have necessitated a 2-fold increase in Warfarin dosage to regain anticoagulant control. Some patients may show a 5-fold fall in plasma Warfarin concentration (Aggeler and O'Reilly, 1969; Antonis et al., 1967; Breckenridge et al., 1971) and one patient recently seen by us showed a 10-fold reduction in Warfarin requirements from 200 to 20 mg per day on cessation of an enzyme-inducing barbiturate hypnotic mixture. Such large changes make the use of any enzyme inducing drug potentially hazardous. Certain alternative drugs are available, however. The benzodiazepine compounds, chlordiazepoxide and diazepam and nitrazepam have no effect on anticoagulant control in man (Breckenridge and Orme, 1971; Lackner and Hunt, 1968; Robinson and Sylvester, 1970; Solomon et al., in press; Breckenridge and Orme, 1973) even though chlordiazepoxide is a potent inducer of hepatic-drug metabolising enzymes in animals (Hooglard et al., 1966). Nitrazepam would appear to be the hypnotic drug of choice for patients on oral anticoagulants.

Meprobamate, although it appears to be an enzyme inducer in animals (Hunningbake and Azarnoff, 1968) has no effect on anticoagulant control in man (Udall, 1970a) and other drugs which have no adverse effect on anticoagulant control in man are diphenhydramine (Hunningbake and Azarnoff, 1968), hydrochlorothiazide (Breckenridge and Orme, 1971a), chlorothiazide (Robinson and Sylvester, 1970) and digoxin, even though under certain circumstances some of them have been reported to cause enzyme induction in animals (Conney, 1967).

TABLE III

Drugs potentiating the pharmacological effect of oral anticoagulants by enzyme inhibition

Phenyramidol	Disulfiram
Methylphenidate	Alcohol
Chloramphenicol	Acetaminophen

3.5 ENZYME INHIBITION (TABLE III)

In contrast to those drugs that accelerate the metabolism of the oral anticoagulants are the drugs that diminish their biotransformation and thereby potentiate the hypoprothrombinaemic action. Enzyme induction takes some days to be manifest, but enzyme inhibition may produce a rise in plasma concentration quite rapidly and the effect may be seen within hours (Christensen and Skovsted, 1969). This mechanism has been little studied compared to enzyme induction although the phenomenon has been known for many years with SKF-525 A (Axelrod et al., 1954).

Bishydroxycoumarin is itself an inhibitor of drug-metabolising enzymes and has been shown to inhibit the metabolism of a number of other drugs. A patient on tolbutamide developed severe hypoglycaemia when given bishydroxycoumarin (Fontana et al., 1968) and other studies have confirmed that the metabolism of tolbutamide is inhibited by bishydroxycoumarin (Kristensen and Hansen, 1967; Solomon and Schrogie, 1967a). Bishydroxycoumarin also inhibits the metabolism of chlorpropamide (Kristensen and Hansen, 1968) and diphenylhydantoin (Hansen et al., 1966). Since bishydroxycoumarin is little used in clinical practice these interactions are of little significance but further substantiate the claim of Warfarin to be used in preference.

Phenyramidol (Analexin) a drug with analgesic and muscle-relaxant properties has been reported to potentiate the pharmacological effect of oral anticoagulants in man (Carter, 1965) and to inhibit the metabolism of bishydroxycoumarin (Solomon and Schrogie, 1966). Methylphenidate (Ritalin) has been reported to potentiate oral anticoagulants in man and to inhibit the metabolism of bishydroxycoumarin and diphenylhydantoin (Garettson et al., 1967) but this report is unconfirmed and animal studies show no effect on Warfarin metabolism (Hunningbake, 1970).

Other drugs that are metabolised by the hepatic enzymes may also inhibit the metabolism of the oral anticoagulants but as yet few have been studied properly. Any agent that interferes with protein synthesis may have the same effect and it is known that chloramphenicol in high doses (2 g daily) will inhibit the metabolism of both bishydroxycoumarin and diphenylhydantoin (Christensen and Skovsted, 1969). Disulfiram, which is used in man as an inhibitor of aldehyde dehydrogenase, probably inhibits the metabolism of oral anticoagulants with the production of excess hypoprothrombinaemia (Rothstein, 1968). Disulfiram has been shown to inhibit the metabolism of diphenylhydantoin (Hansen et al., 1968; Kirboe, 1966).

Alcohol has long been known to potentiate the effect of other drugs such as sedatives. However, in controlled studies a single dose of ethanol of 30–100 g had no effect on the anticoagulant control (Udall, 1970b). It seems unlikely that occasional moderate doses of alcohol will interfere with the anticoagulant control of most patients. However, Breckenridge and Orme (1971), found a marked rise in prothrombin time in 2 patients on Warfarin after taking moderate doses of ethanol in the form of whisky. Both patients had impairment of liver function and in the presence of liver disease, patients on oral anticoagulants should avoid alcohol. Chronic ethanol ingestion will induce the hepatic drug-metabolising enzymes, and chronic alcoholics metabolise Warfarin more rapidly than most normal subjects (Kater et al., 1969). Thus these patients are likely to need a higher dose of Warfarin to achieve anticoagulant control.

Acetaminophen (Tylenol) has been reported to potentiate the effect of Warfarin. Daily doses of 2.6 g of this analgesic increased the prothrombin time of patients on oral anticoagulants by 3–5 sec (Antlitz et al., 1968b). However, in another 10 patients on Warfarin, a daily dose of 3.25 g of acetaminophen for 2 weeks had no effect on the prothrombin time (Udall, 1970b). Any interaction between acetaminophen and oral anticoagulants would appear to be of little clinical importance.

TABLE IV

Drugs that diminish the pharmacological response to oral anticoagulants

By reduced absorption	By stimulation of clotting factor synthesis
Cholestyramine	Vitamin K Oral contraceptives

Drugs that potentiate the pharmacological response to oral anticoagulants

By reducing the availability of vitamin K	By unknown action
Broad spectrum antibiotics	D-Thyroxine Clofibrate Norethandrolone Methandrostenolone Quinidine

3.6 ANTICOAGULANT INTERACTIONS OF UNKNOWN TYPE (TABLE IV)

There are a number of drug interactions with the oral anticoagulants whose exact mechanism is not known, although the effect is usually to potentiate the hypoprothrombinaemia. The anabolic steroids, methandrostenolone, norethandrolone and ethylestrenol increase the pharmacological effect of Warfarin and bishydroxycoumarin (Pyorola and Kekki, 1963; Murakami et al., 1965; Dresdale and Hayes, 1967) and haemorrhagic episodes may occur if the dose of Warfarin is not reduced. The mechanism of this effect is obscure but administration of methandrostenolone or norethandrolone has no effect on the absorption or metabolism of Warfarin (Pyorala et al., 1965) or bishydroxycoumarin (Schrogie and Solomon, 1967) and it may be that these drugs increase the rate of decay of the clotting proteins or they may impair the synthesis of these factors. In contrast, the oral contraceptives have been shown to diminish the pharmacological effect of oral anticoagulants, probably because the oestrogen moiety increases the plasma concentration of factors VII and X, both vitamin K dependent clotting factors (Schrogie et al., 1967; Poller et al., 1969).

D-Thyroxine is used in man for its cholesterol-lowering action. It was first found to potentiate the pharmacological effects of Warfarin in 1962 (Winters and Soloff, 1962) and since then this has been confirmed in most patients studied (Owens et al., 1962; Schrogie and Solomon, 1967). The dose of Warfarin usually has to be reduced by one third to avoid excessive hypoprothrombinaemia (Owens et al., 1962). D-Thyroxine has no effect on the protein binding of Warfarin (Solomon and Schrogie, 1967) and although in high doses it will inhibit the metabolism of bishydroxycoumarin, it has an effect in man at dose levels that have no effect on the metabolism of oral anticoagulants (Schrogie and Solomon, 1967). The current theory is that D-thyroxine increases the receptor site affinity for Warfarin and it has been shown to increase the apparent Michaelis constant (K_m) in man (Solomon and Schrogie, 1967). This is a measure of the apparent affinity of the receptor site for Warfarin.

Quinidine has been shown to be responsible for haemorrhagic episodes in patients on chronic Warfarin therapy (Gazzaniga and Stewart, 1969; Koch-Weser, 1968; Beaumont and Torrit, 1955), although in a group of 10 patients on Warfarin, Udall could find no evidence of potentiation after giving quinidine (Udall, 1969a). Quinine is known to have a hypoprothrombinaemic effect of its own (Pirk and Engleberg, 1945) and it may be that quinidine has a similar effect too small to be noticed in normal subjects, but in susceptible people whose synthesis of vitamin K-dependent clotting factors is already depressed by oral anticoagulants, such an effect could be dangerous (Koch-Weser, 1968; Jarrums, 1954). Quinidine, like quinine is protein-bound (Pirk and Engleberg, 1945) and therefore may displace oral anticoagulants from their binding sites.

Salicylates have a hypoprothrombinaemic action in normal people (Verstraete et al., 1968) and one might expect them to potentiate the effect of oral anticoagulants but this is not the usual experience. Udall found no effect on the prothrombin time of patients on Warfarin given 3 g of aspirin daily (Udall, 1969a). Salicylates, however, should be avoided by patients on oral anticoagulants since they increase the risk of bleeding by affecting platelet function (O'Brien, 1968; Weis and Aledort, 1967).

There are many poorly documented reports of the potentiation of the pharmacological effects of oral anticoagulants by various antibiotics. Many authors have warned that broad spectrum antibiotics, by reducing the number of intestinal bacteria, will reduce the availability of vitamin K. In fact, bacterial synthesis of vitamin K becomes important in man only when the dietary intake is markedly reduced (Frick et al., 1967; Messinger and Samet, 1965). Potentiation of the oral anticoagulants has been shown by only a few controlled studies in man. Penicillin alone has no effect but when combined with oral streptomycin an increase in the prothrombin time of 6–10 sec was seen (Magid, 1962; Noegeli and Matis, 1958). Oxytetracycline (Noegeli and Matis, 1958; Wright et al., 1954), chlortetracycline (Magid, 1962) chloramphenicol (Magid, 1962) and neomycin (Udall, 1969a, b) have all been shown to have a slight potentiating effect on the pharmacological effect of oral anticoagulants. However, this potentiation has not been proved to be due to depression of bacterial synthesis of vitamin K since these antibiotics can enhance the effect of Warfarin by other means (Christensen and Skovsted, 1969). Present evidence suggests that oral antibiotic therapy is unlikely to interfere significantly with the hypoprothrombinaemic response to oral anticoagulants.

4 Digitalis

4.1 DRUG INTERACTIONS THAT ENHANCE DIGITALIS TOXICITY

Digitalis intoxication is a common condition because the drug is widely used in the treatment of cardiac disease and because the margin between its therapeutic and toxic effects is narrow. Digitalis intoxication affects between 7 and 22% of patients on maintenance therapy (Rodensky and Wasserman, 1964; Sodeman, 1965) and the incidence appears to be increasing (Capeller et al., 1959). Apart from overdosage and individual idiosyncracy, factors which increase the liability to toxicity include old age (Hurwitz and Wade, 1969), renal disease and potassium deficiency (Lown et al., 1960). As potassium deficiency is liable to occur in patients who are receiving diuretics, these drugs predispose to digitalis intoxication. Hurwitz and Wade found that 19.8% of 192 patients treated with cardiac glycosides developed adverse reactions. Of the 53 patients who received digitalis alone only 9% showed toxic effects compared with 24% on combined digitalis and diuretic therapy. Potassium supplements or potassium-conserving diuretics such as amiloride, spironolactone or triamterene should normally be given to avoid the harmful effects of this interaction.

There is some evidence that reserpine may increase the susceptibility of patients with atrial fibrillation to the toxic effects of digitalis (Lown et al., 1961). Reserpine also reduces the maximum inotropic response to digitalis (Spann et al., 1966).

4.2 TREATMENT OF DIGITALIS INTOXICATION

In many cases of digitalis intoxication withdrawal of the glycoside is all that is required. However, potassium chloride is a logical treatment particularly if diuretics have been used (Cohen, 1952; Rosenbaum et al., 1960; Sodeman, 1965). Although oral repletion is effective (Goldberg et al., 1960; Page and Real, 1955) it is comparatively slow to act and may be poorly tolerated because of nausea and vomiting. In more urgent cases with cardiac arrhythmias potassium salts can be given intravenously, preferably as an infusion at a rate of 20–40 mEq/hr, but this therapy should be carefully supervised since it may lead to a further increase in atrioventricular block (Fisch et al., 1960; Fisch et al., 1959). As cardiac arrhythmias can provoke a life-threatening situation with little advance warning and cardioversion with synchronised DC shock is contraindicated under these circumstances, reversion by pharmacological methods may be required.

In view of the synergism which exists between digitalis and calcium ions (Goldberg et al., 1960; Page and Real, 1955) one possible approach is to lower serum calcium with chelating agents. Sodium and potassium citrate have been used with some success (Barbieri et al., 1964) but ethylenediamine tetraacetic acid (sodium EDTA) has been used more extensively (Gubner and Kallman, 1957; Rosenbaum et al., 1960; Szekely and Wynne, 1963). Although this acts rapidly its duration of action is short-lived and the injection may cause pain as well as lead to hypotension. Alternatively, most of the standard dysrhythmic agents have been advocated for the treatment of digitalis-induced arrhythmias including diphenylhydantoin (Lang et al., 1965), lignocaine (Sarawicz, 1971), procainamide (DeGraff, 1954; Sodeman, 1965), propranolol (Turner, 1966), and quinidine. There is little indication that any of these agents offers a particular advantage since all are effective in reverting most ventricular dysrhythmias and in high doses can lead to myocardial depression. However, two of these drugs, diphenylhydantoin and propranolol, have theoretical advantages. Diphenylhydantoin unlike the others does not depress A–V conduction (Scherlag et al., 1968) so that bradycardia is less likely to occur (Mosey and Tyler, 1954). Propranolol has advantages because of its additional β-adrenoceptor blocking property which antagonises the effects of circulating catecholamines in digitalis intoxication (Vaughan Williams and Sekeija, 1963). However, profound bradycardia may develop (Watt, 1968) so that extreme caution must be exercised by giving no more than 1 mg intravenously every 5 min to a total of 5 mg.

4.3 INTERACTIONS WITH DIGITOXIN

Digitoxin is well absorbed but is bound to albumin, metabolised by the liver and also undergoes an enterohepatic recirculation. There are therefore several sites at which a drug interaction might occur. Displacement from protein binding by drugs such as phenylbutazone, Warfarin and tolbutamide has been demonstrated in vitro, but is not a problem in practice (Solomon et al., 1971). However, phenylbutazone, phenobarbitone and diphenylhydantoin have been shown to shorten the plasma half-life of digitoxin by induction of liver microsomal enzymes (Solomon and Abrams, 1972). Cholestyramine also reduces the plasma half-life of digitoxin by about 35% (Caldwell and Greenberger, 1970), probably by binding to digitoxin and thereby preventing enterohepatic recirculation. This interaction could be employed in the treatment of digitoxin toxicity.

5 β-Adrenoceptor blocking agents

Since the introduction of the first β-adrenoceptor antagonist, pronethalol, these agents have become widely used in the treatment of angina pectoris, arterial hypertension and cardiac arrhythmias. Their major therapeutic effects, interactions with other drugs, and side effects depend upon their ability to antagonise specifically and reversibly the stimulatory effects of endogenous catecholamines.

5.1 β-ADRENOCEPTOR BLOCKADE AND VASODILATORS IN ANGINA PECTORIS

The beneficial effects of propranolol and similar drugs in angina pectoris are due to a reduction in cardiac work and hence myocardial oxygen consumption (Hamer and Sowton, 1966; Sonnenblick et al., 1965). This is achieved mainly by a reduction in heart rate at rest and on exertion, but also by lowering blood pressure and the force of myocardial contraction. Nitrates also reduce cardiac work (Mason and Braunwald, 1965; Williams et al., 1965) by lowering systemic blood pressure, peripheral resistance and venous pressure. Thus, on theoretical grounds, it might be expected that there would be at least an additive effect of the two treatments. Furthermore, the beneficial effects of nitrates are offset to some extent by a reflex increase in heart rate. Since propranolol antagonises the sympathetic component of the reflex (George et al., in press) a synergistic effect might occur. This interaction has been claimed for propranolol and the long-acting vasodilator, isosorbide nitrate, on the basis of a reduction in the incidence and severity of anginal attacks, improved exercise tolerance and ST segment changes on the electrocardiogram (ECG) (Russek, 1967, 1968). The beneficial effects of the combined treatment on symptomatology have since been confirmed (Battock et al., 1969) but not the additional benefit on exercise tests and on the ECG.

The combined treatment is worthwhile in those patients who fail to derive satisfactory relief of symptoms from β-adrenoceptor blockade alone, and all patients can continue to take glyceryl trinitrate sublingually as required.

5.2 PROPRANOLOL AND QUINIDINE IN CARDIAC ARRHYTHMIAS

Although DC cardioversion is the quickest and most effective method for reverting atrial fibrillation to sinus rhythm – there are circumstances when this treatment is not available – is contraindicated or is ineffective. Quinidine with digitalis was the traditional method of treatment but the high doses of the former which were necessary sometimes resulted in asystole or ventricular fibrillation (Oravetz and Slodki, 1968). Although β-adrenoceptor antagonists are effective in slowing the ventricular rate in atrial fibrillation by increasing the degree of A–V blockade, reversion to sinus rhythm is uncommon (Gibson and Sowton, 1969; Harrison and Griffin, 1967). It is therefore interesting that Stern (1967) achieved reversion to sinus rhythm in 15 of 17 patients with chronic atrial fibrillation by the combined use of propranolol and quinidine. Visioli and Bertaccini (1968) have since reported similar although less spectacular results. Experimentally propranolol antagonises the effect of quinidine in prolonging the effective refractory period (Berger and Mokler, 1969) and the combination has been shown to produce less haemodynamic disturbance than either propranolol or quinidine alone (Stern, 1971). However, further evaluation of this combination is required before it can be widely accepted for reversion of atrial fibrillation since Hillestad and Storstein (1969) have reported fatalities.

Propranolol and procainamide have been given in combination to revert ventricular fibrillation in several patients (Ikram and Nixon, 1966).

5.3 PROPRANOLOL AND NOTROPIC AGENTS

The negative inotropic effects of β-adrenoceptor antagonists, together with the prolongation of ventricular systole, ventricular dilatation and the blockade of normal sympathetic drive may lead to the development of cardiac failure (Chamberlain, 1966; Stephen, 1966). Since propranolol and similar drugs are specific in their actions, they do not interfere with the positive inotropic effects of drugs whose actions are not mediated via stimulation of the β-adrenoceptors. Both digitalis (Gebhardt and Blümchen, 1968) and glucagon (Glick et al., 1968; Lucchesi, 1968) have been shown to counteract the detrimental effects of propranolol on myocardial contractility. β-Adrenoceptor antagonists should be avoided in patients with borderline heart failure or in whom cardiac output is maintained by a rapid heart rate. If, however, mild congestive heart failure should develop it can often be controlled with digitalis or a diuretic. In the more serious situation of acute left ventricular failure developing in a patient on propranolol this should be managed as in acute pulmonary oedema due to other causes. Aminophylline is particularly appropriate in this situation as in propranolol-induced bronchospasm, since it restores cyclic AMP levels by inhibiting the enzyme phosphodiesterase (Butcher and Sutherland, 1962). Routine digitalisation of patients on β-adrenoceptor antagonists however, is both unnecessary and undesirable.

One other complication sometimes seen with β-adrenoceptor antagonists is the development of a bradycardia, especially when the drug is given intravenously. This effect is due mainly to the unopposed action of the vagus nerve after blockade of sympathetic drive and can be counteracted by atropine 1.2 mg given intravenously (Stannard et al., 1968).

5.4 PROPRANOLOL AND INSULIN

Hypoglycaemia has occurred in a number of patients receiving insulin or oral hypoglycaemic agents plus propranolol (Editorial, 1967; Kotler et al., 1966; Reveno and Rosenbaum, 1968) but has also occurred spontaneously in persons who were not receiving drugs other than propranolol (Kotler et al., 1966). β-Adrenoceptor blockade also interferes with many of the normal responses to hypoglycaemia including tachycardia and tremor and may lead to difficulties in diagnosis. Fortunately, propranolol-induced hypoglycaemia is uncommon because in man liver glycogenolysis is mediated by α-adrenergic receptors (Antonis et al., 1967). This interaction is most likely to occur when liver glycogen is depleted by fasting or in the presence of ketoacidosis.

6 Antidepressants and cardiac disease

6.1 MONOAMINE OXIDASE INHIBITORS

Monoamine oxidase inhibitors (MAOI) have both antidepressant and hypotensive effects. However, their clinical use is limited by the problem of interactions with foodstuffs and sympathomimetic drugs. The typical reaction consists of palpitations, pounding headache, profuse sweating and often by nausea and vomiting, 10–90 min after ingestion of the offending food or drug. Physical examination may reveal sinus tachycardia or atrial fibrillation, elevated blood pressure and in some patients, features of a subarachnoid haemorrhage. The symptoms and signs generally resolve over a period of 1–3 hr if left untreated.

6.2 FOODSTUFFS

Many reports have been published concerning the interaction between MAOI and cheese. Blackwell et al. (1964, 1967) reported 20 hypertensive reactions occurring in approximately 740 depressed patients treated at the Maudsley Hospital in London. Most of the patients had taken either cheese or Marmite, an extract made from yeast which contains 1.6 mg of tyramine per g. Horwitz et al. (1964) subsequently showed that patients taking pargyline in a dose of 75–100 mg daily required only about 1/100 of the dose of tyramine to provoke the same hypertensive response as under control conditions. These authors also found considerable differences in the tyramine content of various cheeses, ranging from nil in cottage cheese to 1.4 mg/g in New York State Cheddar.

Although cheese and Marmite are undoubtedly hazardous to patients on MAOI much difficulty has been encountered in warning them of all the possible foodstuffs and drinks (e.g. Chianti and Alicante wine) which contain a dangerous amount of tyramine or other pressor substances. Other foodstuffs which have been reported to provoke 'the cheese reaction' include beef and chicken liver which had deteriorated before or after cooking, and Schmaltz pickled herring (Nuessle et al., 1965). The most likely explanation for these findings is that any foodstuff or beverage that has deteriorated or is normally eaten or drunk after being allowed to undergo partial autolysis may contain significant amounts of tyramine.

This interaction has been exploited by Diamond et al. (1969) in 2 male patients who were disabled by postural hypotension. The treatment given was tranylcypromine 70 mg daily, and cheddar cheese 90 g daily (equivalent to 26 mg tyramine daily) on which blood pressure rose and the patients were able to sit and stand for 6 hr a day.

6.3 MAOI AND OTHER DRUGS

Patients commonly take over-the-counter remedies for minor ailments, and amongst the most popular of these are cough medicines, many of which contain a sympathomimetic agent, phenylpropanolamine. Cuthbert et al. (1969) have reported that 50 mg of this drug taken orally had little effect on blood pressure in normal individuals but caused a severe rise in pressure when given in the same dose to the same individuals while taking a monoamine oxidase inhibitor. A list of a large number of remedies which contain phenylpropanolamine is given by Cuthbert et al. (1969). Hypertensive crisis has also been reported in a patient who was given metaraminol to combat excessive hypotension caused by pargyline (Horler and Wynne, 1965).

Interactions have been reported between MAOI and a number of other drugs such as pethidine and tricyclic antidepressants which are not metabolised by MAO. Some of the reports are contradictory and the mechanisms proposed are unconvincing. There are several reports of patients on MAOI collapsing after administration of normal doses of pethidine. A typical example is a patient who was being treated with phenelzine and was given 100 mg pethidine (Reid and Jones, 1962). She became rigid and comatose within 5 min, developed a fever of 104° F and died 8 hr later. One explanation which has been put forward to account for this interaction is that MAOI also inhibit oxidation by liver microsomes which are responsible for the metabolism of pethidine (Fouts and Brodie, 1956). There are two reasons for doubting the validity of this explanation. First, it is difficult to explain the immediacy of the collapse reported with pethidine as even under normal circumstances very little would have been metabolised in the first few minutes after a dose (Sjöqvist, 1965). Secondly, deliberate administration of increasing doses of pethidine and morphine in 15 patients taking MAOI failed to provoke any adverse effect (Evans-Prosser, 1968). The highest doses used in this study, 40 mg of pethidine and 4 mg of morphine, were not large but should have been sufficient to detect potentiation of the order implied in the published cases. An idiosyncrasy seems possible but the mechanism involved is unknown.

Similar incidents have been reported in some patients taking MAOI who have been given tricyclic antidepressants (Babiak, 1961). Brachfield et al. (1964) reported a patient who was being treated with tranylcypromine in a dose of 10 mg twice daily who collapsed after a single tablet of imipramine. The patient became unconscious with a temperature of 105° F. Chlorpromazine has been used to treat such misadventures with apparent benefit.

These interactions have been reviewed by Sjöqvist (1965) whose article should be consulted for further information. However, some psychiatrists use tricyclic antidepressants and monoamine oxidase inhibitors without encountering serious problems.

6.4 TRICYCLIC ANTIDEPRESSANTS

Since these agents block the uptake of catecholamines into adrenergic neurones (Iversen, 1967) and this process is normally responsible for the termination of their pharmacological effects, the action of noradrenaline and adrenaline may be potentiated by imipramine and similar drugs. Clinically, it has been found that the pressor effects of intravenous adrenaline or noradrenaline may be increased by 2 and by 4–8 times respectively (Barar et al., 1971; Boakes et al., 1973) in volunteers who were at the same time receiving antidepressant drugs of this type. Such an interaction might lead to serious problems if a local anaesthetic containing a catecholamine were inadvertently injected intravenously. Most dentists use local anaesthetics containing adrenaline 1:80,000 or 1:200,000. However, solutions containing 1:25,000 are also available, and should be avoided in patients on tricyclic antidepressants.

A further problem which has been encountered in some patients taking therapeutic doses of these drugs and one which is frequently seen in accidental poisonings is the development of cardiac arrhythmias (Barnes et al., 1968). Electrocardiographic abnormalities have also been reported in patients with and without cardiac disease whilst taking tricyclic antidepressants. Even more alarming was the report by Coull and colleagues (1970) that patients with cardiac disease were subject to an increased risk of sudden death. However, the definition of 'sudden death' given by these authors lacked precision, and a more recent study from The Boston Collaborative Drug Surveillance Program (1972b) failed to show any evidence that tricyclic antidepressants are dangerous in cardiac patients. As cardiac arrhythmias occurring in patients taking these drugs may be related to increased levels of catecholamines (Alexander and Nino, 1969) β-adrenoceptor antagonists should be an effective method of treatment. Propranolol has been shown to revert some arrhythmias in acute poisoning with tricyclic antidepressants (Marshall and Green, 1968).

The interactions between these drugs and the adrenergic neurone blocking agents, bethanidine, debrisoquine and guanethidine are discussed elsewhere in this review.

7 Interactions with anaesthetics

Volatile anaesthetic drugs such as cyclopropane, chloroform, trichloroethylene, halothane and methoxyflurane and propellants used in aerosols have been shown to sensitise the heart to exogenous or endogenous catecholamines and lead to the development of ventricular arrhythmias (Katz and Katz, 1966; Meek et al., 1937; Orth et al., 1939; Bass, 1970; Taylor et al., 1971). This interaction was originally studied in dogs but similar events have been shown to occur in man (Johnstone, 1953). Ether and nitrous oxide do not show this interaction with primary and secondary catecholamines (Katz and Katz, 1966; Meek et al., 1937; Orth et al., 1939).

A number of other factors have been shown to increase the incidence of anaesthetic arrhythmias including elevated arterial pressure (Moe et al., 1948) and raised carbon dioxide tension (Price et al., 1958). Although poor anaesthetic technique predisposes to the development of arrhythmias, they will occur if a sufficiently large dose of catecholamine is given (Katz and Katz, 1966). However, even when there are no anaesthetic problems the dose of catecholamine required to precipitate a disturbance of rhythm is less when certain anaesthetics are being used. The possible mechanisms for these interactions have been fully reviewed by Katz and Epstein (1968).

General anaesthesia and abnormal sympathetic activity appear to be an undesirable combination since it has also been shown that low activity in patients on reserpine may be associated with an increased risk of hypotension. The subject has been reviewed by Ominsky and Wollman (1969) who conclude that there is no evidence that stopping reserpine for 1–2 weeks before elective surgery lessens the risk of this interaction occurring. Furthermore, any drug which interferes with sympathetic nervous control of the heart and blood vessels increases the risk of hypotension during or immediately after anaesthesia.

8 Interactions between antihypertensive drugs

The rationale of combined drug therapy of hypertension rests upon two premises: Firstly, that most drug side-effects are dose-related. Two drugs in small doses will often cause fewer side-effects than one of them in a larger dose having the same effect upon blood pressure; secondly, that interference with blood pressure control mechanisms at more than one point may have a synergistic action and produce a substantially greater fall in pressure than can be obtained with either drug alone.

8.1 BLOOD PRESSURE CONTROL

There is no specific treatment of high blood pressure because it is rarely possible to identify a single factor responsible for the elevation and maintenance of blood pressure. The level of blood pressure is set by the action of several different control systems. Short term pressure changes are regulated by the baroreceptors that provide the brain with sensory information concerning pressure levels in different parts of the circulation. The brain controls the pressure using both sympathetic and parasympathetic afferent pathways to change heart rate and output, and to dilate and constrict peripheral vessels. Drugs are available that interfere with every part of this complex arc. Veratrum increases the rate of baroreceptor discharge and causes pressure reduction as a result of the inaccurate information presented to the brain. Clonidine and methyldopa interfere with central noradrenergic mechanisms and diminish the flow of impulses to the peripheral sympathetic nerves. Ganglion blocking and adrenergic neurone blocking drugs interfere with transmission in the peripheral nervous system either in the autonomic ganglia or at adrenergic terminals. The doses of these drugs used in therapy do not produce maximal inhibition of the pathways upon which they act. Combination of drugs acting at more than one point upon the reflex arc may have an additive effect. Thus methyldopa and bethanidine together have a more favourable effect than either does alone in patients who are resistant to methyldopa (Breckenridge and Dollery, 1966).

The second main control system is concerned with regulating fluid volume and it involves the kidney, the regulation of renal blood flow, the renin–angiotensin–aldosterone system, as well as other mechanisms that regulate mineralocorticoid output. Salt and water overload lead to hypertension if the excess cannot be excreted. The mechanism proposed is that distension of the veins causes an increase in the filling pressure of the heart and a rise in cardiac output. The flow through the tissues rises and ultimately an autoregulatory increase in the resistance of the peripheral arterioles occurs. Salt and water depletion lowers blood volume and cardiac output, but short term changes are buffered by the baro-receptors which increase the peripheral resistance to prevent a fall in pressure. After a time, the baro-receptors tire and re-setting of the level of pressure occurs. Drugs that deplete salt and water are only moderately effective antihypertensive agents by themselves, and have a flat dose–response curve (Cranston et al., 1963).

The main use of diuretics lies in their combination with other drugs. Diuretics potentiate the effects of most other blood pressure-lowering drugs, such as vasodilators, and adrenergic neurone-blocking drugs. The mechanisms involved have occasioned some debate. Diuretics cause an acute reduction of plasma volume which persists for a few days, but is not maintained, and after 6 weeks the plasma volume is only slightly below the pretreatment value (Wilson and Freis, 1959). As diuretics that have no structural features in common all have antihypertensive properties, it seems reasonable to assume that the fall of blood pressure must be mediated by salt and water depletion and not by other pharmacological properties of the drugs. Frusemide, which has a very short duration of action, has less hypotensive effect than some of the other diuretics (Anderson et al., 1971). This may be the result of salt and water retention between the brief periods of drug action.

One of the main problems with the benzothiadiazine diuretics is that they cause potassium loss in the urine, and to minimise potassium depletion it is commonplace for potassium salt to be incorporated in a combined tablet. Enteric coated potassium chloride caused intestinal ulceration and stenosis in some patients (Lindholmer et al., 1964). This problem appears to have been overcome by using formulations in which potassium chloride is embedded in a wax matrix that ensures slow release. However, recently attention has been focused upon combinations of potassium-conserving diuretics such as triamterene, amiloride or spironolactone, with thiazides. These are effective in preventing hypokalaemia in patients with normal renal function, but there is the risk of hyperkalaemia, in patients with renal impairment. A number of fatalities have been reported and such combinations should not be used in patients with an elevated blood urea (Cohen, 1966). The benzothiadiazines and the potassium-conserving diuretics also potentiate one another's saluretic effect. There may be excessive excretion of salt and water unless the dose of both drugs is reduced below the levels usually employed when they are given alone. Amiloride and triamterene when given alone do not elevate serum uric acid as do the benzothiadiazines (Paterson et al., 1968). However, the combination of the two drugs causes a similar degree of hyperuricaemia to a benzothiadiazine alone.

8.2 AUTOREGULATION OF VASCULAR RESISTANCE AND THE USE OF VASODILATORS

The most basic pressure control mechanism lies in the autoregulatory activity of arterioles in the organs. These arterioles alter their resistance to maintain a blood flow appropriate to the local metabolic demands.

There are a number of drugs available that act directly upon the arterioles and lower blood pressure by causing vasodilatation. These include sodium nitroprusside, hydrallazine and diazoxide. These drugs are usually employed by intravenous injection to control blood pressure in hypertensive emergencies. When used in this way they are generally given alone. However, when used as antihypertensive agents by the oral route, vasodilators cause reflex tachycardia and patients often complain of palpitations. The rise in cardiac output has the effect of minimising the fall in blood pressure. Use of an adrenergic neurone-blocking drug or a β-receptor blocking drug prevents the reflex tachycardia and potentiates the fall in blood pressure (Zacest, personal communication; Gilmore et al., 1970).

8.3 COMBINED THERAPY IN PRACTICE

The most widely used drug combinations in the treatment of hypertension rely upon diuretics as one of their basic components. These drugs are often used as 'background therapy' whatever other drugs are to be used to reduce blood pressure. On their own a diuretic such as hydrochlorothiazide and bendrofluazide produces a modest reduction of pressure averaging 10–12 mm Hg and without any significant postural action. If reserpine or hydrallazine in a low dose is added a greater effect can be obtained and such low fixed dose combinations are popular because of their simplicity. In the Veterans Administration Cooperative study (1967) a combination of 100 mg hydrochlorothiazide with 150 mg of hydrallazine and 0.2 mg of reserpine was used and this produced an average reduction of 28 mm Hg of diastolic blood pressure when compared with placebo. If more potent drugs such as methyldopa, bethanidine or guanethidine are added their effect is potentiated by the diuretic and the dose required for equivalent pressure reduction is reduced to about half what it would have been without the diuretic. The regimen has a further advantage that fluid retention wich complicated treatment with these drugs in 15–20% of patients is prevented by administration of the diuretic (Leishman et al., 1959).

Purists may argue that it is better to use only one drug and this is undoubtedly true in the early stages of evaluation of a new therapeutic agent. However, combined therapy has proved to be easier to manage than a single drug in most patients.

The disadvantages are mainly the biochemical abnormalities caused by diuretics such as hypokalaemia, hyperglycaemia and hyperuricaemia. In practice these abnormalities have not proved a major source of difficulty so long as the physician is aware that they may occur (Side Effects of Drugs, vol. 6, 1968).

8.4 DRUG INTERACTIONS THAT CAUSE LOSS OF BLOOD PRESSURE CONTROL IN TREATED HYPERTENSIVES

The most frequent explanation of loss of pressure control in a treated hypertensive patient is that he has failed to take the drug in the dose prescribed. In rare instances, loss of pressure control may be the result of interactions with other drugs.

Depression and hypertension are both common diseases. Depression may be caused or aggravated by antihypertensive therapy with drugs such as reserpine. The most frequently used and effective antidepressant drugs are the tricyclic compounds such as imipramine and amitriptyline. In 1963, Leishman et al. stated that some patients treated with guanethidine lost their side-effects and control of blood pressure when they were given a tricyclic compound treatment for depression. Mitchell and his colleagues (1970) demonstrated that this was a general problem with the adrenergic neurone-blocking drugs, such as guanethidine, bethanidine and debrisoquine and occurred because the antidepressants inhibit the amine pump which concentrates the adrenergic neurone-blocking drugs in adrenergic nerve endings.

In an investigation of 10 patients who had received treatment with both an antidepressant and an adrenergic neurone-blocking drug, Skinner et al.

(1969) found that 6 had poor pressure control. In 4, the tricyclic antidepressant was withdrawn. Two patients showed improved pressure control, and 2 others became hypotensive.

The interaction is a competitive process and if the dose of the adrenergic neurone-blocking drug is increased, blood pressure control can often be restored in the presence of a tricyclic antidepressant. Meyer and his colleagues (1970) reported a patient treated with guanethidine in a dose of 75 mg daily who required 300 mg daily when he was also receiving treatment with amitriptyline. If this situation occurred without the cause being recognised, and the antidepressant was suddenly withdrawn severe hypotension would follow.

The blood pressure-lowering action of adrenergic neurone-blocking drugs is also antagonised by amphetamine and dexamphetamine. This is less of a problem since recognition of the hazards of the use of amphetamines as appetite suppressants has led to a decline in their use. It was originally supposed that the interaction occurred because of a direct effect of amphetamine at the receptor site, but recently Gerkens et al. (1969) have suggested that it occurs because of competition for the neurone pump. A similar mechanism may explain the loss of blood pressure control in some patients on adrenergic neurone-blocking drugs who have treated themselves with cough and cold cures containing phenylpropanolamine. These medicines do not contain a large enough dose of phenylpropanolamine to cause a significant elevation of blood pressure by themselves, but if they are given to patients on adrenergic neurone-blocking drugs, then they may cause complete loss of control.

An interaction between clonidine and desipramine has recently been reported by Briant et al. (1973). Introduction of the tricyclic antidepressant led to loss of blood pressure control in 4 out of 5 patients. The average rise in blood pressure was 22/15 mm Hg in recumbency and 12/11 mm Hg on standing.

Patients who are taking adrenergic neurone-blocking drugs should be warned not to take cough or cold cures without medical advice, and they should not take antidepressants without consideration of the possible interactions that may occur.

Acknowledgement

We wish to thank Miss S. Banks for help in the preparation of this manuscript.

References

Aggeler, P. M. and O'Reilly, R. A. (1966): The pharmacological basis of anticoagulant therapy. *Tromb. diath. haemorr.* (Stuttgart), **21**, 227.

Aggeler, P. M. and O'Reilly, R. A. (1969): Effect of heptabarbital on response to bis-hydroxycoumarin in man. *J. Lab. clin. Med.*, **14**, 229.

Aggeler, P. M., O'Reilly, R. A., Leong, L., and Kowitz, P. E. (1967): *New Engl. J. Med.*, **276**, 496.

Alexander, E. S. and Nino, A. (1969): Cardiovascular complications in young patients taking psychotropic drugs. *Amer. Heart J.*, **78**, 757.

Anderson, J., Godfrey, B. E., Hill, D. M., Munro-Faure, A. D. and Sheldon, J. (1971): A comparison of the effects of hydrochlorothiazide and of frusemide in the treatment of hypertensive patients. *Quart. J. Med.*, **40**, 541.

Antlitz, A. M., Tolentino, M. A. and Kosai, M. F. (1968a): Effect of butabarbital on orally administered anticoagulants. *Curr. Therap. Res.*, **10**, 70.

Antlitz, A. M., Mead, J. A. and Tolentino, M. A. (1968b): Potentiation of oral anti-coagulant therapy by acetaminophen. *Curr. Therap. Res.*, **10**, 501.

Antonis, A., Clark, M. L., Hodge, R. L., Molony, M. and Pilkington, T.R.E. (1967): Receptor mechanisms in the hyperglycaemic response to adrenaline in man. *Lancet*, **1**, 1135.

Avellaneda, M. (1955): Interferencia de los barbituricos en la acción del tromexan. *Medicina* (B. Aires), **15**, 109.

Axelrod, J., Reichental, J. and Brodie, B. B. (1954): The mechanism of the potentiating action of B-diethylaminoethyldiphenylpropylacetate. *J. Pharmacol. exp. Therap.*, **112**, 49.

Babiak, W. (1961): Case fatality due to overdosage of combination of tranylcypromine and imipramine. *Canad. med. Assoc. J.*, **85**, 377.

Barar, F. S. K., Boakes, A. J., Benedikter, L. B., Laurence, D. R., Prichard, B. N. C. and Teoch, P. C. (1971): Interactions between catecholamines and tricyclic and monoamine oxidase inhibitor antidepressive agents in man. *Brit. J. Pharmacol.*, **43**, 472P.

Barbieri, F. F., Gold, H., Lang, T. W., Bernstein, H. and Corday, E. (1964): Sodium and potassium citrate salts for the treatment of digitalis toxicity. *Amer. J. Cardiol.*, **14**, 650.

Barnes, R. J., Kone, S. M. and Wu, R. W. Y. (1968): Electrocardiographic changes in amitriptyline poisoning. *Brit. med. J.*, **3**, 222.

Bass, M. (1970): Sudden sniffing deaths. *J. Amer. med. Ass.*, **212**, 2075.

Battock, D. J., Alvarez, H. and Chidsey, C. A. (1969): Effects of propranolol and iso-sorbide dinitrate on exercise performance and adrenergic activity in patients with angina pectoris. *Circulation*, **39**, 157.

Beaumont, J. L. and Tarrit, A. (1955): Les accidents hémorragiques survenus au de 1500 traitements anticoagulants. *Sang. biol. pathol.*, **26**, 680.

Benjamin, D., Robinson, D. S. and McCormack, J. (1970): Cholestyramine binding of warfarin in man and in vitro. *Clin. Res.*, **18**, 336.

Berger, J. E. and Mokler, C. M. (1969): The interaction of quinidine with alpha and beta adrenergic receptors in the rat myocardium. *J. Pharmacol. exp. Therap.*, **165**, 242.

Blackwell, B. and Marley, E. (1964): Interaction between cheese and monoamine oxidase inhibitors in rats and cats. *Lancet*, **1**, 530.

Blackwell, B., Marley, E., Price, J. and Taylor, D. (1967): Hypertensive interactions between monoamine oxidase inhibitors and foodstuffs. *Brit. J. of Psychiat.*, **113**, 349.

Blank, H. (1967): The actions and interactions of drugs: the therapeutic significance of enzyme induction. *Trans. St. John's Hosp. dermatol. Soc.*, (London), **53**, 1.

Boakes, A. J., Laurence, D. R., Teoh, P. C., Barar, F. S. K., Benedicter, L. T. and Prichard, B. N. C. (1973): Interactions between sympathomimetic amines and antidepressant agents in man. *Brit. med. J.*, **1**, 311.

Boston Collaborate Drug Surveillance Program. (1972a): *New Engl. J. Med.*, **286**, 53.

Boston Collaborate Drug Surveillance Program (1972b): Adverse reactions to the tricyclic antidepressant drugs. *Lancet*, **1**, 529.

Brachfeld, J., Wirtshafter, A. and Wolfe, S. (1964): Imipramine–tranylcypromine incompatibility. *J. Amer. med. Assoc.*, **186**, 1172.

Breckenridge, A. and Dollery, C. T. (1966): Methyldopa and bethanidine: evidence for a synergistic effect. *Lancet*, **1**, 1074.

Breckenridge, A. and Orme, M. (1971): Clinical significance of enzyme induction in man. *Ann. N. Y. Acad. Sci.*, **179**, 421.

Breckenridge, A. and Orme, M. (1971): Proc. Intern. Symp. Benzodiazepine, Milan, 1971. Raven Press, New York.

Breckenridge, A. and Orme, M. (1973): Proc. Symp. Plasma Concentrations of Drugs in Relation to their Biological Effects. Macmillan, p. 145.

Breckenridge, A., Orme, M., Thorgeirsson, S. S., Davies, D. S. and Brooks, R. V. (1971): Drug interactions with warfarin: studies with dichloralphenazone, chloral hydrate and antipyrine. *Clin. Sci.*, **40**, 351.

Briant, R. H., Reid, J. L. and Dollery, C. T. (1973): Interaction between clonidine and desipramine in man. *Brit. med. J.*, **1**, 522.

Brodie, B. B. (1965): Displacement of one drug by another from carrier or receptor sites. *Proc. roy. Soc. Med.*, **58**, 946.

Butcher, R. W. and Sutherland, E. W. (1962): Adenosine 3′5′-phosphate in biological materials. 1. Purification and properties of cyclic 3′5′-nucleotide phosphodiesterase and use of this enzyme to characterize adenosine 3′5′-phosphate in human urine. *J. biol. Chem.*, **237**, 1244.

Caldwell, J. H. and Greenberger, N. J. (1970): Cholestyramine enhances digitalis excretion and protects against lethal intoxication. *J. clin. Invest.*, **49**, 16a.

Capeller, D. V., Copeland, G. D. and Stern, T. N. (1959): Digitalis intoxication: a clinical report of 148 cases. *Ann. intern. Med.*, **50**, 869.

Carter, S. A. (1965): Potentiation of the effect of orally administered anticoagulants by phenyramidol hydrochloride. *New Engl. J. Med.*, **273**, 423.

Catalano, P. M. and Cullen, S. I. (1966): Warfarin antagonism by griseofulvin. *Clin. Res.*, **14**, 266.

Chamberlain, D. A. (1966): Effects of beta-adrenergic blockade on heart size. *Amer. J. Cardiol.*, **18**, 321.

Christensen, L. K. and Skovsted, L. (1969): Inhibition of drug metabolism by chloramphenicol. *Lancet*, **2**, 1397.

Cohen, A. B. (1966): Hyperkalaemic effects of triamterene. *Ann. intern. Med.*, **65**, 521.

Cohen, B. M. (1952), Digitalis poisoning and its treatment. *New Engl. J. Med.*, **246**, 225 and 254.

Conney, A. H. (1967): Pharmacological implications of enzyme induction. *Pharmacol. Rev.*, **19**, 317.

Corn, M. (1966): Effect of phenobarbital and glutethimide on biological half-life of warfarin. *Thromb. diathes. haemorrhag.* (Stuttgart), **16**, 606.

Corn, M. and Rocket, J. F. (1965): Inhibition of bishydroxycoumarin activity by phenobarbital. *Med. Ann., D. C.*, **34**, 578.

Coull, D. C., Crooks, J., Dingwall-Fordyce, I., Scott, A. M. and Weir, R. D. (1970): Amitriptyline and cardiac disease. Risk of sudden death identified by monitoring system. *Lancet*, **2**, 590.

Council on Drugs (1966): An antipruritic for primary biliary cirrhosis and cholestatic jaundice. *J. Amer. med. Assoc.*, **197**, 261.

Cranston, W. I., Juel-Jansen, B. E., Semmence, A. M., Handfield-Jones, R. P. C., Forbes, J. A. and Mutch, L. M. M. (1963): Effects of oral diuretics on raised arterial pressure. *Lancet*, **2** 966.

Cucinell, S. A., Odessky, L., Weiss, M. and Dayton, P. E. (1967): The effect of chloral hydrate on bishydroxycoumarin metabolism. *J. Amer. med. Assoc.*, **197**, 366.

Cunicell, S. A., Conney, A. H., Sansur, M. S. and Burns, J. J. (1965): Drug interactions in man. 1. Lowering effect of phenobarbital on plasma levels of bishydroxycoumarin (Dicumarol) and diphenylhydantion (Dilantin). *Clin. Pharmacol. Therap.*, **6**, 420.

Cullen, S. T. and Catalano, P. M. (1967): Griseofulvin–Warfarin antagonism. *J. Amer. med. Assoc.*, **199**, 582.

Cuthbert, M. F., Greenberg, M. P. and Morley, S. W. (1969): Cough and cold remedies, a potential danger to patients on monoamine oxidase inhibitors. *Brit. med. J.*, **1**, 404.

DeGraff, A. C. (1954): Digitalis Intoxication – clinical conference. *Circulation*, **9**, 115.

Diamond, M. A., Murray, R. H. and Schmid, P. (1969): Treatment of idiopathic postural hypotension with oral tyramine (Ty) and monoamine oxidase inhibitor (MI). *J. clin. Res.*, **17**, 237.

Dresdale, F. C. and Hayes, J. C. (1967): Potential dangers in the combined use of methandrostenolone and sodium warfarin. *J. Med. Soc. N. J.*, **64**, 609.

Editorial (1967): Propranolol. *Lancet*, **1**, 939.

Eisen, M. J. (1964): Combined effect of sodium warfarin and phenylbutazone. *J. Amer. med. Assoc.*, **189**, 64.

Evans-Prosser, C. D. G. (1968): The use of pethidine and morphine in the presence of monoamine oxidase inhibitors. *Brit. J. Anaesthes.*, **40**, 279.

Fisch, C., Martz, B. L. and Priebe, F. H. (1960): Enhancement of potassium-induced atrioventricular block by toxic doses of digitalis drugs. *J. clin. Invest.*, **39**, 1885.

Fisch, C., Steinmetz, E. F., Fasola, A. F. and Martz, B. L. (1959): Effect of potassium and "toxic" doses of digitalis on the myocardium. *Circulat. Res.*, **7**, 424.

Fontana, G., Addarii, F. and Peta, G. (1968): Su di un caso di coma ipoglicenico in corso di terapia con tolbutamide e dicumorolici. *Giornale di Clin. med.*, **49**, 849.

Fouts, J. R. and Brodie, B. B. (1956): On the mechanism of drug potentiation by iproniazid. *J. Pharmacol. exp. Therap.*, **116**, 480.

Fox, S. L. (1964): Potentiation of anticoagulants caused by pyrazole compounds. *J. Amer. med. Assoc.*, **188**, 320.

Frick, P. G., Riedler, G. and Brögh, H. (1967): Dose response and minimal daily requirements for vitamin K in man. *J. appl. Physiol.*, **23**, 387.

Garettson, L. K., Perel, J. P. and Dayton, P. G. (1967): Methylphenidate interactions with both anticonvulsants and ethyl biscoumacetate. *J. Amer. med. Assoc.*, **207**, 2053.

Gazzaniga, A. B. and Stewart, D. R. (1969): Possible quinidine-induced haemorrhage in a patient on warfarin sodium. *New Engl. J. Med.*, **280**, 711.

Gebhardt, W. and Blümchen, G. (1968): Haemodynamic effect of a combined therapy with propranolol and digoxin. *Cardiologia* (Basel), **52**, 190.

George, C. F., Fenyvesi, T. and Dollery, C. T. (1973): Pharmacological effects of propranolol in relationship to plasma levels. In: *Biological Effects of Drugs in Relation to their Plasma Concentrations.* Macmillan, London.

Gerkens, J. F., McCulloch, M. W. and Wilson, J. (1969): Mechanism of the antagonism between guanethidine and dexamphetamine. *Brit. J. Pharmacol.*, **35**, 563.

Gibson, D. and Sowton, E. (1969): The use of beta-adrenergic receptor blocking drugs in dysrhythmias. *Progr. cardiovasc. Dis.*, **12**, 16.

Gilmore, E., Weil, J. and Chidsey, J. C. (1970): Treatment of essential hypertension with a new vasodilator in combination with beta-adrenergic blockade. *New Engl. J. Med.*, **282**, 521.

Glick, G., Parmley, W. W., Wechsler, A. S. and Sonnenblick, E. H. (1968): Glucagon. Its enhancement of cardiac performance in the cat and dog and persistence of its inotropic action despite beta-receptor blockade with propranolol. *Circulat. Res.*, **22**, 789.

Goldberg, L. M., Bristow, J. D., Parker, B. M. and Ritzmann, L. W. (1960): Paroxysmal atrial tachycardia with atrio–ventricular block: its frequent association with chronic pulmonary disease. *Circulation*, **21**, 499.

Goss, J. E. and Dickhouse, D. W. (1965): Increased bishydroxycoumarin requirements in patients receiving phenobarb. *New Eng. J. Med.*, **273**, 1094.

Grilli, H. (1959): Glutethimide y tiempo de prothrombira su aplicación en la terapéutica anticoagulante. *Prensa med. argent.*, **46**, 2867.

Griner, P. F., Reisz, Z. G., Rickler, F. R., Weisner, P. J. and Odoroff, C. L. (1971): Chloral hydrate and warfarin interaction. Clinical significance? *Ann. intern. Med.*, **74**, 540.

Gubner, R. S. and Kallman, H. (1957): Treatment of digitalis toxicity by chelation of serum calcium. *Amer. J. med. Sci.*, **234**, 136.

Hamer, J. and Sowton, E. (1966): Effects of propranolol on exercise tolerance in angina pectoris. *Amer. J. Cardiol.*, **18**, 354.

Hansen, J. M., Kristensen, M., Skovsted, L. and Christensen, L. K. (1966): Dicoumarol-induced diphenyl hydantoin intoxication. *Lancet*, **2**, 265.

Hansen, J. M., Kristensen, M. and Skovsted, L. (1968): Sulthiame (Ospolot) as inhibitor of diphenylhydantoin metabolism. *Epilepsia*, **9**, 17.

Harrison, D. C. and Griffin, J. R. (1967): The antiarrhythmic effects of propranolol. *Ann. N. Y. Acad. Sci.*, **139**, 997.

Hillestadt, L. and Storstein, O. (1969): Conversion of chronic atrial fibrillation to sinus rhythm with combined propranolol and quinidine treatment. *Amer. Heart J.*, **77**, 137.

Hobbs, C. B., Miller, A. L. and Thornley, J. H. (1965): Potentiation of anticoagulant therapy by oxyphenbutazone. *Postgrad. med. J.*, **41**, 563.

Hoffbrand, B. I. and Kininmonth, D. A. (1967): Potentiation of anticoagulants. *Brit. med. J.*, **2**, 838.

Hooglard, D. R., Miya, T. S. and Bousquet, W. F. (1966): Metabolism and tolerance studies with chlordiazepoxide-2-^{14}C in the rat. *Toxicol. appl. Pharmacol.*, **9**, 116.

Horwitz, D., Lovenberg, W., Engelman, K. and Sjoerdsma, A. (1964): Monoamine oxidase inhibitors, tyramine and cheese. *J. Amer. med. Assoc.*, **188**, 1108.

Howard, R. P., Alaupovic, P., Brusco, O. J. and Furmar, R. H. (1963): Effects of ethyl chlorophenoxy isobutyrate, alone or with andosterone (Atromid) on serum lipids, lipoproteins and related metabolic parameters in normal and hyperlipidaemic subjects. *J. Atherosclerosis Res.*, **3**, 482.

Hucker, H. B., Zacchei, A. G., Cox, S. V., Brodie, D. A. and Cantwell, N. H. R. (1966): Studies on the absorption, distribution and excretion of Indomethacin in various species. *J. Pharmacol. exp. Therap.*, **153**, 237.

Hunningbake, D. B. (1970): Studies of the inhibition of drug metabolism by methylphenidate. *Federation Proc.*, **29**, 345.

Hunningbake, D. B. and Azarnoff, D. L. (1968): Drug interactions with warfarin. *Arch. intern. med.*, **121**, 349.

Hurwitz, N. and Wade, O. L. (1969): Intensive hospital monitoring of adverse reactions to drugs. *Brit. med. J.*, **1**, 531.

Ikram, H. and Nixon, P. G. F. (1966): Propranolol in myocardial infarction. *Lancet*, **2**, 1134.

Iversen, L. L. (1967): The uptake and storage of Noradrenaline in sympathetic nerves. Cambridge University Press, London.

Jarrum, S. (1954): Cinchophen and acetylsalicylic acid in anticoagulant treatment. *Scand. J. clin. Lab. Invest.*, **6**, 91.

Johansson, S. A. (1968): Apparent response to oral anticoagulant therapy and influence of hypnotics on some coagulation factors. *Acta med. Scand.*, **184**, 297.

Johnstone, M. (1953): Adrenaline and noradrenaline during anaesthesia. *Anaesthesia*, **8**, 32.

Kater, R. M. H., Roggin, T., Tobin, F., Zieve, P. and Iber, F. L. (1969): Increased rate of clearance of drugs from the circulation of alcoholics. *Amer. J. med. Sci.*, **258**, 35.

Katz, R. L. and Epstein, R. A. (1968): The interaction of anaesthetic agents and adrenergic drugs to produce cardiac arrhythmias. *Anesthesiology*, **29**, 763.

Katz, R. L. and Katz, G. J. (1966): Surgical infiltration of pressor drugs and their interaction with volatile anaesthetics. *Brit. J. Anaesthesia*, **38**, 712.

Kirboe, E. (1966): Phenytoin intoxication during treatment with Antabuse (disulfiram). *Epilepsia*, **7**, 246.

Koch-Weser, J. (1968): Quinidine-induced hypoprothrombinaemic haemorrhage in patients on chronic warfarin therapy. *Ann. intern. Med.*, **68**, 511.

Koch-Weser, J. (1971): Chloral hydrate and warfarin therapy. *Ann. intern. Med.*, **75**, 141.

Kotler, M. N., Berman, L., and Rubenstein, A. H. (1966): Hypoglycaemia precipitated by propranolol. *Lancet*, **2**, 1389.

Kristensen, M. and Hansen, J. M. (1967): Potentiation of the tolbutamide effect by dicoumarol. *Diabetes*, **16**, 211.

Kristensen, M. and Hansen, J. M. (1968): Accumulation of chlorpropamide caused by dicoumarol. *Acta med. Scand.*, **183**, 83.

Kurin, C. M. and Finland, M. (1961): Clinical pharmacology of the tetracycline antibiotics. *Clin. Pharmacol. Therap.*, **2**, 51.

Lackner, H. and Hunt, V. E. (1968): The effect of Librium on hemostasis. *Amer. J. med. Sci.*, **256**, 368.

Lang, T. W., Bernstein, H., Barbieri, F., Gold, H. and Corday, E. (1965): Digitalis toxicity. Treatment with diphenylhydantoin. *Arch. intern. Med.*, **116**, 573.

Lasagna, L. (1965): Drug toxicity in man – the problem and the challenge. *Ann. N. Y. Acad. Sci.*, **123**, 312.

Leishman, A. W., Matthews, H. L. and Smith, A. J. (1959): Guanethidine. Hypotensive drug with prolonged action. *Lancet*, **2**, 1044.

Leishman, A. W., Matthews, H. L. and Smith, A. J. (1963): Antagonism of guanethidine by imipramine. *Lancet*, **1**, 112.

Levy, G., O'Reilly, R. A., Aggeler, P. M. and Keech, G. M. (1970); Pharmacokinetic analysis of the effect of barbiturate on the anticoagulant action of warfarin in man. *Clin. Pharmacol. Therap.*, **11**, 372.

Lindholmer, B., Nyman, E. and Raf, L. (1964): Nonspecific stenosing ulceration of the small bowel. A preliminary report. *Acta Chir. Scand.*, **128**, 310.

Lown, B., Black, H., and Moore, F. D. (1960): Digitalis, electrolytes and the surgical patient. *Amer. J. Cardiol.*, **6**, 309.

Lown, B., Ehrlich, L., Lipschultz, B. and Blake, J. (1961): Effect of digitalis in patients receiving reserpine. *Circulation*, **24**, 1185.

Lucchesi, B. R. (1968): Cardiac actions of glucagon. *Circulation Res.*, **22**, 777.

MacDonald, M. G., Robinson, D. S., Sylwester, D., and Jaffe, J. J. (1969): Effects of phenobarbitone, chloral betaine and glutethimide administration on warfarin plasma levels and hypoprothrombinaemic responses in man. *Clin. Pharmacol. Therap.*, **10**, 80.

Magid, E. (1962): Tolerance to anticoagulants during antibiotic therapy. *Scand. J. clin. lab. Invest.*, **14**, 565.

Marshall, L. J. and Green, V. A. (1968): Propranolol and diazepam for imipramine poisoning. *Lancet*, **2**, 1249.

Mason, D. T. and Braunwald, E. (1965): Effects of nitroglycerin and amyl nitrite on arteriolar and venous tone in the human forearm. *Circulation*, **32**, 755.

Meek, W. J., Hathaway, H. R. and Orth, O. S. (1937): The effects of ether, chloroform and cyclopropane on cardiac automaticity. *J. Pharmacol. exp. Therap.*, **61**, 240.

Messinger, W. J. and Samet, C. M. (1965): The effect of a bowel sterilizing antibiotic on blood coagulation mechanisms: the anti cholesterol effect of paromomycin. *Angiology*, **16**, 29.

Meyer, J. F., McAllister, C. K. and Goldberg, L. I. (1970): Insidious and prolonged antagonism of guanethidine by amitriptyline. *J. Amer. med. Assoc.*, **213**, 1487.

Mitchell, J. R., Cavanaugh, J. H., Arias, A. and Oates, J. A. (1970): Guanethidine and related agent. III. Antagonism by drugs which inhibit the norepinephrine pump in man. *J. clin. Invest.*, **49**, 1596.

Moe, G. K., Malton, S. D., Rennick, B. R. and Freyburger, W. A. (1948): The role of arterial pressure in the induction of idioventricular rhythm under cyclopropane anaesthesia. *J. Pharmacol. exp. Therap.*, **94**, 319.

Mosey, L. and Tyler, M. D. (1954): The effect of diphenyl hydantoin sodium (Dilantin), procaine hydrochloride, procaine amide hydrochloride, and quinidine hydrochloride on ouabain-induced ventricular tachycardia in unanaesthetised dogs. *Circulation*, **10**, 65.

Murakami, M., Odake, K., Matsuda, T., Onchi, K., Umeda, T. and Nishino, T. (1965): Effects of anabolic steroids on anticoagulant requirements. *Jap. Circulat. J.*, **29**, 243.

Nagashima, R., O'Reilly, R. A. and Levy, G. (1969): Kinetics of the pharmacologic effects in man; the anticoagulant action of warfarin. *Clin. Pharmacol. Therap.*, **10**, 22.

Noegeli, T. and Matis, P. (1958): Die Bedeutung zusatzlicher exogene Faktoren bei der therapeutischen Gerinnungshemmung. *Langenbecks Arch. klin. Chirur.*, **288**, 36.

Nordy, S. (1959): Combined treatment with phenylbutazone and anticoagulants. *T. den Norske Laegefor.*, **79**, 143.

Nuessle, W. F., Norman, F. C. and Miller, H. E. (1965): Pickled herring and tranylcypromine reaction. *J. Amer. med. Assoc.*, **192**, 726.

Oakley, D. P. and Lautch, H. (1963): Haloperidol and anticoagulant treatment. *Lancet*, **2**, 1231.

O'Brien, J. R. (1968): The effect of salicylates on human platelets. *Lancet*, **1**, 779.

Oliver, M. F., Roberts, S. D., Hayes, D., Pantridge, J. F., Suzaan, M. M. and Bersohn, I. (1963): Effect of atromid and ethyl chlorophenoxy isobutyrate on anticoagulant requirements. *Lancet*, **1**, 143.

Ominsky, A. J. and Wollman, H. (1969): Hazards of general anaesthesia in the reserpinized patient. *Anesthesiology*, **30**, 443.

O'Reilly, R. A. and Aggeler, P. M. (1969): Effect of barbiturates on oral anticoagulants in man. *Clin. Res.*, **17**, 153.

O'Reilly, R. A. and Aggeler, P. M. (1968): Phenylbutazone potentiation of anticoagulant effect: fluorometric assay of warfarin. *Proc. Soc. exp. Biol. Med.*, **128**, 1080.

O'Reilly, R. A., Aggeler, P. M. and Leong, L. S. (1963): Studies on the coumarin anticoagulant drugs: the pharmacodynamics of warfarin in man. *J. clin. Invest.*, **42**, 1542.

Orth, O. S., Leigh, M. D., Mellish, C. H. and Stutzman, J. W. (1939): Action of sympathomimetic amines in cyclopropane, ether and chloroform anaesthesia. *J. Pharmacol. exp. Therap.*, **67**, 1.

Owens, J. C., Nealy, W. B. and Owen, W. R. (1962): Effect of sodium dextrothyroxine in patients receiving anticoagulants. *New Engl. J. Med.*, **266**, 76.

Page, E. and Real, J. D. (1955): Interrelationships between cardiac effects of ouabain, hypocalcaemia and hyperkalaemia. *Circulat. Res.*, **3**, 501.

Paterson, J. W., Dollery, C. T. and Haslam, R. M. (1968): Amiloride hydrochloride in hypertensive patients. *Brit. med. J.*, **1**, 422.

Pirk, L. A. and Engleberg, R. (1945): Hypoprothrombinaemic action of quinine sulphate. *J. Amer. med. Assoc.*, **128**, 1093.

Poller, L., Thomson, J. M., Tabiowo, A. and Priest, C. M. (1969): Progesterone oral contraception and blood coagulation. *Brit. med. J.*, **1**, 554.

Price, H. L., Lurie, A. A., Jones, R. E., Price, M. L. and Linde, H. W. (1958): Cyclopropane anaesthesia. II. Epinephrine and norepinephrine in initiation of ventricular arrhythmias by carbon dioxide inhalation. *Anesthesiology*, **19**, 619.

Pyorola, K. and Kekki, M. (1963): Decreased anticoagulant tolerance during methandrostenolone therapy. *Scand. J. clin. Lab. Invest.*, **15**, 367.

Pyorola, K., Myllyla, G. and Kekki, M. (1965): Metabolism of warfarin during methandrostenolone treatment. *Ann. Med. exp. Biol. Fenn.*, **43**, 95.

Pyorola, K., Ristola, P. and Myllyla, G. (1968): Warfarin metabolism during ethyl chlorphenoxy isobutyrate treatment. *Ann. Med. intern. Fenn.*, **57**, 157.

Reid, N. C. R. W. and Jones, D. (1962): Pethidine and phenelzine. *Brit. med. J.*, **1**, 408.

Reveno, W. S. and Rosenbaum, H. (1968): Propranolol hypoglycaemia. *Lancet*, **1**, 920.

Reverchon, R. and Sapir, M. (1961): Clinical verification of an antagonism between barbiturates and anticoagulants. *Presse med.*, **69** 1570.

Roberts, S. J. and Pantridge, J. F. (1963): Effect of Atromid on requirements of warfarin. *J. Atheroscl. Res.*, **3**, 671.

Robinson, D. S., Benjamin, D. M. and McCormack, J. J. (1971): Interaction of warfarin and nonsystemic gastrointestinal drugs. *Clin. Pharmacol. Therap.*, **12**, 491.

Robinson, D. S. and MacDonald, M. G. (1966): The effect of phenobarbital administration on the control of coagulation achieved during warfarin therapy in man. *J. Pharmacol. exper. Therap.*, **153**, 250.

Robinson, D. S. and Sylwester, D. (1970): Interaction of commonly prescribed drugs and warfarin. *Ann. intern. Med.*, **72**, 853.

Rodensky, P. L. and Wasserman, F. (1964): The possible role of sex in digitalis tolerance. *Amer. Heart J.*, **68**, 325.

Rosenbaum, J. L., Mason, D. and Seven, M. J. (1960): The effect of disodium EDTA on digitalis intoxication. *Amer. J. med. Sci.*, **240**, 77.

Rothstein, E. (1968): Warfarin effect enhanced by disulfiram. *J. Amer. med. Assoc.*, **206**, 1574.

Russek, H. I. (1967): Propranolol and isosorbide dinitrate synergism in angina pectoris. *Amer. J. med. Sci.*, **254**, 406.

Russek, H. I. (1968): Propranolol and isosorbide dinitrate synergism in angina pectoris. *Amer. J. Cardiol.* **21**, 44.

Sarawicz, B. (1971): Current status of digitalis in therapeutics. In: *Cardiovascular Therapy*. Editors: H. I. Russek and B. C. Zohlman. The William and Wilkins Co., Baltimore.

Scherlag, B. J., Helfant, R. H. and Damato, A. N. (1968): The contrasting effects of diphenylhydantoin and procainamide on A–V conduction in the digitalis-intoxicated and the normal heart. *Amer. Heart J.*, **75**, 200.

Schrogie, J. J. and Solomon, H. M. (1967): The anticoagulant response to bishydroxy coumarin. II. The effect of D-thyroxine, clofibrate and norethandrelone. *Clin. Pharmacol. Therap.*, **8**, 70.

Schrogie, J. J., Solomon, H. M. and Zieve, P. D. (1967): Effect of oral contraceptives on vitamin K-dependent clotting activity. *Clin. Pharmacol. Therap.*, **8**, 670.

Seiler, K. and Duckert, F. (1968): Properties of 3-(1-phenylpropyl)-4-oxycoumarin (marcoumarine) in the plasma when tested in normal cases and under the influence of drugs. *Thromb. Diathes. Haemorrh.* (Stuttgart), **19**, 389.

Sellers, E. M. and Koch-Weser, J. (1970a): Potentiation of warfarin induced hypoprothrombinaemia by chloral hydrate. *New Engl. J. Med.*, **283**, 827.

Sellers, E. M. and Koch-Weser, J. (1970b): Displacement of warfarin from human albumin by diazoxide and ethacrynic, mefenamic and nalidixic acids. *Clin. Pharmacol. Therap.*, **11**, 524.

Sellers, E. M. and Koch-Weser, J. (1971): Kinetics and clinical importance of displacement of warfarin from albumin by acidic drugs. *Ann. N. Y. Acad. Sci*, **179**, 213.

Side effects of drugs, Vol. VII (1968): Editors: L. Meyler and A. Herxheimer. Excerpta Medica, Amsterdam.

Sjöqvist, F. (1965): Psychotropic drugs (2). Interaction between monoamine oxidase (MAO) inhibitors and other drugs. *Proc. roy. Soc. Med.*, **58**, 967.

Skinner, C., Coull, D. C. and Johnston, A. W. (1969): Antagonism of the hypotensive action of bethanidine and debrisoquine by tricyclic antidepressants. *Lancet*, **2**, 564.

Smith, J. W., Seidl, L. G. and Cluff, L. E. (1966): Studies on the epidemiology of adverse drug reactions. *Ann. intern. Med.*, **65**, 629.

Sodeman, W. A. (1965): Current concept – diagnosis and treatment of digitalis toxicity. *New Engl. J. Med.*, **273**, 35.

Solomon, H. M. and Abrams, W. B. (1972): Interactions between digitoxin and other drugs in man. *Amer. Heart J.*, **83**, 277.

Solomon, H. M., Barakat, M. J. and Ashley, C. J. (in press): Failure of diazepam and chlordiazopoxide to influence the response to warfarin in man. *J. Amer. med. Assoc.*

Solomon, H. M., Reich, S., Spirt, N. and Abrams, W. B. (1971): Interactions between digitoxin and other drugs in vitro and in vivo. In: *Drug metabolism in man. Ann. N. Y. Acad. Sci.*, **179**, 338.

Solomon, H. M. and Schrogie, J. J. (1966): Effect of phenyramidol on metabolising bishydroxycoumarin. *J. Pharmacol. exp. Therap.*, **154**, 660.

Solomon, H. M. and Schrogie, J. J. (1967a): Effect of phenyramidol and bishydroxycoumarin on the metabolism of tolbutamide in human subjects. *Metabolism*, **16**, 1029.

Solomon, H. M. and Schrogie, J. J. (1967b): Change in receptor site affinity: a proposed explanation for the potentiating effect of D-thyroxine on the anticoagulant response to warfarin. *Clin. Pharmacol. Therap.*, **8**, 797.

Solomon, H. M. and Schrogie, J. J. (1967c): The effect of various drugs on the binding of ^{14}C warfarin to human albumin. *Biochem. Pharmacol.*, **16**, 1219.

Solomon, H. M., Schrogie, J. J. and Williams, D. (1968): The displacement of phenylbutazone-^{14}C and warfarin-^{14}C from human albumin by various drugs and fatty acids. *Biochem. Pharmacol.*, **17**, 143.

Sonnenblick, E. H., Ross, J., Covell, J. W., Kaiser, G. A. and Braunwald, E. (1965): Velocity of contraction as a determinant of myocardial oxygen consumption. *Amer. J. Physiol.*, **209**, 919.

Spann, J. F., Sonnenblick, E. H., Cooper, T., Chidsey, C. A., Willman, V. L. and Braunwald, E. (1966): Studies on digitalis XIV. Influence of cardiac norepinephrine stores on the response of isolated heart muscle to digitalis. *Circulat. Res.*, **19**, 326.

Stannard, M., Sloman, G. and Sangster, L. (1968): The haemodynamic effects of atropine combined with propranolol in acute myocardial infarction. *Med. J. Aust.*, **1**, 333.

Starr, K. J. and Petrie, J. C. (1972): Drug interactions in patients on long term oral anticoagulant and antihypertensive adrenergic neurone-blocking drugs. *Brit. med. J.*, **4**, 133.

Stephen, S. A. (1966): Unwanted effects of propranolol. *Amer. J. Cardiol.*, **18**, 463.

Stern, S. (1967): Conversion of chronic atrial fibrillation to sinus rhythm with combined propranolol and quinidine treatment. *Amer. Heart J.*, **74**, 170.

Stern, S. (1971): Haemodynamic changes following separate and combined administration of beta-blocking drugs and quinidine. *Europ. J. clin. Invest.*, **1**, 432.

Szekely, P. and Wynne, N. A. (1963): Effects of calcium chelation on digitalis-induced cardiac arrhythmias. *Brit. Heart J.*, **25**, 589.

Taylor, G. J., Harris, W. S. and Bogdonoff, M. D. (1971): Ventricular arrhythmias induced in monkeys by the inhalation of aerosol propellants. *J. clin. Invest.*, **50**, 1546.

Turner, J. R. B. (1966): Propranolol in the treatment of digitalis induced and digitalis-resistant tachycardias. *Amer. J. Cardiol.*, **18**, 450.

Udall, J. A. (1969a): Drug interference with warfarin. *Amer. J. Cardiol.*, **23**, 143.

Udall, J. A. (1969b): Drug interference with warfarin therapy. *Clin. Res.*, **17**, 104.

Udall, J. A. (1970a): Warfarin therapy not influenced by meprobromate. A controlled study in nine men. *Curr. Therap. Res.*, **12**, 724.

Udall, J. A. (1970b): Drug interference with warfarin therapy. *Clin. Med.*, **77**, 20.

Van Dam, F. E. and Gribnau-Overkamp, M. J. H. (1967): The effect of some sedatives (phenobarbital, glutethimide, chlordiazepoxide, chloral hydrate) on the rate of disappearance of ethyl biscoumacetate from the plasma. *Folia med. neerland.*, **10**, 141.

Van Dam, F. E., Overkamp, M. and Haanen, C. (1966): The interaction of drugs. *Lancet*, **2**, 1027.

Vaughan Williams, E. M. and Sekeija, A. (1963): Prevention of arrhythmias due to cardiac glycosides by block of sympathetic beta receptors. *Lancet*, **1**, 420.

Verstraete, M., Vermylen, J. and Claeys, H. (1968): Dissimilar effect of two antianginal drugs belonging to the benzofuran group on the action of coumarin derivatives. *Arch. intern. Pharmacodynam.*, **176**, 33.

Vessell, E. S., Passananti, T. and Greene, F. E. (1970): Impairment of drug metabolism in man by Allopurinol and Nortriptyline. *New Engl. J. Med.*, **283**, 1484.

Veterans Administration Cooperative Study Group on Antihypertensive Agents (1967): Effects of treatment on morbidity in hypertension. *J. Amer. med. Assoc.*, **202**, 1028.

Visioli, O. and Bertaccini, G. (1968): Combined propranolol and quinidine treatment in cardiac arrhythmias. *Amer. Heart J.*, **75**, 719.

Watt, D. A. L. (1968): Sensitivity to propranolol after digoxin intoxication. *Brit. med. J.*, **3**, 413.

Weiner, M., Siddiqui, A. A., Bostanci, N. and Dayton, P. G. (1965): Drug interaction – the effect of combined administration on the half-life of coumarin and pyrazolone drugs in man. *Federation Proc.*, **24**, 153.

Weis, H. J. and Aledort, L. M. (1967): Impaired platelet-connective tissue reaction in man after aspirin ingestion. *Lancet*, **2**, 495.

Williams, J. F., Glick, G. and Braunwald, E. (1965): Studies on cardiac dimensions in intact unanesthetised man. *Circulation*, **32**, 767.

Wilson, I. M. and Freis, E. D. (1959): Relationship between plasma and extracellular fluid volume depletion and the antihypertensive effect of chlorothiazide. *Circulation*, **20**, 1028.

Winters, W. L. and Soloff, L. A. (1962): Observations on sodium D-thyroxine as a hypocholesterolaemic agent in persons with hypercholesterolaemia with and without ischeamic heart disease. *Amer. J. med. Sci.*, **243**, 458.

Wright, I. S., Bourgain, R. H., Foley, W. T., McDevitt, E., Grass, C., Burke, G., Simon, E., Liebermann, J., Symons, C. and Huebrer, R. (1954): Long term anticoagulant therapy. *Circulation*, **9**, 748.

CHAPTER 8

Drug interactions in respiratory disease

K. N. V. PALMER AND J. W. PATERSON

1 Introduction

Drug combinations are deliberately used in respiratory medicine to increase or potentiate a therapeutic response, for example atropine may be added to isoprenaline to prolong its bronchodilator effect. On the other hand, additional drugs prescribed for coincident disease may result in dangerous interactions, for example tricyclic antidepressants greatly increase the cardiovascular response to adrenaline.

Drugs are used in respiratory medicine with 3 main objects:

(1) Reduction in airways obstruction;
(2) Stimulation of respiration;
(3) Easing of expectoration.

The treatment of pulmonary infection is dealt with elsewhere.

2 Reduction in airways obstruction

2.1 GENERAL

Diffuse airway obstruction occurs mainly in bronchial asthma and chronic obstructive bronchitis. The major changes are bronchoconstriction, swelling and oedema of the bronchial mucous membrane, changes in sputum properties and sputum retention. In addition bronchial narrowing occurs because of fibrotic changes in the airway walls secondary to chronic infection, and loss of elastic retraction of the peripheral airways caused by emphysema. Bronchoconstriction and vascular changes may result from the release of chemical mediators from mast cells in the lung. The multiple factors involved in causing airway obstruction mean that drug interaction can be used to advantage in its treatment. Thus a bronchodilator might be combined with an antiinflammatory agent such as as a corticosteroid, and disodium cromoglycate which prevents the release of bronchoconstrictor compounds.

Although bronchoconstriction is not the only cause of airway obstruction, the control of bronchial muscle tone provides a basis for understanding drug interactions. The tone of bronchial smooth muscle is modified by the autonomic nervous system and humoral factors.

2.2 AUTONOMIC NERVOUS SYSTEM

The parasympathetic nervous system causes bronchoconstriction, and the sympathetic nervous system bronchodilatation. The parasympathetic nervous system releases acetylcholine at its nerve endings in the bronchial smooth muscle. This transmitter combines with cholinergic receptors to produce bronchoconstriction (Fig. 1). Bronchoconstriction may be prevented by atropine. The sympathetic nervous system opposes the parasympathetic and produces bronchodilatation. Noradrenaline is released at sympathetic nerve endings, and adrenaline circulates from the adrenal medulla. Both combine with adrenergic receptors in the bronchial smooth muscle.

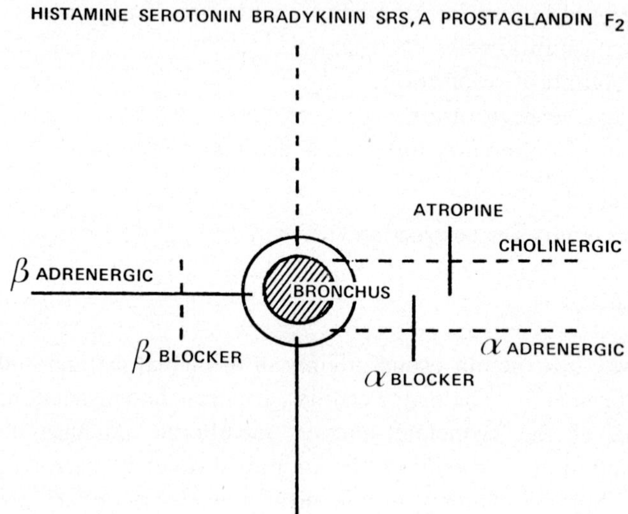

Fig. 1. Factors affecting bronchial tone.

TABLE I

Adrenergic receptors

Alpha	$Beta_1$	$Beta_2$
Vasoconstriction	Heart	Bronchodilatation
Arteries	Chronotropic	Vasodilatation
Veins	Inotropic	Arteries
Bronchoconstriction		Veins
Enhancement of histamine release		Inhibition of histamine release
		Skeletal muscle tremor

Ahlquist in 1948 first proposed a sub-classification of adrenergic receptors into alpha and beta. The bronchodilator receptors in bronchial smooth muscle are β-receptors. More recently, the β-receptors have been sub-divided into β_1 and β_2 (Lands et al., 1967). The results of stimulating these adrenergic receptor systems in man are shown in Table I. Stimulation of β_2-receptors causes bronchodilatation and vasodilatation in the systemic and pulmonary circulation. Stimulation of β_1-receptors leads to a rise in heart rate, cardiac output, and pulmonary blood flow. This is important clinically because an increase in pulmonary blood flow in patients with ventilation perfusion imbalance in the lung may increase this imbalance, and therefore reduce arterial oxygen tension. Drugs with selective β_2-stimulant properties may also increase cardiac output in man at doses higher than required for bronchodilatation by causing an increase in central blood volume through peripheral vasodilatation (Gibson and Coltart, 1971). Even in therapeutic dosage they may cause pulmonary vasodilatation. Thus even drugs with less effect on cardiac receptors may cause an increase in pulmonary blood flow.

There is now substantial evidence that there are also α-adrenergic receptors in human bronchial muscle (Simonsson et al., 1970; Bianco et al., 1972; Gaddie et al., 1972b). Thus it seems that the autonomic control of bronchial tone reflects a balance between cholinergic receptors and α- and β-adrenergic receptors. Normally the α-receptors have a very minor role. In pulmonary disease however, there may be a disturbance of the balance between α- and β-adrenergic receptors and cholinergic receptors, leading to bronchoconstriction.

It has been suggested that the effects of adrenergic receptors may be mediated by 3′,5′-cyclic adenosine monophosphate (AMP) (Robison et al., 1967; Leading Article, 1970). Adenyl cyclase in the presence of magnesium catalyses the conversion of adenosine triphosphate (ATP) to the highly active molecule adenosine 3′,5′-cyclic monophosphate (3′,5′-cyclic AMP, Fig. 2). 3′,5′-Cyclic AMP is gradually broken down to the biologically

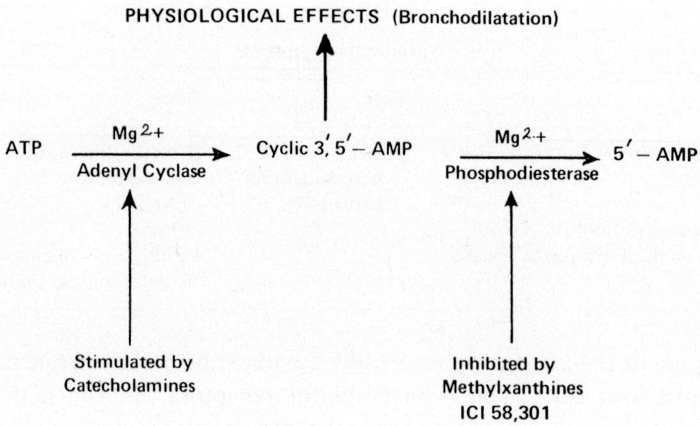

Fig. 2. Factors controlling cyclic AMP levels.

inactive 5′-AMP. This is catalysed by the enzyme phosphodiesterase. The breakdown of cyclic 3′,5′-AMP is inhibited by the methyl xanthine group of drugs, and in particular theophylline (Fig. 2). It is thought that β-stimulation increases adenyl cyclase activity and thus intracellular cyclic AMP levels, and that α-stimulation has the reverse effect. It can be seen how methylxanthines could interact with β-stimulants in the treatment of airway obstruction. Recently it has been suggested that the release of chemical mediators of bronchoconstriction from mast cells in the lung is also affected by the adrenergic system. Thus β-stimulant drugs increase the level of cyclic 3′,5′-AMP and inhibit the release of substances such as histamine and SRS-A which cause bronchoconstriction, whereas α-stimulation reduces the levels of cyclic 3′,5′-AMP and increases the release of bronchoconstrictors (Lichtenstein and Bourne, 1971; Orange and Austen, 1971).

2.3 HUMORAL FACTORS

The various humoral mediators of importance in controlling bronchomotor tone and vascular permeability in the lung have been reviewed recently (Brocklehurst, 1971; Vane, 1971a). Histamine produces bronchoconstriction and also increases vascular permeability and secretions. It is known that asthmatics are abnormally sensitive to this substance. Bradykinin causes bronchoconstriction and an increase in vascular permeability and bronchial secretions. Slow reacting substance of anaphylaxis (SRS-A) has been shown to cause bronchconstriction. 5-Hydroxytryptamine also causes an increase in bronchial muscle tone. The prostaglandins are naturally occurring fatty acids which are widely distributed in the body. Prostaglandins E_1 and E_2 are bronchodilator. Prostaglandin $F_{2\alpha}$ is a powerful bronchoconstrictor (Sweatman and Collier, 1968; Horton, 1969). In man inhaled prostaglandin E_1 is a more powerful bronchodilator weight for weight than isoprenaline (Cuthbert, 1969). The bronchodilator effect of prostaglandin E_1 is not reduced by β-adrenergic receptor blocking drugs, whereas the bronchodilator action of isoprenaline is (Large et al., 1969). Horton (1969) has outlined the possible ways in which prostaglandins could influence airway obstruction. It is possible that there could be overproduction of the bronchoconstrictor $F_{2\alpha}$ at the expense of the E series, or that bronchial smooth muscle could be over sensitive to the bronchoconstrictor prostaglandins. The metabolism of $F_{2\alpha}$ might be abnormal, or prostaglandin E could be converted to prostaglandin F in the abnormal lung. At present there is no evidence that there is any difference in how prostaglandins are handled or that the balance between the E and F series is any different between asthmatic and normal subjects. If such differences were found, a possible approach to therapy would be to alter the balance of the different prostaglandins. Intravenous prostaglandins are currently widely used to induce labour or therapeutic abortion. Smith (1973) has reported the effects of intravenous prostaglandin $F_{2\alpha}$ and E_2 on lung resistance in normal subjects. These patients were receiving the compounds for termination of pregnancy. A small but significant elevation in lung resistance which was reversible occurred following both prostaglandin $F_{2\alpha}$ and prostaglandin E_2. Bronchoconstriction following prostaglandin E_2 was an unexpected finding. The use of prostaglandins for termination of pregnancy may therefore represent a serious hazard in asthmatic patients.

It has already been mentioned that asthmatics are hypersensitive to drugs stimulating cholinergic receptors. Eye drops containing parasympathomimetics such as carbachol or anticholinesterase agents such as prostigmine are used in the treatment of glaucoma. When these eye drops are used, sufficient may be inhaled via the nose to cause an asthmatic attack in an asthmatic patient, and therefore such preparations should be used with caution.

Atropine and other anticholinergic drugs have an important diagnostic and therapeutic value in patients with airway obstruction. Altounyan (1966) showed that allergic asthmatic and non-allergic obstructive bronchitic airway obstruction reacted differently to atropine. In bronchial asthma atropine did not increase the FEV_1 as much as isoprenaline did, whereas in patients with non-allergic airway obstruction there was a good response to atropine, and not much additional response after isoprenaline. The patients who showed a poor response to atropine usually improved greatly with corticosteroid drugs. Clinical improvement in cases responding to corticosteroids was often accompanied by an increase in the response to atropine. Confirmation of Altounyan's findings has come from Crompton (1968) and Alliott et al. (1972). In both these studies the FEV_1 increase in obstructive bronchitics was much greater with atropine than it was with adrenaline. In Crompton's study the patients showing a good response to atropine did not respond to corticosteroids, whereas those showing a small response to atropine as compared to adrenaline showed a good response to corticosteroids. Atropine and related drugs appear to be less effective than β-stimulants in the treatment of airways obstruction responsive to steroids. Following successful treatment with steroids the atropine response increases, and Altounyan (1966) suggested it could indicate a suitable maintenance dose of corticosteroid. Thus the response to atropine is similar in both groups when the asthmatics are in remission. In an exacerbation of asthma a different mechanism of airway obstruction occurs resistant to atropine but sensitive to corticosteroids.

It is important to realise that patients presenting with airways obstruction late in life may be thought to have obstructive bronchitis when in fact they are suffering from asthma, and will therefore gain considerable benefit from treatment with corticosteroids, and here the atropine test may be useful.

An additional use of atropine is in combination with short-acting β-stimulant drugs such as isoprenaline. Chamberlain et al. (1962) showed that if isoprenaline and atropine were mixed in the same aerosol, then the bronchodilator effect of isoprenaline was prolonged. Although deptropine, another anti-cholinergic drug has little effect on airway obstruction in asthma given orally, when given by inhalation in combination with isoprenaline in general it potentiated and prolonged the effect of the isoprenaline. Nevertheless one asthmatic developed severe asthma after the inhalation of isoprenaline combined with deptropine citrate. Thus combinations of drugs may lead to a paradoxical increase in airway resistance in susceptible patients (Kennedy, 1965).

Mixtures of atropine and a sympathomimetic are no longer indicated purely for an increased duration of action, as the newer drugs orciprenaline, salbutamol and isoetharine have a much longer duration of effect. The response to atropine in asthma responding to steroids is small, and therefore it is not used often in the management of airways obstruction.

2.4 DRUGS AFFECTING ADRENERGIC RECEPTORS

For many years asthma was treated mainly with adrenaline or ephedrine. These drugs are relatively non-specific, with effects on both α- and β-adrenergic receptors. In view of recent work suggesting the presence of bronchoconstrictor α-receptors in bronchial smooth muscle, and in addition the effects of α-stimulation on histamine release, it is probable that the use of drugs with an α-effect may have more disadvantages than advantages. The most commonly used β-stimulant drug until recently was isoprenaline. This is a powerful stimulant of β_1- and β_2-receptors, and thus has a powerful effect on the heart as well as on the bronchial smooth muscle. The duration of action of adrenaline is dependent on uptake 1, that is uptake into sympathetic nerve endings, and in addition circulating adrenaline will be taken up into other tissues such as vascular smooth muscle, uptake 2 (Iversen, 1971). Following uptake the adrenaline may be metabolised by monoamine oxidase and catechol-*o*-methyltransferase. Isoprenaline is rapidly removed from the circulation by uptake 2 and is metabolised by catechol-*o*-methyltransferase, and after oral administration is conjugated to an ethereal sulphate (Davies et al., 1969; Paterson and Conolly, 1970).

Tricyclic antidepressants such as protriptyline block uptake into sympathetic nerve endings, and cause marked potentiation of the cardiovascular effects of noradrenaline and adrenaline in man (Svedmyr, 1968). Thus in patients receiving tricyclic antidepressants, drugs such as adrenaline must be given with extreme caution. In contrast patients taking monoamine oxidase inhibitors (MAOI) are not at great risk from infusion of adrenaline or isoprenaline (Barar et al., 1971) as the pharmacological effects are rapidly terminated by the uptake process and not by the action of the enzyme MAO. Cuthbert and Vere (1971) found however that cardiac stimulation from injections of adrenaline and isoprenaline were potentiated after the MAOI tranylcypromine, and so one should be cautious with any sympathomimetic in a patient receiving MAOIs.

Following MAOIs there is loss of MAO in the gastrointestinal tract and at sympathetic nerve endings. Drugs such as tyramine and phenylephrine which are destroyed by MAO in the gut wall become more effective orally. Loss of MAO at sympathetic nerve endings causes an increase in intraneuronal noradrenaline. Thus the effect of so-called 'indirect' (i.e. act by releasing noradrenaline) sympathomimetic drugs is increased. Following a MAOI the effects of oral and intravenous ephedrine were potentiated to a similar extent (Elis et al., 1967). Phenylephrine was also potentiated but the effect of an oral dose was increased much more than the effect of an intravenous dose as phenylephrine is metabolised by MAO in the gut wall (Elis et al., 1967).

Treatment of coincident hypertension with adrenergic neurone-blocking drugs such as guanethidine and bethanidine can lead to important interactions. The antihypertensive effect of these drugs can be reversed by sympathomimetics like ephedrine (see Chapter 7, p. 141).

The rise in asthma mortality which was seen in the United Kingdom appeared to be related to the overuse of pressurised aerosols containing mainly isoprenaline. The subsequent fall in mortality appeared to be related to a reduction in the use of such aerosols (Inman and Adelstein, 1969). While there may have been other factors to explain this correlation, the possibility of drug interaction is very relevant. The pressurised aerosols in addition to containing an active bronchodilator, also contained a mixture of fluorinated analogues of methane and ethane as propellant gases. These were known under the trade names 'Arcton' in Great Britain and 'Freon' in the United States. These compounds are structurally related to chloroform and halothane, the compounds of which are known to sensitise the hypoxic myocardium to the effect of sympathomimetic drugs. It was reported that a blood level of 20–25 μg/ml of fluorocarbon-11 and a blood level of 40–50 μg/ml of fluorocarbon-12 was necessary to sensitise the conscious dog to the injection of adrenaline (Jack, 1971). Paterson et al. (1971b) studied the blood level of fluorocarbon-11 in patients known to overuse broncho-dilator aerosols. In such subjects no fluorocarbon-11 could be detected in the blood except immediately after two puffs from a pressurised salbutamol aerosol (equivalent to 50 mg of fluorocarbon-11). A peak level of from 0.13 to 2.6 μg/ml was seen, and the half-life was from 0.3 to 1.5 min. These levels were considerably lower than those required to sensitise the dog heart to adrenaline. Clark and Tinston (1971) found that a blood level of fluoro-carbon-11 20 times greater than the peak level seen in patients did *not* sensitise the dog heart to isoprenaline, at an oxygen tension of approximately 50 mm Hg. It seems unlikely that interaction between fluorocarbons and β-stimulants is a major problem in the use of bronchodilator aerosols, although this assumes no species difference and that lower oxygen tensions would not greatly alter the response.

Although isoprenaline reduces airway obstruction in asthma it does not always improve the reduced arterial oxygen tension (Knudson and Constantine, 1967; Palmer and Diament, 1967). This is thought to be due to an intensification of the already existing ventilation perfusion imbalance in the lung. When isoprenaline is administered, bronchodilatation will result from stimulation of β_2-receptors in bronchial smooth muscle. However, there will also be cardiac stimulation which will lead to an increase in cardiac output and in addition there may be a reversal of pulmonary vasoconstriction caused by hypoxia. In this way an increase in blood flow through poorly ventilated areas of the lung would cause a further drop in oxygen tension. Studies using a selective β_1-receptor-blocking drug showed that the major effect of isoprenaline on oxygen tension is the effect on the heart, as following practolol the drop in oxygen tension seen with isoprenaline was completely prevented (Palmer et al., 1969).

Attempts have been made to reduce the effects of β_1-stimulation by adding phenylephrine to isoprenaline in a pressurised aerosol. Phenylephrine predominantly affects α-receptors, and therefore it was hoped that it would lead to pulmonary vasoconstriction, and therefore diminish the ventilation perfusion imbalance occurring as a result of pulmonary vasodilatation following isoprenaline. It was also hoped that the drug would delay the absorption of isoprenaline from the bronchial mucosa because of its vasoconstrictor effect, and so prolong the duration of action of isoprenaline. No evidence was found to suggest that the bronchodilator action of isoprenaline could be prolonged in this way. There is no indication for giving such mixtures to prolong duration of action, as the selective β_2-drugs such as salbutamol and terbutaline have a much longer duration of action in any case. It would also seem undesirable to give a drug with α-receptor-stimulating properties, in view of the recent demonstration of α-receptors in bronchial smooth muscle. Indeed in one study it was found that in a significant number of patients the FEV_1 either did not change or dropped after the administration of this preparation (Pflug et al., 1970).

Keighley (1966) reported a small group of asthmatic patients who did not respond to treatment with steroids or other agents until isoprenaline was withdrawn. Thus isoprenaline prevented an adequate response to other drugs. The patients were studied when they had recovered and showed a normal bronchodilator response to isoprenaline. However after the bronchodilator effect had worn off bronchoconstriction ensued. This rebound bronchoconstriction following isoprenaline was also demonstrated after intravenous isoprenaline by Paterson et al. (1971a). They found that in two such patients the bronchoconstriction could be overcome by giving much larger doses of a selective β_2-stimulant drug, salbutamol, but in one patient administration of aminophylline was necessary. Keighley (1966) suggested that in patients ceasing to respond to large doses of adrenergic drugs these agents should be withdrawn and treatment with theophylline, and, if necessary corticosteroids, instituted.

One explanation of the phenomenon was that isoprenaline was metabolised to 3-o-methylisoprenaline which has weak β-blocking properties (Paterson et al., 1968; Paterson and Conolly, 1970). Asthmatics develop frank asthma when given a β-blocker (McNeill and Ingram, 1966) and so a β-blocking metabolite would prevent the action of β-stimulants if it reached sufficient concentrations. Bassett (1971) subsequently showed that 3-o-methylisoprenaline has very weak β-blocking properties. In addition Blackwell et al. (1970) showed that only a very small fraction of an aerosol dose of isoprenaline was converted to 3-o-methylisoprenaline. It is therefore unlikely that isoprenaline resistance was due to β-blocking metabolite. An alternative explanation is that prolonged β-stimulation by any β-adrenergic drug would eventually lead to resistance, not only to exogenous sympathomimetic drugs but to the natural transmitter (Paterson and Conolly, 1970; Conolly et al., 1971; Paterson et al., 1971a). Resistance to isoprenaline has been produced in man and dog by prolonged exposure to the same, or pharmacologically similar compounds, terbutaline and isoetharine. In guinea-pigs, pretreatment with these agents increases asthma mortality provoked by histamine which suggests that this resistance may reduce the effectiveness of endogenous sympathetic drive to the bronchi. Drug-induced cross resistance to endogenous sympathetic stimulation could lead to a deterioration of the asthmatic state in patients using pressurized aerosols of sympathomimetic bronchodilators.

Tothill et al. (1971a) found in animal experiments that resistance to isoprenaline coincided with the liberation of prostaglandins, and she suggested (Tothill, 1972) that following overusage of isoprenaline in asthma, resistance may be due to the release of prostaglandins, inducing bronchoconstriction. Vane (1971b) has shown that aspirin and indomethacin — anti-inflammatory drugs — inhibit the synthesis of prostaglandins E_2 and $F_{2\alpha}$ in the guinea-pig lung. This raises the theoretical possibility that in patients who have become resistant to β-adrenergic stimulant drugs antiinflammatory agents such as aspirin and indomethacin might be useful. However in so-called 'aspirin allergic' cases of asthma aspirin and indomethacin provoke severe attacks. These patients develop asthma at the age of 30–40 years and have nasal discharge and nasal polyps. Severe attacks are also provoked by nasal polypectomy. No immunological basis for the aspirin allergy has been shown (Smith, 1971). In practice these patients respond to the withdrawal of adrenergic drugs and treatment with theophylline and steroids, as suggested by Keighley (1966). Tothill et al. (1971b) have also pointed out that the release of prostaglandins may be inhibited by psychotropic drugs such as promazine and chlorpromazine, but in the treatment of acute asthma the effects of these drugs on the respiratory centre and the cardiovascular system contraindicate their use.

The finding that α-receptor stimulation causes bronchoconstriction raises the possibility that α-blockade may be useful in the treatment of airway obstruction. Kerr et al. (1970) showed that the α-blocking drugs, phentolamine and phenoxybenzamine inhibited histamine-induced airway obstruction in asthmatic patients. Both these α-blocking drugs have other pharmacological properties. Thus phenoxybenzamine leads to the release of catecholamines, and phentolamine has antihistamine properties. Also these agents inhibit the uptake 1 process and thus would potentiate the effects of endogenous noradrenaline and adrenaline. A new α-blocking drug thymoxamine has virtually no antihistaminic properties, and this drug significantly affected airway obstruction induced by histamine in asthmatic patients (Gaddie et al., 1972b). In the same study the drug was given without histamine to asthmatics with mild airway obstruction, but these patients showed no significant increase in FEV_1. No formal trial has been carried out to see whether an α-blocking drug might potentiate the action of a β-stimulant drug. It would certainly seem worthwhile to try the effect of an α-blocking drug in a situation where the patient is no longer responsive to β-stimulant drugs.

β-Adrenergic blocking drugs are used in the treatment of a variety of conditions, such as arrhythmias, angina and hypertension. In patients with a past history of asthma or bronchitis, a β-blocking drug can produce an increased airway obstruction. β-Blocking drugs with cardioselective properties such as practolol (MacDonald and McNeill, 1968) or intrinsic activity such as alprenolol (Conolly and Batten, 1970) may produce a lesser fall in airway resistance than propranolol, but no β-blocking drug is free from this side-effect (Paterson, 1971).

Bronchoconstriction produced by a β-blocker can be reversed with aminophylline (McNeill and Ingram, 1966) which bypasses the blocked β-receptor, or atropine intravenously (MacDonald et al., 1967). As β-blockade is competitive, the bronchoconstriction can also be overcome by using an increased dose of a β-stimulant, such as isoprenaline or orciprenaline (Meier et al., 1966).

In patients with allergic asthma or rhinitis, the increase in airways resistance caused by histamine or methacholine is greatly increased by pretreatment with propranolol (Zaid and Beall, 1966). Ouellette and Reed (1966) challenged hay fever patients sensitive to ragweed with ragweed aerosol, and showed that β-blockade increased the fall in FEV_1 caused by ragweed. These latter nteractions are of importance to workers carrying out bronchial reactivity tests.

2.5 METHYL XANTHINE DRUGS

These drugs are thought to act by inhibiting phosphodiesterase, and thus in common with adrenergic drugs increase the concentration of 3′,5′-cyclic AMP. The major drug in this group is theophylline. It may be used in the treatment of acute asthma as aminophylline, either by suppository or intravenous injection. Aminophylline consists of a mixture of theophylline and ethylenediamine, which is used to increase the solubility of the theophylline. Theophylline is a potent bronchodilator, and causes vasodilatation, increased cardiac output, and an increase in heart rate. In the management of an acute attack it may be given intravenously but should be given slowly because of its cardiovascular effects. Oral theophylline is available in a multiplicity of different preparations, choline theophyllinate being the oldest, no other having been shown to be more effective. In general it seems that oral theophyllines are less effective than adrenergic drugs such as salbutamol or terbutaline (Palmer et al., 1971). Proprietary preparations of theophylline and ephedrine were introduced because it was thought that lower doses of each agent would potentiate one another and so reduce side-effects due to each drug. However these preparations also contain barbiturates, and because of the depressant effect of these drugs on respiration, tablets of this nature may well be dangerous in the treatment of severe asthma, especially if the patient's condition is worsening and the dose is increased. In two studies potentiation of the bronchodilator effects of inhaled isoprenaline by intravenous aminophylline were shown (Cander and Comroe, 1955; Hume and Rhys-Jones, 1961). Because of their different sites of action (Fig. 2) it would seem reasonable that β-stimulants and theophylline should have a synergistic bronchodilator effect. Apart from the studies referred to, there is a lack of objective data to substantiate this. When the β-receptors are blocked aminophylline will still cause bronchodilatation (McNeill and Ingram, 1966), and in patients unresponsive to β-stimulants aminophylline may be effective (Paterson et al., 1971a). Other compound proprietary preparations of methyl xanthines contain iodides, and this is not desirable because if taken for a long time such combinations can lead to a block in thyroxine formation, and in some patients hypothyroidism.

ICI 58,301 (3 acetamido-6-methyl-8-*n*-propyl-*s*-triazolo[4,3-a]pyrazine) is a new compound which has been shown to inhibit the enzyme cyclic AMP phosphodiesterase (Somerville et al., 1970). Experiments in vitro and in vivo suggest that greater inhibition of phosphodiesterase is produced by this compound than by theophylline (Davies et al., 1971). In vitro ICI 58,301 had only a very weak bronchodilator effect at concentrations of 1–5 μg/ml whereas in guinea pigs at plasma levels of 0.3 μg/ml it was highly effective in preventing bronchoconstriction produced by various stimuli, including histamine (G. E. Davies, F. L. Rose and A. R. Somerville, to be published). In 10 asthmatic subjects whilst the drug was well absorbed when given by mouth producing maximum plasma levels at 3 hours, no significant changes occurred in FEV_1, pulse rate or blood pressure (Richards et al., 1971) and no effect from the drug could be demonstrated on histamine and exercise induced bronchoconstriction in asthmatic subjects (Legge et al., 1972). It should be noted that the effects of ICI 58,301 on phosphodiesterase were studied in vitro in ox heart tissue. It is probable that more than one phosphodiesterase exists, and that there may be organ to organ and interspecies variation. This could well explain why a drug which was effective in inhibiting phosphodiesterase in ox heart had much less effect in human bronchus, and does not necessarily invalidate the cyclic AMP theory.

2.6 CORTICOSTEROIDS

These drugs are very important in the treatment of airway obstruction in asthma. Their mode of action in relieving airway obstruction is still debated. The effect may be due to the non-specific antiinflammatory properties of the drug, or it may prevent reaccumulation of histamine in mast cells. It has been suggested that in large doses corticosteroids have direct smooth muscle relaxant effects.

Of interest is the possibility that the corticosteroids interact with adrenergic drugs including endogenous catecholamines. They could possibly restore the response of adenyl cyclase to β-stimulation. Certainly in animals pharmacological β-blockade can be overcome by a large dose of glucocorticoid (Szentivanyi et al., 1963).

Another way in which steroids could affect the response to adrenergic drugs is by altering the uptake process. Nicol and Rae (1972) found that corticosterone inhibited uptake 2 of noradrenaline and adrenaline into vascular smooth muscle and potentiated their pharmacological effect. Foster (1969) showed that the relaxant effect of isoprenaline on the isolated trachea was potentiated by drugs which blocked uptake 2, although steroids were not specifically studied. Thus there is more than one possible mechanism by which steroids could interact with adrenergic drugs in relieving airway obstruction in asthma. The important practical implication of this is that when corticosteroid drugs are started in an individual asthmatic patient, bronchodilator drugs of the adrenergic group should be continued.

It is common practice when withdrawing corticosteroids to give a course of ACTH in order to stimulate the adrenals and restore the hypothalamic pituitary adrenal axis more rapidly, and so the response to stress. Recent animal work (Hodges and Mitchley, 1971) has shown that in fact this practice prolongs the time taken for the animal to recover its response to stress. Thus in rats treated with β-methasone alone, adrenocortical response to stress recovered fairly quickly, but if the animals were given ACTH after withdrawal of the β-methasone, the recovery of the response to stress was delayed. Carreon et al. (1960) certainly found that ACTH caused an increased excretion of corticosteroid, following cessation of long-term steroids in patients. However when ACTH was stopped there was immediate and persistent regression to a 'hypoadrenal' state. Thus the administration of ACTH as an 'aid' to the withdrawal of corticosteroids may be harmful.

Patients having corticosteroid drugs for asthma must not be given phenobarbitone or other sedatives such as dichloralphenazone or glutethimide, as these drugs are potent microsomal enzyme inducers and may contribute to clinical worsening, deterioration of spirometric tests and increased eosinophil counts (Brooks et al., 1972).

2.7 DISODIUM CROMOGLYCATE

This drug has no direct bronchodilator activity. Its principal action is to block the release of bronchoconstrictors from mast cells in the lung. It thus prevents bronchoconstriction rather than causing bronchodilatation (Cox, 1971). The drug is only active when given by inhalation, and any drug swallowed is not absorbed. It can be given alone or in combination with isoprenaline which was included in an attempt to offset possible increases in airway obstruction due to the inhalation of a dry powder. However this happens extremely rarely. A consequence of giving the drug with isoprenaline is that the patient experiences bronchodilatation, due to the isoprenaline content which is equivalent to that in commercially available pressurised portable aerosols containing isoprenaline. Thus it is very difficult to educate the patient in the proper prophylactic use of the drug, and for this reason the drug should be given without isoprenaline. However, if the patient is wheezy it is beneficial to allow the use of a bronchodilator aerosol — preferably of salbutamol or terbutaline, 10 min before taking disodium cromoglycate, in order that bronchodilation will cause a greater amount of the drug to be inhaled into the lung.

Not all patients with classical allergic airway obstruction respond to the drug, and a proportion of intrinsic asthmatics do show some beneficial effect (Kidner et al., 1968; Gaddie et al., 1972a). Disodium cromoglycate can reduce the responsiveness of the airways in asthma to histamine (Inoue and Nishima, 1969), and it is possible that it may have some blocking effect on α-adrenergic receptors. Kerr et al. (1970) have shown that prior inhalation of disodium cromoglycate abolished the reduction in FEV_1 and FVC produced by intravenous histamine in asthmatics. The drug also reduces bronchoconstriction induced by exercise (Davies, 1968). When it is combined with salbutamol, an adrenergic drug, it completely prevents the post-exercise fall in FEV_1, whereas both drugs singly are less effective (Palmer and Legge, 1969).

When it is successful in the treatment of asthma, it reduces the need for bronchodilator drugs and corticosteroid therapy (Moran et al., 1968; Morrison-Smith and Devey, 1968; Gaddie et al., 1972a).

3 Respiratory stimulants

Normally chemical control of respiration is achieved by feed-back from peripheral and central chemoreceptors, which are stimulated by changes in $PaCO_2$, PaO_2 or pH. In the normal subject the change in $PaCO_2$ tends to be the dominant factor. The changes in $PaCO_2$, PaO_2 or pH lead to an increase in ventilation which tends to restore the status quo. In lung disease, either acute or chronic but especially chronic, changes occurring in blood gas tensions and pH are not corrected by the corresponding increases of ventilation. Moreover, in patients with lung disease with hypercapnia the respiratory centre becomes more sensitive than normal to the depressant effect of drugs, and this hypersensitivity of the respiratory centre to sedatives may be present in the absence of hypercapnia, asthmatics for example being extremely sensitive to sedative drugs, tranquillisers and morphine derivatives, all of which may lead to profound depression of ventilation. This can be counteracted by respiratory stimulants such as aminophylline, nikethamide, ethamivan or amiphenazole. If depression is due to morphine or its derivatives, the specific antagonist nalorphine will be preferred.

In patients who have or have had a raised arterial $PaCO_2$ tension, i.e. hypercapnia, the respiratory centre becomes relatively insensitive to increases in $PaCO_2$ and the control of respiration is maintained more by hypoxic stimulation. If these patients are given uncontrolled oxygen therapy, especially if combined with sedatives, there is profound depression of respiration with $PaCO_2$ rising to anaesthetic levels. In such patients the clinical response to a respiratory stimulant, especially nikethamide, may be dramatic, consciousness returning within a moment or so. Nikethamide is probably the most effective respiratory stimulant drug. Part of the beneficial effect of such agents, in addition to changes in minute ventilation, is due to their central arousal effects allowing coughing and the carrying out of physiotherapy (Dulfano and Segal, 1963; McNicol et al., 1963; Murray and Grant, 1966). In patients with ventilatory failure no sedative drug is safe; even nitrazepam which causes no depression of respiration in normal subjects, even after overdosage, readily produces carbon dioxide narcosis in hypercapnic subjects receiving oxygen (Clark et al., 1971).

4 Easing of expectoration

4.1 EXPECTORANTS

Expectorant mixtures are intended to increase the volume of sputum and to make it less viscid. Traditionally and for many years mixtures of ammonium salts and ipecacuanha, ammonium salts and iodides, sodium chloride and sodium bicarbonate, iodides and stramonium, have been given for this purpose, but controlled trials have indicated that these mixtures do not increase the volume of sputum in chronic bronchitis (Alstead, 1939, 1941), and so their popularity has waned. Since oral expectorants were ineffective, attempts were made to reduce sputum viscosity and increase its volume by aerosol inhalation of various substances. Many of these compounds appeared to act simply by hydrating the viscid sputum (Palmer, 1957). Ascorbic acid in the presence of molecular oxygen was shown in vitro to cause depolymerisation of mucopolysaccharides (the main component of mucoid sputum), and a marked reduction in viscosity. This reaction is enhanced by cupric ions (Robertson et al., 1940). When this mixture is given by aerosol to patients with chronic bronchitis, there is a decrease in sputum viscosity (Palmer, 1961) and an increase in sputum volume (Fisher and Ten Pas, 1966), and improvement in airflow rates (Sabath et al., 1965). Controlled trials have shown this mixture to cause a statistically significant improvement in ventilatory tests, and increase in sputum volume and decrease in sputum viscosity (Dulfano and Glass, 1969).

N-Acetyl cysteine has been reported to be an effective mucolytic in vitro (Scheffner, 1963) and during short-term administration to patients by aerosol (Webb, 1962; Hirsch and Kory, 1967). However the drug increased airway obstruction in many patients. A controlled study in chronic obstructive bronchitis where nebulised N-acetyl cysteine was combined with adrenaline showed the mixture to be highly effective in thinning sputum, and the bronchial obstruction which was previously reported with N-acetyl cysteine alone did not occur (Kory et al., 1968).

TABLE II

Some proprietary cough and cold medicines containing phenylpropanolamine

Tablets and capsules	Syrups and linctuses
Mucron	Delexin
Rinurel	Dimotane
Contac 400	Rinurel
Procol	Salaton
Triogesic	Syrtusser
Triominic	Tixylix
Triotussic	Triogesic
Eskornade	Triotussic
	Vallex
	Eskornade

4.2 COLD CURES AND COUGH MIXTURES

Many proprietary cold cures and cough mixtures contain sympathomimetic drugs which can cause alarming interactions if given to patients taking other medicines. Thus Cuthbert et al. (1969) showed that phenylpropanolamine (norephedrine) produced marked rises in blood pressure in doses contained in proprietary mixtures, when given to normal subjects after MAOI. This substance is present in a large variety of popular cold cures (Table II). Moreover Misage and McDonald (1970) showed that phenylpropanolamine antagonised the hypotensive effects of bethanidine.

References

Ahlquist, R. P. (1948): A study of the adrenotropic receptors. *Amer. J. Physiol.*, **153**, 586.

Alliott, R. J., Lang, B. D., Rawson, D. R. W. and Leckie, W. J. H. (1972): Effects of salbutamol and isoprenaline/phenylephrine in reversible airways obstruction. *Brit. med. J.*, **1**, 539.

Alstead, S. (1939): Potassium iodide and ipecacuanha as expectorants. *Lancet*, **2**, 932.

Alstead, S. (1941): Ammonium chloride and ammonium carbonate in chronic bronchitis. *Lancet*, **1**, 308.

Altounyan, R. E. C. (1966): Measurement of factors influencing bronchoconstriction. *Proc. roy. Soc. Med.*, **59**, 56.

Barar, F. S. K., Boakes, A. J., Benedikter, L. B., Laurence, D. R., Prichard, B. N. C. and Teoh, P. C. (1971): Interactions between catecholamines and tricyclic and monoamine oxidase inhibitor antidepressive agents in man. *Brit. J. Pharmacol.*, **43**, 471P.

Bassett, J. R. (1971): Beta-adrenoceptor antagonist activity of 3-methoxyisoprenaline. *Brit. J. Pharmacol.*, **41**, 113.

Bianco, S., Griffin, J. P., Kamburoff, P. L. and Prime, F. J. (1972): The effect of thymoxamine on histamine-induced bronchospasm in man. *Brit. J. Dis. Chest*, **66**, 27.

Blackwell, E. W., Conolly, M. E., Davies, D. S. and Dollery, C. T. (1970): The fate of isoprenaline administered by pressurized aerosols. *Brit. J. Pharmacol.*, **39**, 194P.

Brocklehurst, W. E. (1971): The pharmacology of asthma and possible therapeutic developments. In: *Identification of Asthma* (Ciba Foundation Study Group No. 38) p. 132. Editors: Ruth Porter and Joan Birch. Churchill Livingstone, Edinburgh and London.

Brooks, S. M., Werk, E. F., Ackermann, S. J., Sullivan, I. and Thraser, K. (1972): Adverse effects of phenobarbital on corticosteroid metabolism in patients with bronchial asthma. *New Engl. J. Med.*, **286**, 1125.

Cander, L. and Comroe, J. H. (1955): A method for the objective evaluation of bronchodilator drugs. *J. Allergy Appl. Immunol.*, **26**, 210.

Carreon, G. G., Canary, J. J., Meyer, R. J. and Kyle, L. H. (1960): Adrenocortical function after long term corticoid therapy. *J. Lab. clin. Med.*, **56**, 235.

Chamberlain, D. A., Muir, D. C. F. and Kennedy, K. P. (1962): Atropine methylnitrate and isoprenaline in bronchial asthma. *Lancet*, **2**, 1019.

Clark, D. G. and Tinston, D. J. (1971): Sniffing syndrome. *Brit. med. J.*, **3**, 113.

Clark, T. J. H., Collins, J. V. and Tong, D. (1971): Respiratory depression caused by nitrazepam in patients with respiratory failure. *Lancet*, **2**, 737.

Connolly, C. K. and Batten, J. C. (1970): Comparison of the effect of alprenolol and propranolol on specific airway conductance in asthmatic subjects. *Brit. med. J.*, **2**, 515.

Conolly, M. E., Davies, D. S., Dollery, C. T. and George, C. F. (1971): Resistance of beta adrenoreceptor stimulants. *Brit. J. Pharmacol.*, **43**, 389.

Cox, J. S. G. (1971): Disodium cromoglycate – mode of action and its possible relevance to the clinical use of the drug. *Brit. J. Diseases Chest.*, **65**, 189.
Crompton, G. K. (1968): A comparison of responses to bronchodilator drugs in chronic bronchitis and chronic asthma. *Thorax*, **23**, 46.
Cuthbert, M. F. (1969): Effect on airways resistance of prostaglandin E_1 given by aerosol to healthy and asthmatic volunteers. *Brit. med. J.*, **4**, 723.
Cuthbert, M. F., Greenberg, M. P. and Morley, S. W. (1969): Cough and cold remedies: a potential danger to patients on monoamine oxidase inhibitors. *Brit. med. J.*, **1**, 404.
Cuthbert, M. F. and Vere, D. W. (1971): Potentiation of the cardiovascular effects of some catecholamines by a monoamine oxidase inhibitor. *Brit. J. Pharmacol.*, **43**, 471P.
Davies, D. S., Morgan, C. D., Conolly, M. E., Paterson, J. W., Sandler, M. and Dollery, C. T. (1969): The metabolic fate of d,l-isoproterenol-7-^{3}H in man and dog. *Federation Proc.*, **28**, 797.
Davies, S. E. (1968): Effect of disodium cromoglycate on exercise-induced asthma. *Brit. med. J.*, **3**, 593.
Dulfano, M. J. and Glass, P. (1969): An effective mucolytic aerosol in chronic bronchitis. *J. Amer. med. Assoc.*, **207**, 1310.
Dulfano, M. J. and Segal, M. S. (1963): Nikethamide as a respiratory analeptic. *J. Amer. med. Assoc.*, **185**, 69.
Elis, J., Laurence, D. R., Mathie, H. and Prichard, B. N. C. (1967): Modification by monoamine oxidase inhibitors of the effect of some sympathomimetics on blood pressure. *Brit. med. J.*, **2**, 75.
Fisher, A. J. and Ten Pas, R. H. (1966): Clinical evaluation of ascoxyl – a new mucolytic drug. *Anaesthesia Analgesia*, **45**, 531.
Foster, R. W. (1969): An uptake of radioactivity from ($\pm$)-^{3}H-isoprenaline and its inhibition by drugs which potentiate the responses to ($-$) isoprenaline in the guinea-pig isolated trachea. *Brit. J. Pharmacol.*, **35**, 418.
Gaddie, J., Legge, J. S. and Palmer, K. N. V. (1972a). The effect of disodium cromoglycate on pulmonary function in asthma. *Brit. J. Diseases Chest.* **66**, 254.
Gaddie, J., Legge, J. S., Petrie, G. and Palmer, K. N. V. (1972b). The effect of an alpha receptor adrenergic blocking drug on histamine sensitivity in bronchial asthma. *Brit. J. Diseases Chest.* **66**, 141.
Gibson, D. G. and Coltart, D. J. (1971): Haemodynamic effects of intravenous salbutamol in patients with mitral valve disease: comparison with isoprenaline and atropine. *Postgrad. med. J.*, **47**, 40.
Hirsch, S. R. and Kory, R. C. (1967): An evaluation of the effect of nebulised N-acetyl-L-cysteine on sputum consistency. *J. Allergy Appl. Immunol.*, **39**, 265.
Hodges, J. R. and Mitchley, S. (1971): Effect of prolonged treatment with tetracosactrin on hypothalamo–pituitary–adrenal function in the rat. *Brit. J. Pharmacol.*, **43**, 804.
Horton, E. W. (1969): Hypotheses on physiological roles of prostaglandins. *Physiol. Rev.*, **49**, 122.
Hume, K. M. and Rhys-Jones, E. (1961): The response of bronchodilators in intrinsic asthma. *Quart. J. Med.*, **30**, 118.
Inman, W. H. W. and Adelstein, A. M. (1969): Rise and fall of asthma mortality in England and Wales in relation to the use of pressurised aerosols. *Lancet*, **2**, 279.
Inoue, S. and Nishima, S. (1969): Effect of disodium cromoglycate on asthmatic children. *Allergy (Tokyo)*, **18**, 692.
Iversen, L. L. (1971): Role of transmitter uptake mechanisms in synaptic neurotransmission. *Brit. J. Pharmacol.*, **41**, 571.
Jack, D. (1971): Sniffing syndrome. *Brit. med. J.*, **2**, 708.
Keighley, J. F. (1966): Iatrogenic asthma associated with adrenergic aerosols. *Ann. intern. Med.*, **65**, 985.
Kennedy, M. C. S. (1965): Bronchodilator action of deptropine citrate with or without isoprenaline by inhalation. *Brit. med. J.*, **2**, 916.
Kerr, J. W., Govindaraj, M. and Patel, K. R. (1970): Effect of alpha receptor blocking

drugs and disodium cromoglycate on histamine hypersensitivity in bronchial asthma. *Brit. med. J.*, **2**, 139.

Kidner, P. H., Meisner, P., Pride, N. B. and Pearson, R. S. B. (1968): Disodium cromoglycate in the treatment of bronchial asthma. *Lancet*, **2**, 655.

Knudson, R. J. and Constantine, H. P. (1967): An effect of isoproterenol on ventilation/perfusion in asthmatic versus normal subjects. *J. appl. Physiol.*, **22**, 402.

Kory, R. C., Hirsch, S. R. and Giraldo, J. (1968): Nebulisation of N-acetyl-cysteine combined with a bronchodilator in patients with chronic bronchitis. *Diseases Chest*, **54**, 504.

Lands, A. M., Arnold, A. McAuliff, J. P. M., Luduena, F. P. and Brown, T. G. (1967): Differentiation of receptor systems activated by sympathomimetic amines. *Nature*, **214**, 597.

Large, B. J., Leswell, P. F. and Maxwell, D. R. (1969): Bronchodilator activity of an aerosol of prostaglandin E_1 in experimental animals. *Nature*, **224**, 79.

Leading Article (1970): Cyclic AMP: the second messenger. *Lancet*, **2**, 1119.

Legge, J. S., Gaddie, J. and Palmer, K. N. V. (1972): The effect of phosphodiesterase-inhibiting drugs on histamine-induced bronchoconstriction in asthmatic subjects (resumé). *Bull. Physio-pathol.*, **8**, 488.

Lichtenstein, L. M. and Bourne, H. R. (1971): Inhibition of allergic histamine release by histamine and other agents which stimulate adenyl cyclase. In: *Biochemistry of the Acute Allergic Reactions.* Editors: K. F. Austen and E. L. Becker, p. 161. Blackwell, London.

MacDonald, A. G., Ingram, C. G. and McNeill, R. S. (1967): The effect of propranolol on airway resistance. *Brit. J. Anaesthes.*, **39**, 919.

MacDonald, A. G. and McNeill, R. S. (1968): A comparison of the effect on airway resistance of a new beta-blocking drug ICI. 50, 172 and propranolol. *Brit. J. Anaesthes.*, **40**, 508.

McNeill, R. S. and Ingram, C. G. (1966): Effect of propranolol on ventilatory function. *Amer. J. Cardiol.*, **18**, 473.

McNicol, M. W., Pride, N. B., Reynolds, E. O. R. and Semple, S. J. G. (1963): Nikethamide for severe carbon dioxide retention in exacerbations of chronic bronchitis. *Brit. med. J.*, **1**, 646.

Meier, J., Lydtin, H. and Zöllner, N. (1966): The action of adrenergic beta receptor blockers on ventilatory functions in obstructive lung disease. *Ger. med. Monthly*, **11**, 1.

Misage, J. R. and McDonald, R. H. (1970): Antagonism of hypotensive action of bethanidine by "common cold" remedy. *Brit. med. J.*, **4**, 347.

Moran, F., Bankier, J. D. H. and Boyd, G. (1968): Disodium cromoglycate in the treatment of allergic bronchial asthma. *Lancet*, **2**, 137.

Morrison-Smith, J. and Devey, G. F. (1968): A clinical trial of disodium cromoglycate in bronchial asthma in children. *Brit. med. J.*, **2**, 340.

Murray, W. D. and Grant, I. W. B. (1966): Nikethamide and aminophylline in ventilatory failure. *Scot. med. J.*, **11**, 89.

Nicol, C. J. M. and Rae, R. M. (1972): Inhibition of accumulation of adrenaline and noradrenaline in arterial smooth muscle by steroids. *Brit. J. Pharmacol.*, **44**, 361P.

Orange, R. P. and Austen, F. K. (1971): Immunological release of the chemical mediators of anaphylaxis. In: *Identification of Asthma* (Ciba Foundation Study Group No. 38). Editors: Ruth Porter and Joan Birch, p. 99. Churchill Livingstone, Edinburgh and London.

Ouellette, J. J. and Reed, C. E. (1966): Effect of partial beta-adrenergic blockade on bronchial response of hay fever subjects to ragweed aerosol. *J. Allergy Appl. Immunol.*, **37**, 102.

Palmer, K. N. V. (1957): The effect of an aerosol detergent in chronic bronchitis. *Lancet*, **1**, 611.

Palmer, K. N. V. (1961): A new mucolytic agent by aerosol for inhalation in chronic bronchitis. *Lancet*, **2**, 802.

Palmer, K. N. V. and Diament, M. L. (1967): Effect of aerosol isoprenaline on blood gas tensions in severe bronchial asthma. *Lancet*, **2**, 1232.

Palmer, K. N. V. and Legge, J. S. (1969): Disodium cromoglycate in exercise-induced asthma. *Lancet*, **2**, 219.

Palmer, K. N. V., Legge, J. S., Hamilton, W. F. D. and Diament, M. L. (1969): Effect of a selective beta adrenergic blocker in preventing falls in arterial oxygen tension following isoprenaline in asthmatic subjects. *Lancet*, **2**, 1092.

Palmer, K. N. V., Legge, J. S. and Gaddie, J. (1971): Comparison of drugs for asthma. *Brit. med. J.*, **1**, 727.

Paterson, J. W. (1971): Beta-adrenergic blocking drugs. *Brit. med. J.*, **2**, 652.

Paterson, J. W. and Conolly, M. E. (1970): The clinical pharmacology of inhaled isoprenaline. Excerpta Medica International Congress Series No. 220. Proceedings of the Twelfth Meeting of the European Society for the Study of Drug Toxicity, Uppsala, June 1970, p. 138. Excerpta Medica, Amsterdam.

Paterson, J. W., Conolly, M. E., Davies, D. S. and Dollery, C. T. (1968): Isoprenaline resistance and the use of pressurised aerosols in asthma. *Lancet*, **2**, 426.

Paterson, J. W., Courtney Evans, R. J. and Prime, F. J. (1971a): Selectivity of bronchodilator action of salbutamol in asthmatic patients. *Brit. J. Dis. Chest*, **65**, 21.

Paterson, J. W., Sudlow, M. F. and Walker, S. R. (1971b): Blood levels of fluorinated hydrocarbons in asthmatic patients after inhalation of pressurised aerosols. *Lancet*, **2**, 565.

Pflug, A. E., Cheney, F. W. and Butler, J. (1970): The effects of an ultrasonic aerosol on pulmonary mechanics and arterial blood gases in patients with chronic bronchitis. *Amer. Rev. resp. Disease*, **101**, 710.

Robertson, W. V., Ropes, M. W. and Bauer, W. (1940): Mucinase bacterial enzyme which hydrolyses synovial fluid mucin and other mucines. *J. biol. Chem.*, **133**, 261.

Robison, G. A., Butcher, R. W. and Sutherland, E. W. (1967): Adenyl cyclase as an adrenergic receptor. *Ann. N. Y. Acad. Sci.*, **139**, 703.

Sabath, L. D., Sasahara, A. A. and Burlesen, V. A. (1965): Evaluation of a new mucolytic agent. *Diseases Chest.*, **50**, 47.

Scheffner, A. L. (1963): The reduction in vitro of mucoprotein solution by a new mucolytic agent – *N*-acetyl-L-cysteine. *Ann. N. Y. Acad. Sci.*, **106**, 298.

Simonsson, B. G., Anderson, R., Bergh, N. P., Skoogh, B. E. and Svedmyr, N. (1970): In vivo and in vitro studies of pharmacological effects on different receptors regulating bronchial tone in man. In: *Bronchitis III*, p. 334. Editors: N. G. M. Orie and B. van der Lande. Charles C. Thomas, Springfield, Ill.

Smith, A. P. (1971): Response of aspirin-allergic patients to challenge by some analgesics in common use. *Brit. med. J.*, **2**, 494.

Smith, A. P. (1973): The effect of intravenous infusion of graded doses of prostaglandins $F_{2}\alpha$ and E_2 on lung resistance in patients undergoing termination of pregnancy. *Clin. Sci.*, **44**, 17.

Somerville, A. R., Rabouhans, M. L. and Smith, A. A. (1970): Adenosine 3′, 5′-cyclic monophosphate phosphodiesterase: kinetic and inhibitor studies. *Biochem. J.*, **120**, 11P.

Svedmyr, N. (1968): The influence of a tricyclic antidepressive agent (protriptyline) on some of the circulatory effects of noradrenaline and adrenaline in man. *Life Sci.*, **7**, 77.

Sweatman, W. J. F. and Collier, H. O. J. (1968): Effect of prostaglandins on human bronchial muscle. *Nature*, **217**, 69.

Szentivanyi, A., Fishel, C. W. and Talmage, D. W. (1963): Adrenaline mediation of histamine and serotonin hyperglycaemia in normal mice and the absence of adrenaline-induced hyperglycaemia in pertussis sensitised mice. *J. infect. Diseases*, **113**, 86.

Tothill, A. (1972): Resistance to beta adrenoceptor stimulants. *Brit. med. J.*, 689.

Tothill, A., Bamford, D. and Draper, J. (1971a): Inhibition of prostaglandin release and the control of threatened abortion. *Lancet*, **2**, 381.

Tothill, A., Rathbone, L. and Willman, E. (1971b): Relation between prostaglandin E_2 and adrenaline reversal in the rat uterus. *Nature*, **233**, 56.

Vane, J. R. (1971a): Mediators of the anaphylactic reaction. In: *Identification of Asthma* (Ciba Foundation Study Group No. 38). Editors: Ruth Porter and Joan Birch, p. 121. Churchill Livingstone, Edinburgh and London.
Vane, J. R. (1971b): Inhibition of prostaglandin synthesis as a mechanism of action for aspirin-like drugs. *Nature New Biol.*, **231**, 232.
Webb, W. R. (1962): Clinical evaluation of a new effective mucolytic agent. *J. thorac. cardiovasc. Surg.*, **44**, 330.
Zaid, G. and Beall, G. N. (1966): Bronchial response to beta-adrenergic blockade. *New Engl. J. Med.*, **275**, 580.

CHAPTER 9

Drug interactions in the management of infections

JAMES R. PHILP

1 Introduction

When considering interactions between drugs in relation to the management of infections it is essential to remember the pre-existence of another set of interactions, i.e. the *host–parasite–drug triangle* (Fig. 1a). When another drug is introduced it may interact with any, or all, of the three corners of this triangle as shown in Fig. 1b. It can be seen that, apart from direct interactions, Drug II may also interfere indirectly with Drug I via the host or parasite. The result may be beneficial or adverse. Significant interactions can also occur outside the body if the two drugs are mixed in a bottle or syringe for simultaneous parenteral administration. In addition there are a number of important interactions which occur in the laboratory which influence the accuracy of antibiotic sensitivity reports. An awareness of these can assist the physician in the initiation and assessment of antimicrobial therapy.

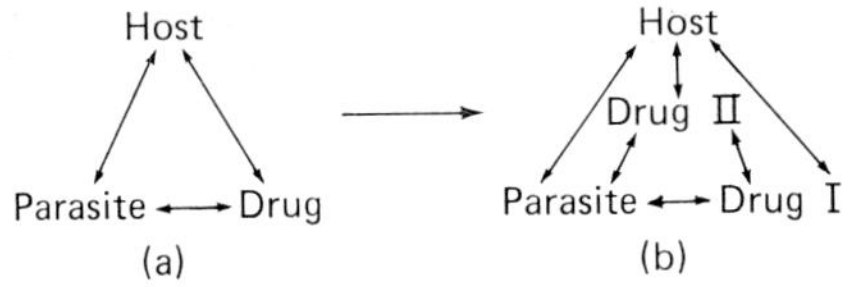

Fig. 1. The interactions of the host–parasite–drug triangle.

2 Interactions between antimicrobials and other classes of drugs

2.1 GENERAL

The two interacting drugs need not be antibiotics. Steroids and immunosuppressants, by impairing host defences, may adversely influence the response to antimicrobial therapy even when the organism is fully sensitive (Remington, 1971). In contrast, steroids may be employed in conjunction with specific chemotherapy in the management of acute iridocyclitis, superficial mixed skin infections (Davis et al., 1968) and possibly tuberculous meningitis (Lorber, 1960). In these, a beneficial effect may derive from suppression of an inflammatory response which is disadvantageous to the patient. These contrasting effects illustrate that no general rules can be applied to this problem.

Drug interactions may be intentionally manipulated with advantage to the patient.

Probenecid inhibits the tubular secretion of both the penicillins and the cephalosporins and can be used to increase the blood and tissue levels of these drugs (Medical Letter, 1971b). In the case of oral or parenteral penicillins probenecid can increase peak serum levels by 50–300% and prolong the period of active blood levels. This manoeuvre has mostly been applied to those situations where sensitive organisms such as staphylococci are sequestered in situations where diffusion is poor e.g. endocarditis, osteomyelitis and meningitis. Probenecid has also been used to increase and prolong penicillin levels in the 'one shot' treatment of gonorrhoea. This regimen may become more widely used if the spread of gonococci of increasing resistance to penicillin continues. In one series (Cobbold et al., 1970), the failure rate of combined therapy was 7% compared to 13% with penicillin alone. Probenecid may also be used in the treatment of *Pseudomonas* infections in order to permit a reduced dose of carbenicillin. When used along with a penicillin it should always be remembered that probenecid itself may give rise to adverse reactions such as skin rashes!

TABLE I

A selection of antimicrobial agents influenced by urinary pH

Activity increased	
In alkaline pH	In acid pH
Aminoglycosides	Tetracyclines
Streptomycin	Nitrofurantoin
Neomycin	Nalidixic acid
Kanamycin	Mandelamine
Gentamicin	(Hexamine mandelate)
Erythromycin	
Cephaloridine	

Agents which influence urinary pH can be important in the management of urinary tract infections. Alkalinisation can be achieved using sodium bicarbonate or acetazolamide. Acidification can be effected by giving ammonium chloride. A selection of agents influenced by urinary pH is shown in Table I. Unfortunately in the case of urinary infections with urease splitting organisms (e.g. *Proteus* species) it is impossible to acidify the urine by this means *even in the presence of a profound induced systemic acidosis.* (See Table I).

Mandelamine only releases formaldehyde at pH < 5 and checking of urinary pH several times each day is necessary to avoid futile therapy.

There are a number of important adverse effects resulting from drug interactions between antibiotics and non-antimicrobial agents.

Frusemide enhances the nephrotoxicity of cephaloridine (Lawson et al., 1970; Brown et al., 1970).

Adverse interactions also occur in patients on anticoagulants (Medical Letter, 1971a; Formiller and Cotton, 1969; Koch-Weser and Sellers, 1971; Editorial Brit. Med. J., 1971a). Griseofulvin reduces the anticoagulant effect of Warfarin and may lead to an increased dosage of the latter. This may result in hypocoagulability when griseofulvin therapy is stopped. Over a longer period of administration, oral ampicillin and tetracycline, by interfering with the normal gut flora, may decrease the endogenous production of vitamin K with enhancement of anticoagulant activity. Clearly, any hepatotoxic antimicrobial may increase prothrombin time (Philp, 1971). At another point of interaction, sulphonamides displace Warfarin from its binding sites on plasma proteins thereby potentiating its effect.

For the same reason, diabetic patients on oral hypoglycaemic agents such as tolbutamide and chlorpropamide may experience hypoglycaemic episodes if treated with sulphonamides (Tucker and Hirsch, 1972).

Some interactions result in diminished absorption from the gut. Because of chelation, blood levels of tetracycline may be reduced by 50–90% if given orally along with ferrous sulphate (Editorial Brit. Med. J., 1970a; Neuvonen et al., 1970). Calcium, aluminium and magnesium containing antacids and even food have a similar effect. Because of this effect of food on absorption, most oral penicillins are also best given on an empty stomach. In this context, it is worth noting that rifampicin reduces the absorption of *p*-aminosalicylic acid (PAS) (Boman et al., 1971). Consequently these two antituberculous agents should not be given orally at the same time but separated by several hours. Conversely, the absorption of isoniazid (INH) can be deliberately slowed by incorporation in a matrix to allow once weekly administration (Ellard et al., 1972). In this event special attention should be paid to the interference of INH with pyridoxine metabolism and the possibility of a resulting neuropathy or pellagra-like syndrome.

Another clinically important interaction is the prolonged muscular paralysis and apnoea which may follow the intraperitoneal administration of large doses of kanamycin at operations for peritoneal soilage. This is due to neuromuscular blockade with potentiation of muscle relaxants (Craig et al., 1966; Pindell, 1966). The same effect, which can also be produced by intrapleural instillation, has also been observed with streptomycin, neomycin and the polymyxins. It has not been observed, to date, with gentamicin.

Before proceeding to a discussion proper of antibiotic interactions in vivo it is important to consider three other groups of interactions which can be of prime importance in deciding the outcome of therapy: interactions in the mind of the prescriber; interactions in the laboratory, and interactions in mixtures for parenteral infusion.

2.2 INTERACTIONS IN THE MIND OF THE PRESCRIBER

This group is undoubtedly the most important category. It arises from the pressure on the physician to do his very best for his patient along with the tendency to think of clinical syndromes such as 'pneumonia' and 'urinary infection' instead of the specific organism likely to be responsible in any one case. Some quantitative measure of the importance of this phenomenon can be obtained from the estimate that fixed combinations of antimicrobial drugs to the value of approximately $200,000,000 are consumed in the United States each year. This does not take account of patients who receive several antibiotics at the same time, each administered separately. As very few doctors deliberately prescribe irresponsibly (Maronde, Burks, Lee, 1969) this phenomenon must re present one of the most significant failures in medical education (Philp, 1970). Having once accepted the philosophy that a suspected infection must enjoy any possible benefit of chemotherapy, it is an easy step to the position where, if one antimicrobial is not effective then one or two or more are added until the desired effect is attained. Another temptation is to prescribe several antibiotics when there is uncertainty about the identity of the infecting agent. Drug companies exploit this insecurity by marketing products such as the combination of tetracycline and novobiocin (Hewlitt and Kunin, 1969; Editorial, Lancet, 1969), although there is no evidence to support their efficacy and much to condemn them. There is, for example, no evidence that amphotericin B or nystatin diminishes the incidence of fungal superinfections consequent on tetracycline therapy (Report, Brit. Med. J., 1968). The only gain with this combination is cost and the false sense of security deriving from this type of prescribing carries obvious dangers for the patient. Also, the patient who receives two antibiotics is at least twice as likely to experience an adverse reaction than the patient who receives only one. Another danger is the selective encouragement of multiply resistant bacteria in the environment (Anderson, 1968) and in the patient's own indigenous flora (Gaya et al., 1970). This phenomenon, judging by their prescribing behaviour, is frankly disbelieved by many doctors despite objective proof of its actuality. In one hospital the routine employment of prophylactic ampicillin plus cloxacillin led to the repeated closure of a neurosurgical unit (Price and Sleigh, 1970). The problem was finally solved by prohibiting *all* antibiotics in the unit. Another measure of the importance of this phenomenon can be gauged by the existence of large (52 %) numbers of multiply resistant *E. coli* in some communities. As many (60 %) of these bacteria have the ability to transfer this resistance to other enterobacteria by means of *Resistance Transfer Factors* the potential dangers are clear (Datta, 1969).

2.3 INTERACTIONS IN THE LABORATORY

There are a number of important interactions which, although laboratory phenomena, can affect the accuracy of antibiotic sensitivity reports and therefore influence both the choice and outcome of therapy. It is impossible for the majority of physicians to become familiar with the technical minutiae of antibiotic sensitivity testing. Nonetheless there is an unhealthy acceptance of the veracity of laboratory reports. Two recent reviews on this subject (Medical Letter, 1971c; Editorial, Brit. Med. J., 1971b) directed at a general medical audience are therefore worthy of attention.

The strict performance of antibiotic disc sensitivity tests so as to yield results comparable with tube dilution techniques necessitates a degree of control which a busy diagnostic laboratory would find impossible to implement. Nonetheless, errors can be reduced by the concurrent testing of control cultures and it seems justified to insist on the universal application of this measure.

The composition of the medium on which tests are carried out is important. For example, the addition of blood will reduce the zone of inhibition if the antibiotic in question is significantly protein bound (e.g. fucidin and novobiocin). Again, it is futile to test for sulphonamide sensitivity on media containing blood or other sulphonamide antagonists such as *p*-aminobenzoic acid (PABA). For this purpose special media such as that of Mueller and Hinton should be employed. The assessment of gentamicin sensitivity is influenced by the magnesium content of the medium and electrolyte content can also affect the activity of fucidin and the penicillins against *Proteus* (Garrod and Waterworth, 1969).

The pH of the medium is very important and although this should not be altered to favour the antibiotics the changes which influence their effectiveness should be kept in mind. Streptomycin is approximately 500 times more active at pH 8.5 than pH 5.5. Gentamicin and kanamycin are similarly affected although to a lesser extent. The macrolide antibiotics (e.g. erythromycin) also have an increased effect at alkaline pH. Tetracyclines are more active in an acid medium as is mandelamine. Sensitivities to the latter are not routinely carried out in laboratories because mandelamine is not effective above pH 5 (see above).

A few other specific problems may be mentioned. For instance, a penicillin resistant *Staphylococcus* may exhibit a significant inhibition zone around a penicillin or ampicillin disc. However, the full size colonies at the edge of the zone of inhibition give a clue to the resistance of these organisms. Again, staphylococcal resistance to methicillin may not be obvious if the organism is grown on a normal medium and incubated at 37° C overnight. Incubation at 30° C for 18 hr will reveal the true resistance of these organisms (Hewitt et al., 1969).

Because of possible synergy, the combination of sulphonamide and trimethoprim (cotrimoxazole) has recently become a very popular therapeutic agent for respiratory and urinary infections. It should be kept in mind that this synergy cannot be demonstrated by a single disc containing both drugs, and the value of such a single disc test is under debate. It is therefore preferable to test both drugs separately with the two discs placed apart at a distance which enables the presence or absence of synergy to be demonstrated (Waterworth, 1969).

2.4 INTERACTIONS IN MIXTURES FOR PARENTERAL INFUSION

Interactions between drugs placed in the same bottle (or syringe) for parenteral infusion is now a well-documented difficulty. In clinical practice it is frequently overlooked! The problem is compounded by the fact that physical evidence of incompatability, such as precipitation, need not mean therapeutic inactivation since buffers or other additives may be incompatible rather than the drugs themselves. If the mixture shows evidence of such precipitation it should, of course, be discarded. Conversely, some chemical interactions may result in clinically significant changes without any visible evidence of deterioration. This type of incompatability presents a greater hazard than those resulting in a visible change.

One of the chief causes of incompatability is alteration in pH of which the inactivation of potassium penicillin G by vitamin C is an example. Penicillin is most stable in the pH range 6–7. As tetracycline hydrochloride

TABLE II

Antibiotic incompatibilities for parenteral administration

Antibiotic	pH	Incompatibilities
Amphotericin B	5	Avoid adding any drugs: e.g. potassium chloride, results in precipitation, as does the ascorbic acid in "parentrovite" or in tetracycline preparations
Cephalosporins*		Barbiturates, calcium chloride and gluconate, erythromycin, polymixins, tetracyclines, trometamol (Tham, Tris). Hydrocortisone sodium succinate, aminophylline, chloramphenicol, kanamycin, penicillin G, sulfisoxazole
Cephaloridine	3.5–6	
Cephalothin		
Chloramphenicol	6–7.5	Ascorbic acid (included in parentrovite), erythromycin, penicillins, phenothiazines, hydrocortisone solutions, sulphonamides, tetracyclines, aminophylline, cephalothin, sulfisoxazole
Erythromycin	7.5	Acid and alkaline solutions, barbiturates, cephalosporins, chloramphenicol, heparin, metaraminol, penicillin, phenothiazines, streptomycin, tetracycline, aminophylline
Lincomycin	6	Penicillins, sulphonamides
Penicillins	8–10	Ascorbic acid, barbiturates, chloramphenicol, heparin, phenothiazines, sulphonamides, tetracyclines, sodium bicarbonate, Amphotericin B
Ampicillin	5–7	
Benzylpenicillin	5–7	
Carbenicillin	6–8	
Cloxacillin	5–7	
Flucloxacillin	5–7	
Methicillin	7–8	As above plus aminophylline, hydrocortisone sodium succinate
Polymyxins	6.5–7.5	Do not mix with drugs of very high or low pH, e.g. ascorbic acid, barbiturates, cephalosporins, penicillins, sulphonamides, tetracyclines. Also avoid amphotericin B, chlorothiazide, heparin, hydrocortisone, sodium succinate, thiopentone, vitamins
Colistin		
Polymyxin B		
Aminoglycosides		Amphotericin B, ampicillin, barbiturates, chloramphenicol, heparin, sulphonamides, tetracyclines, calcium salts
Gentamicin	4.5	
Kanamycin	6	
Streptomycin	5–5.5	
Sulphonamides	8.5–10.5	Chloramphenicol, iron dextran, lignocaine, lincomycin, methyldopa, phenothiazines, streptomycin group, tetracyclines, vitamins (parentrovite)
Tetracyclines		Aminophylline, barbiturates, calcium salts, cephalosporins, chloramphenicol, erythromycin, heparin, hydrocortisone, penicillins, polymyxins, riboflavine (in pabrinex and parentrovite), sulphadiazine, methyldopa
Chlortetracycline	3–4	
Oxytetracycline	2–3	
Tetracycline	2–3	

* May be added to saline or dextrose without significant loss of potency over 12 hr.

solutions for intravenous administration may contain vitamin C as a buffer, penicillin G will be inactivated if the two are mixed. In one such experiment the loss was 37% in 6 hr (Medical Letter, 1968).

It has also been shown that penicillin, ampicillin, oxacillin, dicloxacillin and nafcillin in the presence of sucrose and bicarbonate lose approximately 90% of their activity in 24 hr. A similar effect is observed with 6% dextran (Editorial, Brit. Med. J., 1970b; Simberkoff et al., 1970). For a more detailed review of interactions involving the penicillins reference should be made to the publications of Lynn (1970, 1971; Lynn and Jones, 1971).

There has been a great deal of recent interest in the inactivation of gentamicin in the presence of high concentrations of carbenicillin (McLaughlin and Reeves, 1971; Jackson and Riff, 1971; Noone and Pattison, 1971). Although some evidence has been published to suggest that this may have an adverse effect on therapy, this is not sufficient to lead to the abandonment of this combination. However, it does seem wise to administer the two agents separately.

A summary of some of the more significant incompatibilities is contained in Table II (Drugs, 1969; Guide to i.v. Additives, 1971). The only reasonable practical advice is that, if at all possible, therapeutic agents should not be mixed and that intravenous therapy should be carried out using a T-tube drip so that the drugs can be infused separately. Occasionally it may be necessary to mix drugs in which case their compatibilities should be checked from the manufacturers label prior to administration.

3 Therapeutic antibiotic combinations

3.1 GENERAL

One reason sometimes given to justify the use of several drugs is the reduction of toxic effects by using a lower dose of each individual drug. This manoeuvre has not entered the author's experience. Mixed infections may sometimes necessitate more than one antimicrobial but with the exception of superficial skin infections where various combinations of bacitracin, neomycin and polymyxins are often employed it is usually possible to choose a single agent with effect. Several antibiotics have been used with justification in serious infections such as septic shock or neonatal pneumonia before the responsible organism has been determined (Medical Letter, 1972a). Even in these circumstances the choice can be narrowed by an intelligent assessment of the probable organisms and their current sensitivities (the antibiogram) (Medical Letter, 1972b). For example, in septic shock following genito-urinary instrumentation, treatment with gentamicin alone will suffice at the present time. As the antibiogram changes this policy may need to be modified.

3.2 ANTIMICROBIAL INTERACTIONS WITH HETEROGENEOUS BACTERIAL POPULATIONS

A universally accepted reason for the use of several antibiotics is to prevent the emergence of resistant bacteria during the course of treatment. This involves a rather complex group of interactions of the drugs with what is, in effect, a non-homogeneous population of organisms. The best example is antituberculous chemotherapy when the patient is infected with a *large* population of tubercle bacilli. The resistance mutation rate of *Mycobacterium tuberculosis* to streptomycin is approximately 10^{-5}. If standard therapy with three effective drugs is employed there would need to be more than 10^{15} tubercle bacilli present in the patient for there to be a statistical chance of a resistant mutant emerging. It is unlikely that this weight of infection is ever encountered (10^{15} tubercle bacilli weight >1 kg) and in many regimens only two drugs are now employed for this reason (Newman et al., 1971). At the other extreme, in persons whose only evidence of tuberculous infection is a positive skin test, the total population of bacilli is so small that it is safe to employ only one drug. The usual choice is isoniazid because of its high antituberculous activity and low toxicity. It must be emphasised that while the emergence of drug resistant mutants is often blamed for failure of therapy this is seldom true in acute infections. Emergence of resistance usually occurs in chronic infections treated for more than seven days with aminoglycosides or bacteriostatic antibiotics (Sanders and Cluff, 1968; Wright and Harper, 1970).

There are some other interesting examples of interactions of several antibiotics with 'large' heterogeneous bacterial populations. There is the unusual type of 'pseudo synergy' between penicillin G and fucidin against staphylococci producing *small* amounts of penicillinase (Waterworth, 1963). The majority of the staphylococci are inhibited by the fucidin while the small numbers of mutants resistant to fucidin are too few to exert a significant penicillinase effect and are killed by the penicillin. In contrast, fucidin may be shown to be antagonistic to both methicillin and cloxacillin in vitro (Waterworth, 1963). Despite this and the tendency to the emergence of fucidin resistant mutants in clinical trials, the combination of fucidin plus methicillin has been used with success in the treatment of infections due to multiply-resistant staphylococci (Jensen and Lassen, 1969). In these studies no organism developed resistance to methicillin, and only one to fucidin. Unfortunately this may not obtain in the case of chronic infections and resistant mutants were more commonly observed when erythromycin plus novobiocin were employed in a burns unit (Lowbury, 1957) and fucidin and lincomycin in patients with cystic fibrosis (Wright and Harper, 1970).

In recent years yet another fascinating set of interactions between mixed bacterial populations and the penicillins have been described. Penicillinase-producing staphylococci if present in the urethra may provide a 'penicillinase umbrella' for gonococci and prevent their eradication by penicillin (Sanders et al., 1962). It has also been suggested that penicillinase-producing staphylococci (Massell et al., 1966) and enterobacteria (Maddocks and May, 1969) in the upper respiratory tract may reduce the efficacy of ampicillin in the treatment of streptococcal and *Haemophilus* infections respectively. In this situation methicillin may be useful, in the first two cases to kill off the staphylococci and in the third to bind the enterobacterial penicillinase. Certainly methicillin in vitro can bind and inactivate *Pseudomonas* penicillinase and allow the Pseudomonad to be killed by penicillin G (Sabath et al., 1970). One obstacle to the application of this type of therapeutic manipulation is in its identification by the laboratory.

4 Indifference, antagonism and synergy between antimicrobials acting on a single bacterial population

4.1 GENERAL

Jawetz and Gunnison (1952) suggested that two bactericidal antibiotics might be synergistic, combinations of bacteriostatic agents indifferent, and bactericidal plus bacteriostatic possibly antagonistic. Jawetz himself points out that this hypothesis has not been substantiated and that no general rules can now be drawn. For example, two bactericidal agents, penicillin and carbenicillin, have been shown to be antagonistic against a strain of *Enterobacter cloacae* (Seligman, 1968), and nalidixic acid and nitrofurantoin are antagonistic when tested against some *Proteus* species (Garrod and O'Grady, 1971). Then there is the bactericidal synergy between the sulphonamides and trimethoprim which singly are bacteriostatic (Reeves, 1971). Finally, while penicillin plus sulphonamides seem to be indifferent, the polymyxins are synergistic with both sulphonamides (Russell, 1963; Holmgren and Möller, 1970) and trimethoprim (Noall et al., 1962) against *Proteus* species, and polymyxins and sulphonamides against *Pseudomonas* (Simmons, 1969).

4.2 INDIFFERENCE

Indifference is, by far, the commonest (70–90 %) result when two or more antibiotics are tested in combination against a single microbial population. In some cases a rational explanation for this can be advanced. For example, cycloserine inhibits the incorporation of D-alanine into the bacterial cell wall. As the penicillins act at a later stage in cell wall synthesis, by preventing cross linkage of the preformed glycopeptide, their effect is irrelevant if cycloserine has already done its work.

4.3 ANTAGONISM

Many cases of antagonism between antibiotics have been demonstrated. The antagonism between nitrofurantoin and nalidixic acid in relation to *Proteus* species has already been referred to (Garrod and O'Grady, 1971). In the presence of erythromycin, *Staphylococcus aureus* becomes resistant to lincomycin and these two agents should not be used together. The explanation may be that erythromycin induces an enzyme which confers resistance to lincomycin (Barber and Waterworth, 1964). Because of the complexity of these types of effects their role in clinical practice is difficult to assess. It is probably minor in the majority of cases.

In contrast, antagonism between penicillin and tetracycline or chloramphenicol is of great clinical significance. Mice with experimental streptococcal infections have a higher (50%) mortality when treated with penicillin and tetracycline than if they are treated with penicillin alone (0%) (Jawetz, 1971a or b). Similarly, Wallace et al. (1965) showed that penicillin-killed pneumococci when given before but not if given after or at the same time as chloramphenicol. This was true in vitro and also in experimental meningitis in dogs. When patients with pneumococcal meningitis were treated with penicillin (12 Munits/day for 14 days) the mortality was 30%. When chloramphenicol was added in dosage of 50 mg/kg/day the mortality was 79% (Lepper and Dowling, 1951). Similarly, Mathies et al. (1967) at the Los Angeles General Hospital showed that when patients with several types of meningitis (e.g. *Haemophilus*, pneumococcal and meningococcal) were treated with ampicillin alone, the mortality was 4.3% (43 patients). When chloramphenicol (100 mg/kg/day) and streptomycin (for 2 days) were added, the mortality was 10.5%. Again, Strom (1955) showed that the addition of chlortetracyline to penicillin in the treatment of streptococcal pharyngitis interfered with the elimination of the streptococci from the throat. The probable explanation for all these phenomena is that penicillin is most effective in preventing cell wall synthesis in a rapidly dividing bacterial population. If cell division is arrested by the action of tetracycline or chloramphenicol, penicillin loses its bactericidal effect.

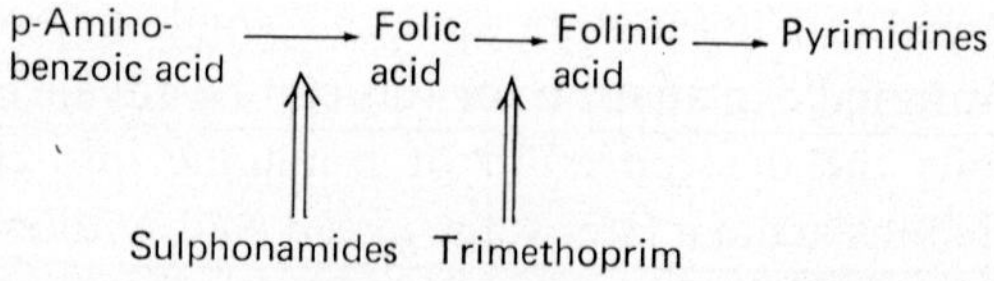

Fig. 2. The sites of action of the sulphonamides and trimethoprim in relation to folate metabolism.

4.4 SYNERGY

Synergy between antimicrobial agents is, unfortunately, rare. One spectacular exception to this is the bactericidal synergy between trimethoprim and the sulphonamides (cotrimoxazole). The two agents act at sequential points on the biochemical pathway which synthesises PABA into nucleic acids (Fig. 2). The therapeutic role of this combination has been reviewed by Reeves (1971) and, unlike most synergistic combinations, cotrimoxazole finds application in many common clinical situations, particularly respiratory and urinary infections. It has also been used, with apparent effect, in a variety of other conditions such as gonorrhoea, nocardiosis (Baikie et al., 1970), Q fever (Freeman and Hodson, 1972), serious staphylococcal infections, typhoid and brucellosis. Unfortunately *Haemophilus* (Garrod and O'Grady, 1971) and coliforms (Lacey et al., 1972) resistant to trimethoprim have already been described, and in this event synergy with the sulphonamides is improbable. Like the sulphonamides, trimethoprim is also synergistic with the polymyxins (Noall et al., 1962). Trimethoprim has also been used with sulphonamides in the treatment of drug resistant falciparum malaria (Leading article, 1971). In this context of drugs interfering with folate metabolism it is also appropriate to mention the combination of pyrimethamine and the sulphonamides in the treatment of falciparum and vivax malaria and in toxoplasmosis (Nolan and Rosen, 1968).

While the bacterial enzyme, dihydrofolate reductase, which converts folic to folinic acid (Fig. 2) is 10^4 times more sensitive to trimethoprim than its mammalian counterpart, it is not surprising that cotrimoxazole can interfere with folate metabolism in man causing a reduction in serum folate levels. However, folate depletion is not so marked as with the less selective pyrimethamine and few related haematological abnormalities have actually been observed (Allison et al., 1969; Whitman, 1969). One possible exception is that trimethoprim may prevent a satisfactory response to vitamin B12 in patients with megaloblastic haemopoiesis (Chanarin and England, 1972). Clearly, cotrimoxazole will share the untoward effects of the sulphonamides and unique adverse reactions may be difficult to prove. Hulme and Reeves (1971) have, however, described a leucopenia in renal transplant patients which they feel, on statistical grounds, may be specific. Leucopenia has also been reported in patients with typhoid treated with cotrimoxazole (Stamps and Wicks, 1972). Large doses of trimethoprim are teratogenic in rats (Udall, 1969) and, although cotrimoxazole has been used in all trimesters of pregnancy without any effect on the foetus (Williams et al., 1969), it seems reasonable to maintain vigilance in this regard particularly as, like thalidomide, trimethoprim may have immunosuppressive properties (Ghilchik et al., 1970).

TABLE III

Some antimicrobial combinations worthy of trial for bactericidal synergy

Streptococci		
Penicillin, cephaloridine or erythromycin	plus	Aminoglycosides* or vancomycin
Staphylococci		
Methicillin or cephaloridine	plus	Aminoglycosides or vancomycin
Erythromycin or novobiocin	plus	Aminoglycosides
Erythromycin or fucidin	plus	Rifamide
Gram-negative bacilli		
Ampicillin, carbenicillin or cephaloridine	plus	Aminoglycosides

* Aminoglycosides (streptomycin, kanamycin, neomycin, gentamicin).

Apart from the examples already given and the few serious infections with resistant organisms, such as endocarditis and osteomyelitis, the search for and application of synergistic interactions between antimicrobial drugs is seldom necessary. Such treatment must be tailored to the individual patient, and should only be initiated and can only be carried through in the closest liaison with the microbiologist. A list of some combinations worthy of test for synergy is contained in Table III (Garrod and O'Grady, 1971). The archetype of this problem is the synergy between penicillin and streptomycin in the management of enterococcal endocarditis. In one case, neither penicillin (16 μg/ml) nor streptomycin (10 μg/ml) alone had a significant effect on the enterococcus. When the two agents were combined in the same concentrations a complete bactericidal effect was achieved in vitro (Garrod and O'Grady, 1971). This phenomenon in vitro corresponds to therapeutic efficacy in patients. In a review presented by Jawetz (1971a or b) all of six patients with enterococcal endocarditis failed to respond to penicillin (6–12 g) or ampicillin (4–8 g) alone. When streptomycin was added to this regimen only 1 patient out of 6 failed to respond. The dose of streptomycin should probably be of the order of 0.5 g 4 times daily in an effort to keep the peak levels of streptomycin low relative to the mean level. If there is renal impairment this dose should be reduced. Other combinations which have been used in the treatment of enterococcal endocarditis include penicillin + kanamycin (Garrod and Waterworth, 1962), penicillin + neomycin, penicillin + erythromycin and/or bacitracin (Jawetz and Sonne, 1966) and penicillin + gentamicin (Watananakuakorn, 1971). Such combinations are occasionally necessary in the treatment of endocarditis due to '*Streptococcus viridans*' (Dormer, 1960).

Staphylococcal endocarditis seems to be on the increase and can present a difficult management problem. In cases due to 'penicillin sensitive' *Staphylococcus aureus* the addition of streptomycin and kanamycin may be needed to achieve a complete bactericidal effect. If the organism is resistant to methicillin, kanamycin + methicillin or kanamycin + cephalothin may be effective (Bulger, 1967). Another possibility is fucidin + methicillin although Jensen and Lassen (1969) reported two failures when this combination was used. Staphylococcus albus endocarditis can occur with or without pre-existing heart disease or post cardiotomy. Penicillin + streptomycin seems to be effective if the organism is sensitive to penicillin. If the organism is resistant to penicillin the course is less clear and depends on testing the organism against various combinations including vancomycin (Dowling, 1952; Lerner and Weinstein, 1966; Quinn and Cox, 1970).

5 Conclusions

Antibiotic combinations have only a small place in antimicrobial chemotherapy. With some exceptions such as cotrimoxazole, which has found an important role in the management of respiratory and urinary infections, and the administrative convenience of PAS–INH cachets, fixed combinations are to be condemned. Apart from tuberculous chemotherapy the need for several agents to prevent the emergence of resistant mutants is rare. In most other situations the disadvantages of cost and cumulative adverse effects exist without any counter gains. The rational application of antimicrobial synergy is confined to hospital practice and then only in close liaison with the microbiologist.

References

All'son, M. E. M., Kennedy, A. C., McGeachie, J. and McDonald, G. A. (1969): Sulphamethoxazole-trimethoprim therapy in urinary tract infection with reference to its haematological effects. *Scot. med. J.*, **14**, 355.

Anderson, E. S. (1968): Drug resistance in *salmonella typhimurium* and its implication. *Brit. med. J.*, **3**, 333.

Baikie, A. G., MacDonald, C. B. and Mundy, G. R. (1970): Systemic nocardiasis treated with trimethoprim and sulphamethoxazole. *Lancet*, **2**, 261.

Barber, M. and Waterworth, P. M. (1964): Antibacterial activity of lincomycins and pristinamycin: A comparison with erythromycin. *Brit. med. J.*, **2**, 603.

Boman, G., Hanngren, A., Malmborg, A-S., Borgå, O. and Sjöqvist, F. (1971): Decreased serum concentrations of rifampin when given with PAS. *Lancet*, *ii*, 800.

Brown, J. J., Gleadle, R. I., Lawson, D. H. et al. (1970): Renin and acute renal failure: studies in man. *Brit. med. J.*, **1**, 253.

Bulger, R. J. (1967): In-vitro activity of cephalothin–kanamycin and methicillin–kanamycin combinations against methicillin-resistant *Staphylococcus aureus*. *Lancet*, **1**, 17.

Chanarin, I. and England, J. M. (1972): Toxicity of trimethoprim–sulphamethoxazole in patients with megaloblastic haemopoiesis. *Brit. med. J.*, **1**, 651.

Cobbold, R. J. C., Morrison, G. D., Spitzer, R. J. and Willcox, R. R. (1970): One-session treatment of gonorrhoea in males with procaine penicillin plus probenecid. *Postgrad. med. J.*, **46**, 142.

Craig, H. V., Guillet, G. G., Walker, J. A. and Artz, C. P. (1966): Respiratory depression related to intraperitoneal neomycin. *Amer. Surg.*, **32**, 27.

Datta, N. (1969): Drug resistance and R factors in the bowel bacteria of London patients before and after admission to hospital. *Brit. med. J.*, **2**, 407.

Davis, C. M., Fulghum, D. D. and Taplin, D. (1968): The value of neomycin in a neomycin steroid cream. *J. Amer. med. Assoc.*, **203**, 298.

Dormer, A. E. (1960): The treatment of bacterial endocarditis. *Brit. med. Bull.*, **16**, 61.

Dowling, H. F. (1952): Staphylococci endocarditis: an analysis of 25 cases treated with antibiotics along with a review of the literature. *Medicine*, **31**, 155.

Drugs. Drug incompatibilities for parenteral administration. Drugs Aug. 1969. Publ. Dept. Pharmaceutical and Central Supply Services, Shands Teaching Hospital, University of Florida.

Editorial (1969): Fixed dose antibiotic combinations. *Lancet*, *iii*, 365.

Editorial (1970a): Another drug interaction (tetracyclines). *Brit. med. J.*, **4**, 509.

Editorial (1970b): Penicillin instability in infusions. *Brit. med. J.*, **4**, 571.

Editorial (1971a): Drugs altering anticoagulants. *Brit. med. J.*, **1**, 360.

Editorial (1971b): Antibiotic sensitivity testing. *Brit. med. J.*, **2**, 416.

Ellard, G. A., Gammon, P. T. *et al.* (1972): Pharmacology of some slow-release preparations of isoniazid of potential use in intermittent treatment of tuberculosis. *Lancet*, *i*, 340.

Formiller, M. and Cotton, M. S. (1969): Coumarin and inandione anticoagulants: potentiators and antagonists. *Amer. J. hosp. Pharm.*, **26**, 574.

Freeman, R. and Hodson, M. E. (1972): Q Fever endocarditis treated with trimethoprim and sulphamethoxazole. *Brit. med. J.*, **1**, 419.

Garrod, L. P. and O'Grady, F. (1971): In: *Antibiotics and Chemotherapy*. Livingstone, Edinburgh.

Garrod, L. P. and Waterworth, P. M. (1962): Methods of testing combined antibiotic bactericidal action and the significance of the results. *J. clin. Pathol.*, **15**, 328.

Garrod, L. P. and Waterworth, P. M. (1969): Effect of medium composition on the apparent sensitivity of *Pseudomonas aeroginosa* to gentamicin. *J. clin. Pathol.*, **22**, 534.

Gaya, H., Adnitt, P. I. and Turner, P. (1970): Changes in gut flora after Cephalexin treatment. *Brit. med. J.*, **3**, 624.

Ghilchik, M. W., Morris, A. S. and Reeves, D. S. (1970): Immunosuppressive powers of the antibacterial agent trimethoprim. *Nature*, **227**, 393.

Guide to i.v. additives (1971): Pharmacy Department, St. Mary's Hospital, London W.2.

Hewitt, J. H., Coe, A. W. and Parker, M. T. (1969): The detection of methicillin resistance in *Staphylococcus aureus*. *J. med. Microbiol.*, **2**, 443.

Hewlitt, W. L. and Kunin, C. M. (1969): Fixed combinations of antimicrobial agents. *New Engl. J. Med.*, **280**, 1149.

Holmgren, J. and Möller, O. (1970): Studies on the sensitivity of *Proteus mirabilis* and

Proteus vulgaris to sulphonamide and colistin, alone and in combination. *Scand. infect. Diseases*, **2**, 121.

Hulme, B. and Reeves, D. S. (1971): Leucopenia associated with trimethoprim–sulphamethoxazole after renal transplantation. *Brit. med. J.*, **3**, 610.

Jackson, G. G. and Riff, L. (1971): Gentamicin plus carbenicillin. *Lancet*, **1**, 592.

Jawetz, E. (1971a): Problems of antimicrobial combinations. In: *Changing Patterns of Bacterial Infections and Antibiotic Therapy*, p. 47. Editor: H. C. Neu. Excerpta Medica, Amsterdam.

Jawetz, E. (1971b): See Jawetz (1971a), p. 49.

Jawetz, E. and Gunnison, J. B. (1952): Studies on antibiotic synergism and antagonism: a scheme of combined antibiotic action. *Antibiot. Chemotherap.*, **2**, 243.

Jawetz, E. and Sonne, M. (1966): Penicillin–streptomycin treatment of enterococcal endocarditis. A re-evaluation. *New Engl. J. Med.*, **274**, 710.

Jensen, K. and Lassen, H. C. A. (1969): Combined treatment with antibacterial chemotherapeutical agents in staphylococcal infections. *Quart. J. Med.*, **38**, 91.

Koch-Weser, J. and Sellers, E. M. (1971): Drug interactions with coumarin anticoagulants. *New Engl. J. Med.*, **285**, 487 and 547.

Lacey, R. W., Brutten, D. M., Gillespie, W. A. and Lewis, E. L. (1972): Trimethoprim resistant coliforms. *Lancet*, **1**, 409.

Lawson, D. H., Macadam, R. F., Singh, H. et al. (1970): The nephrotoxicity of cephaloridine. *Postgrad. med. J., Suppl.*, **46**, 36.

Leading article (1971): Drug resistance in malaria. *Lancet*, **3**, 855.

Lepper, N. H. and Dowling, H. F. (1951): Treatment of pneumococcal meningitis with penicillin compared with penicillin plus aureomycin. *Arch. int. Med.*, **88**, 489.

Lerner, P. I. and Weinstein, L. (1966): Infective endocarditis in the antibiotic era. *New Engl. J. Mea.*, **274**, 199.

Lorber, J. (1960): Treatment of tuberculous meningitis. *Brit. med. J.*, **1**, 1309.

Lowbury, E. J. L. (1957): Chemotherapy for *Staphylococcus aureus*. Combined use of novobiocin and erythromycin in the treatment of burns. *Lancet*, *ii*, 305.

Lynn, B. (1970): Pharmaceutical aspects of semi-synthetic penicillins. *J. hosp. Pharm.*, March 1970.

Lynn, B. (1971): Recent work on parenteral penicillins. *J. hosp. Pharm.* July 1971.

Lynn, B. and Jones, A. (1971): Interactions between penicillins and aminoglycoside antibiotics in parenteral solution, 7th Internat. Congr. Chemother. (Prague 1971). To be published.

Maddocks, J. L. and May, J. R. (1969): "Indirect pathogenicity" of penicillinase-producing enterobacteria in chronic bronchial infections. *Lancet*, **2**, 793.

Maronde, R. F., Burks, D. and Lee, P. V. (1969): Physician prescribing practices. A computer based study. *Amer. J. hosp. Pharm.*, **26**, 566.

Massell, B. F., Michael, J. G., Michael, T. and Amezcua, J. (1966): Temporary suppression of penicillinase producing staphylococci by oxytetracycline. *Amer. J. med. Sci.*, **252**, 314.

Mathies, A. W., Leedom, J. M., Ivler, D., Wehrle, P. F. and Portnoy, B. (1967): Antibiotic antagonism in bacterial meningitis. In: *Antimicrob. Agents Chemotherap.*, p. 218.

McLaughlin, J. E. and Reeves, D. S. (1971): Clinical and laboratory evidence for inactivation of gentamicin by carbenicillin. *Lancet*, **1**, 261.

Medical Letter (1968): Continuous versus intermittent intravenous antibiotics. *Med. Letter Drugs, Therap.*, **10**, 57.

Medical Letter (1971a): Principal toxic, allergic and other adverse effects of antimicrobial drugs. *Med. Letter, Drugs Therap.*, **13**, 53.

Medical Letter (1971b): Use of probenecid in antimicrobial therapy. *Med. Letter, Drugs Therap.*, **13**, 88.

Medical Letter (1971c): Interpretation of antimicrobial susceptibility tests. *Med. Letter, Drugs Therap.*, **13**, 89.

Medical Letter (1972a): Pathogens most likely to cause acute infections. *Med. Letter, Drugs Therap.*, **14**, 20.

Medical Letter (1972b): The choice of systemic antimicrobial drugs. *Med. Letter, Drugs Therap.*, **14**, 8.

Neuvonen, P. J., Gothoni, G., Hackman, R. and Björksten, K.af. (1970): Interference of iron with absorption of tetracyclines in man. *Brit. med. J.*, **4**, 532.

Newman, R., Doster, B., Murray, F. J. and Ferebee, S. (1971): Rifampin in initial treatment of pulmonary tuberculosis. *Amer. Rev. resp. Dis.*, **103**, 461.

Noall, E. W. P., Sewards, H. F. G. and Waterworth, D. M. (1962): Successful treatment of a case of *Proteus* septicaemia. *Brit. med. J.*, **2**, 1101.

Nolan, J. and Rosen, E. S. (1968): Treatment of active toxoplasmic retino-choroiditis. *Brit. J. Ophthal.*, **52**, 396.

Noone, P. and Pattison, J. R. (1971): Therapeutic implications of interaction of gentamicin and penicillins. *Lancet*, **3**, 575.

Philp, J. R. (1970): Rational prescribing and drug usage. *Amer. J. hosp. Pharm.*, **27**, 659.

Philp, J. R. (1971): Untoward effects of antimicrobial drugs. *Postgrad. Med. J.*, **50**, 193.

Pindell, M. H. (1966): The pharmacology of kanamycin – a review and new developments. *Ann. N.Y. Acad. Sci.*, **132**, 805.

Price, D. J. and Sleigh, J. D. (1970): Control of infection due to *Klebsiella aerogenes* in a neurosurgical unit by withdrawal of all antibiotics. *Lancet*, **2**, 1213.

Quinn, E. L. and Cox, F. (1970): Bacterial endocarditis based upon experience with 203 patients. In: *Antimicrobial Therapy*, p. 260. Editor: Kagan. Saunders, Philadelphia, London, Toronto.

Reeves, D. S. (1971): Sulphamethoxazole–trimethoprim: the first two years. *J. clin. Pathol.*, **24**, 430.

Remington, J. S. (1971): Infection in transplant patients. Proc. Internat. Conf. Nosocamial Infections, p. 95. Editors: P. S. Brachman and T. C. Eickhoff. Publ. Amer. Hosp. Assoc. Chicago.

Report (1968): Comparison of side effects of tetracycline and tetracycline plus nystatin. *Brit. med. J.*, **4**, 411.

Russell, F. E. (1963): Synergism between sulphonamide drugs and antibiotics of the polymyxin group against *Proteus* sp. in vitro. *J. clin. Pathol.*, **16**, 362.

Sabath, L. D., Gerstein, D. A., Leaf, C. D. and Finland, M. (1970): Increasing the usefulness of antibiotics. Treatment of infections caused by Gram-negative bacilli. *Clin. Pharm. Therap.*, **11**, 161.

Sanders, E. and Cluff, L. E. (1968): Mechanism of action of antimicrobial agents. *Paediat. clin. N. Amer.*, **15**, 3.

Sanders, A. C., Pelczar, M. J. and Hoefling, A. F. (1962): Interactions of staphylococcus and *Neisseria gonorrhoeae* in "penicillin resistant" gonorrhoea. *Antibiot. Chemother.*, **12**, 1.

Seligman, S. J. (1968): Resistance of *Klebsiella* and *enterobacter* to the penicillins. *Proc. Soc. exp. med. Biol.*, **127**, 915.

Simberkoff, M. S., Thomas, L., McGregor, D. et al. (1970): Inactivation of penicillins by carbohydrate solutions at alkaline pH. *New Engl. J. Med.*, **283**, 116.

Simmons, N. A. (1969): Potentiation of Inhibitory Activity of colistin on *Pseudomonas aeroginosa* by Sulphamethoxazole and sulphamethizole. *Brit. med. J.*, **3**, 603.

Stamps, T. J. and Wicks, A. C. B. (1972): Trimethoprim–sulphamethoxazole in typhoid fever. *Brit. med. J.*, **1**, 176.

Strom, J. (1955): The question of antagonism between penicillin and chlortetracycline. Illustrated by therapeutical experiments in scarlatina. *Antibiot. Med.*, **1**, 6.

Tucker, H. St. G. and Hirsch, J. I. (1972): Sulfonamide–sulfonylurea interaction. *New Engl. J. Med.*, **286**, 110.

Udall, V. (1969): Toxicology of sulphonamide–trimethoprim combinations. *Postgrad. med. J.*, **45**, *Suppl.*, 42.

Wallace, J. F., Smith, R. H., Garcia, M. and Petersdorf, R. G. (1965): Antagonism between penicillin and chloramphenicol in experimental pneumococcal meningitis. *Antimicrob. Agents Chemotherap.*, **5**, 439.

Watananakuakorn, C. (1971): Penicillin combined with gentamicin or streptomycin: synergism against enterococci. *J. infect. Dis.*, **124**, 581.

Waterworth, P. M. (1963): Apparent synergy between penicillin and erythromycin or fusidic acid. *Clin. Med.*, **70**, 941.

Waterworth, P. M. (1969): Practical aspects of testing sensitivity to trimethoprim and sulphonamide. *Postgrad. med. J.*, **45**, *Suppl.*, 21.

Whitman, E. W. (1969): Effects in man of prolonged administration of trimethoprim and sulfisoxazole. *Postgrad. med. J.*, **45**, *Suppl.*, 46.

Williams, J. D., Brumfitt, W., Condie, A. P. and Reeves, D. S. (1969): The treatment of bacteriuria in pregnant women with sulphamethoxazole and trimethoprim. A microbiological clinical and toxicological study. *Postgrad. med. J.* **45**, *Suppl.*, 71.

Wright, G. L. T. and Harper, J. (1970): Fusidic acid and lincomycin therapy in staphylococcal infections in cystic fibrosis. *Lancet*, **1**, 9.

CHAPTER 10

Drug interactions and the kidney

M. D. MILNE

1 Introduction

Interactions between drugs in relation to the kidney can be conveniently classified as follows:

(i) There may be a potentiation or an inhibition of a desirable effect of a drug on renal function or disease;

(ii) There may be potentiation or prevention of undesirable toxic effects on kidney structure or function;

(iii) The effects of one drug may alter the excretion rate in the urine of another drug, and thus affect the half-life of the compound within the body.

Interactions relating to the kidney are both numerous and complex, and therefore this account will make no attempt to be comprehensive but will detail the more important and frequent interactions in current practice.

2 Desirable actions of drugs on renal function and disease

The main classes of drugs which are prescribed primarily for therapy of renal disease or for desirable effects on renal function are:

Diuretic drugs;
Drugs used in the control of urinary infections;
Uricosuric drugs;
Immunosuppressive drugs;
Anticoagulant drugs in glomerular disease.

2.1 DIURETICS

Diuretics increase the rate of sodium excretion in the urine in states of constant sodium intake, and thereby reduce the body sodium content. This will cause a secondary rise of urinary volume by increase of the solute load. Increase of urinary sodium is almost invariably due to reduction of sodium reabsorption by the renal tubular epithelial cells, but this process is extremely complex and still poorly understood. It may, however, be sub-divided as follows:

(i) Proximal tubular isosmotic reabsorption of Na^+ and Cl^-;

(ii) Proximal tubular reabsorption of Na^+ in exchange for H^+, production of hydrogen ion being dependent on the activity of carbonic anhydrase. By progressive acidification of the tubular fluid, this mechanism also reduces urinary content of HCO_3^-;

(iii) Sodium reabsorption at or very near Henle's loop;

(iv) Sodium reabsorption in the deeper parts of the ascending limb where osmolality of the tubular fluid is progressively reduced to a level equal to that of plasma and other major body fluids;

(v) Sodium reabsorption in more superficial parts of the ascending limb with progressive dilution of the tubular fluid below the isosmotic value;

(vi) Further sodium absorption in the distal convoluted tubule;

(vii) Ion exchange under the control of aldosterone whereby H^+ and K^+ are directly exchanged for Na^+;

(viii) Similar distal tubular ion exchange which, however, is not under the control of aldosterone.

Much progress has been made in defining the exact sites of action of the major diuretic drugs both in man and in the experimental animal. Obviously, if two diuretic agents administered together act on separate areas of the renal tubule they are more likely to be additive than if they act on the same site. In the latter case the effects of the drugs will only be additive if both are given at a sub-maximal dose, and in fact the apparent potentiation could equally be achieved by increasing the dose of either drug in isolation.

2.1.1 *Mercurial diuretics*

These drugs have been largely superseded by agents active by mouth, but are still used on occasions. All effective organic mercurial diuretics possess acid labile-carbon to mercury bonds, and release ionized mercury within the renal parenchyma (Clarkson et al., 1965). This explains the well-known potentiation of mercurial action by the metabolic acidosis produced by ingestion of ammonium chloride or acetazolamide, and the corresponding depression of diuretic action in states of metabolic alkalosis (Farah et al., 1959), e.g. after ingestion of sodium or potassium bicarbonate. Mercurial diuresis can be prevented or terminated by injection of the dithiol compound, dimercaprol, but monothiol compounds, e.g. cysteine, are inactive (Cafruny and Farah, 1956; Farah and Kruse, 1960). This suggests that dimercaprol has a greater affinity for mercury ions than the tubular receptor site, whereas cysteine has less affinity. Organic mercurials which have acid stable-carbon to mercury bonds have no diuretic action (Kessler et al., 1957), but may reduce or prevent the diuretic action of the active mercurials by a competitive interaction at the receptor site.

The simultaneous injection of different mercurial diuretics merely produces an additive effect without any true potentiation of activity. Other types of diuretics act on different sites of the nephron and may, therefore, increase sodium output by true potentiation of mercurial action, e.g. thiazides, acetazolamide, frusemide, ethacrynic acid, spironolactone, triamterene and amiloride. Continued administration of mercurial diuretics alone will rapidly produce a refractory state by at least two separate mechanisms. Increased urinary output of hydrogen ion, which is an unavoidable effect of mercurial action, causes a metabolic alkalosis which itself reduces mercurial action, and progressive sodium loss together with retention of mercury within the renal cortex will reduce the glomerular filtration rate and also produce secondary hyperaldosteronism. Such undesirable mercury retention occurs whenever injections of organic mercurials are continued despite a refractory state without any increase of urinary volume and sodium output, and especially when associated with a significant reduction of the glomerular filtration rate (Burch et al., 1950; Grossman et al., 1951). The exact site of action of mercurial diuretics in inhibition of sodium reabsorption is still uncertain. The most likely area is at the loop of Henle and the inner portion of the ascending limb, proximal to the medullary diluting site.

2.1.2 *Acetazolamide*

This drug owes its weak diuretic action to inhibition of the enzyme carbonic anhydrase. Less hydrogen ion is, therefore, available for exchange for sodium in the proximal tubular ion exchange site, and consequently more sodium and bicarbonate are excreted in the urine. As it acts on a separate reabsorptive area of the nephron than most other diuretics, it has a weak potentiating action on the activity of mercurials, thiazides, frusemide and ethacrynic acid. When given as the sole diuretic agent, its effect is weak and transitory. Increased output of bicarbonate causes a metabolic acidosis with a fall of plasma bicarbonate. As the filtered load of bicarbonate falls the diuretic effect is rapidly reduced, the drug therefore having a self-inhibitory action (Maren et al., 1961; Counihan et al., 1954). Metabolic acidosis produced by other agents, e.g. ammonium chloride, has a similar inhibitory effect. Acetazolamide is now little used as a diuretic and has been almost completely superseded.

2.1.3 *Benzothiadiazine diuretics*

These drugs are structurally similar, and are usually referred to by the abbreviated name of 'thiazides'. Quinethazone and chlorthalidone differ considerably in chemical structure and are, therefore, not strictly thiazide drugs, but have an identical type of pharmacological action. These drugs are only weak carbonic anhydrase inhibitors, their main effect being an inhibition of sodium and chloride reabsorption in the cortical segment of the ascending limb of Henle's loop (Earley and Orloff, 1964; Sullivan and Pirch, 1966). Other types of diuretic drugs in combination will, therefore, potentiate the action of thiazides, but different members of the thiazide group merely have a simple additive effect on sodium output. Structural analogues of thiazide drugs which themselves are devoid of diuretic activity can block the diuretic effect of potent thiazide drugs, by competition at renal tubular receptor sites (Ross and Cafruny, 1963).

In addition to their action as diuretics, these drugs are widely used as antihypertensive agents, either alone or as adjuvants of other more potent compounds.

They are also prescribed to reduce urinary volume in cases of diabetes insipidus (Crawford and Kennedy, 1959) and to reduce urinary calcium in cases of idiopathic hypercalcuria (Yendt et al., 1966; Harrison and Rose, 1968). Thiazides are useful in the control of polyuria in both nephrogenic diabetes insipidus and in the pituitary type of the disease, although obviously antidiuretic hormone is the most effective therapy in the latter. Chlorpropamide is active only in the pituitary type of the disease as it owes its effect to mobilization of antidiuretic hormone or to potentiation of the action of low subnormal levels of endogenous ADH (Miller and Moses, 1970). Thiazides are, therefore, chiefly useful in control of nephrogenic diabetes insipidus where other agents are ineffective.

Most diuretic drugs increase calcium output in addition to that of sodium (Parfitt, 1969; Tambyah and Lim, 1969). Thiazides, however, strongly reduce urinary calcium in previously hypercalciuric patients (Lamberg and Kühlback, 1959) and are, therefore, useful in the treatment of cases of idiopathic hypercalciuria causing nephrocalcinosis or urinary calculi. The effect is potentiated by drugs reducing calcium absorption from the gut, e.g. sodium phytate, inorganic phosphates, or sodium cellulose phosphate.

2.1.4 *Ethacrynic acid and frusemide*

Although these two highly potent diuretic drugs are completely dissimilar chemically, their pharmacological effects are almost, but not completely identical. Both drugs inhibit sodium and chloride absorption in the diluting segment of the medullary portion of the ascending limb of the loop of Henle (Goldberg et al., 1964; Suki et al., 1965; Morrin, 1966), and thus reduce the capacity of the kidney both to concentrate and to dilute urine. Given together they merely have an additive effect if the dosage of each is low, without any true potentiation of sodium output (Hook and Williamson, 1965). Other types of diuretic drugs including thiazides will, however, have a slight potentiating effect on the already powerful diuresis produced by either compound (Olesen and Sigurd, 1971). Frusemide is a weak carbonic anhydrase inhibitor, due to the $SO_2{\cdot}NH_2$ radicle, but this is not present in the molecule of ethacrynic acid. Urinary pH, therefore, increases after frusemide, but falls after ethacrynic acid (Puschett and Goldberg, 1968). Both drugs diminish free water clearance (C_{H_2O}), and reduce urinary diluting capacity, but ethacrynic acid is more potent than frusemide in this respect. Deafness, usually temporary but very occasionally permanent, may occur on overdose with either drug, especially if large amounts are given rapidly to patients suffering from severe renal failure (Wigand and Heidland, 1971). The main effect is on the organ of Corti, producing a mid-tone deafness. Presumably this toxic effect would be additive if both drugs were given together. Some antibiotics, e.g. streptomycin, neomycin and kanamycin, may damage the auditory tract by a more central action, and again this is more likely to occur in cases of renal failure. The risk of ototoxicity in patients suffering from renal failure can be minimized by reduced dosage of the drugs concerned and by avoidance of prescription of ototoxic agents simultaneously.

All diuretic drugs which increase urinary chloride will also inhibit tubular reabsorption of other halides, especially bromide and iodine. Thus, mercurials, thiazides, frusemide and ethacrynic acid combined with sodium chloride infusions are useful in the management of bromide poisoning by greatly increasing urinary output of this anion (McCarthy et al., 1967). In addition, long continued administration of these diuretics may produce mild iodine depletion by increasing its urinary excretion (Mehbod et al., 1967).

2.1.5 *Drugs acting on the distal tubular exchange site*

These diuretics include spironolactone acting as a competitive inhibitor of aldosterone, and triamterene and amiloride, which inhibit K^+–Na^+ exchange independently of aldosterone action (Liddle, 1966). They are the only diuretics which simultaneously reduce K^+ output and increase that of Na^+.

These drugs are weak diuretics when used alone, but are useful in the potentiation of action of all other types of diuretics and in the counteraction of potassium loss in the urine, an effect especially prominent after thiazide compounds. They should rarely, if ever, be given together with oral or parenteral potassium salts, as excretion of K^+ is prevented or delayed, and dangerous hyperkalaemia may occur (Cohen, 1966; McNay and Oran, 1970). All diuretics tend to reduce the glomerular filtration rate and cause a rise of blood urea because of sodium depletion and consequent lowering of plasma volume. Triamterene, however, tends to reduce the glomerular filtration rate by an amount disproportionate to the concurrent sodium loss (Shaldon and Ryder, 1962; Ginsberg et al., 1964). Amiloride does not suffer from these particular disadvantages, and is probably the most potent member of this group of diuretic drugs (Antcliff et al., 1971).

2.2 DRUGS USED IN URINARY INFECTIONS

Drugs used in urinary infections include sulphonamides, trimethoprim, ampicillin, carbenicillin, cephalosporins, streptomycin, kanamycin, gentamicin, tetracyclines, chloramphenicol, polymyxins, nitrofurantoin, nalidixic acid, mandelamine and antifungal drugs. Many of these compounds have important toxic effects in relation to kidney structure and function. Their interactions are, therefore, best discussed in relation to their separate anti-infective and nephrotoxic actions. Drug interactions relating to antiinfective action are difficult to predict, as combinations of drugs may be synergistic, indifferent, or even antagonistic, and the effects may vary with the organism concerned, and with the dosage of the drugs. In particular, in vivo effects cannot always be predicted from in vitro observations in bacterial cultures. Combinations of bactericidal agents are often synergistic, but those of bacteriostatic compounds are more usually merely additive in their effects. Use of the two types of drug together is often inhibitory to the more important action of bactericidal drugs which, with the exception of polymyxins, are only active against multiplying bacteria (Jawetz and Gunnison, 1952).

2.2.1 *Sulphonamides*

These drugs are still widely used in urinary infections, although a large number of strains of *E. coli* isolated from infected urine are now sulphonamide resistant. They are all bacteriostatic drugs which act by the competitive inhibition of the incorporation of *p*-aminobenzoic acid (PABA) in bacterial folate synthesis (Hutner et al., 1959; Brown et al., 1961). Obviously, their action is antagonised by PABA itself, a compound which has been recommended on somewhat inadequate evidence for the treatment of scleroderma, and by injections of some local anaesthetics, e.g. procaine, which are hydrolysed in vivo to PABA (Brodie et al., 1948). Sulphonamides have an additive effect with other bacteriostatic drugs, e.g. tetracyclines, and may also be used in combination with bactericidal drugs, e.g. ampicillin, without inhibition of the bactericidal effect. The choice of sulphonamides for urinary tract infections is influenced by their toxicity, rate of absorption from the gut, plasma protein binding, rate of urinary excretion or of acetylation, and particularly by the solubility of the unaltered drug and of its acetylated derivative. Those most often used in urinary tract infections include sulphadimidine, Sulphatriad, sulphasomidine, sulphamethizole and sulphafurazole. Sulphatriad is a proprietary name for a mixture of equal amounts of sulphathiazole, sulphadiazine and sulphamerazine. Any one of these drugs does not affect the solubility in urine of the other two (Lehr, 1947, 1957), and thus an identical antibacterial effect can be attained at a dosage of approximately one third of any one of the three drugs, with a corresponding reduction of the liability to crystal formation and obstructive uropathy. Such mixtures may be especially indicated in patients with cardiac decompensation or hypertension, where large doses of sodium bicarbonate to alkalinize the urine would be undesirable. Sulphasomidine, sulphamethizole, and sulphafurazole are highly soluble compounds and thus complications from crystalluria are most unlikely to occur.

2.2.2 *Trimethoprim*

This is a bacteriostatic drug which inhibits the bacterial enzyme, dihydrofolate reductase. With large doses of the drug, i.e. more than 1 g/day, some evidence of human folate deficiency may occur (Kahn et al., 1968). This is easily treated by oral folate supplements which do not affect the antibacterial activity, as sensitive bacteria are unable to utilize preformed folate in the surrounding medium.

Trimethoprim and sulphonamides are highly synergistic as they separately inhibit sequential processes in bacterial synthesis of tetrahydrofolate, necessary for nucleoprotein production (Darrell et al., 1968). Maximum potentiation of the antibacterial activities occurs when the two drugs are at separate concentrations proportionate to their minimum inhibitory concentrations against the relevant organism. For many bacteria the most effective concentration ratio is trimethoprim–sulphonamide = 1:20, and this ratio should be maintained as long as possible in body fluids. A sulphonamide with similar pharmacokinetic properties to those of trimethoprim is, therefore, the most effective synergist, and sulphamethoxazole is the drug nearest to the theoretical optimum. The acetyl derivative of this sulphonamide is relatively insoluble in acidic urine and is formed in considerable amounts. A water diuresis, preferably combined with urinary alkalinization by sodium bicarbonate is, therefore, safer to avoid the risks of crystalluria. Available preparations of trimethoprim and sulphamethoxazole, e.g. cotrimoxazole (Septrin; Bactrim), contain five times as much of the sulphonamide relative to trimethoprim, a proportion which usually maintains the maximum synergistic ratio in body fluids. Trimethoprim is, however, a weak base of pK_a 7.3 and is excreted more rapidly in acidic than in alkaline urine. Sharpstone (1969) found that the clearance varied from 19 to 148 ml/min, the highest values occurring in urines of maximal acidity. Acidosis will, therefore, cause lower plasma concentrations of trimethoprim and will increase the urinary content. Obviously, the most effective ratio of the concentrations of the two drugs cannot always be maintained. In addition, if used in cases of renal failure, the plasma concentration ratio of the two drugs may alter as excretion rates of the two drugs fall by different amounts with reduction of the glomerular filtration rate.

Further potentiation of the antibacterial action of the two drugs can be obtained by purine antagonists (Hitchings, 1961), as these compounds inhibit a still later sequence in the chain of reactions involving folate and purine synthesis. This may explain the potentiation of both sulphonamides and trimethoprim by polymyxins (Noall et al., 1962; Russell, 1963). These antibiotics damage membranous structures in bacteria (Merrick, 1965), possibly by interference with purine synthesis.

2.2.3 *Penicillins*

The penicillins used most frequently in urinary infections are ampicillin and carbenicillin. Antibiotics of the penicillin group are only bactericidal to dividing cells, as their mode of action is an inhibition of synthesis of cell wall mucopeptide, with no similar effect on protein synthesis (Park, 1958; Madelstam and Rogers, 1959). This failure of cell wall production leads to cell death by osmotic lysis. Therefore, bacteriostatic drugs which prevent cell growth and multiplication often inhibit the bactericidal effect of penicillins, an antagonism which is seen particularly with tetracyclines and chloramphenicol, but not with sulphonamides.

Ampicillin is bactericidal to a wide range of Gram-positive and Gram-negative bacteria (Sutherland and Robinson, 1964) which are common causes of urinary infection. Carbenicillin is active against many species of pseudomonas and indole producing strains of proteus. All penicillins are excreted by glomerular filtration and proximal tubular secretion, and therefore their renal clearance is reduced by probenecid. Carbenicillin has a short half-life and is still a very expensive drug. Except when used in cases of moderate or severe renal failure, carbenicillin should always be given together with oral probenecid. The action of the antibiotic is thus considerably prolonged, and the interval between successive doses may be correspondingly increased.

2.2.4 *Cephalosporins*

The action of these antibiotics is somewhat similar to the penicillins (Abraham, 1962). Cephaloridine and cephalothin, must be given parenterally, whereas cephalexin is acid-stable and can be given orally. Hypersensitivity reactions to cephalothin are common but, unlike cephaloridine, this drug is not apparently nephrotoxic. All the cephalosporins are excreted by tubular secretion, and their potential toxicity is increased in patients suffering from renal failure (Braun et al., 1968; Perkins et al., 1969).

2.2.5 *Streptomycin, kanamycin and gentamicin*

These antibiotics are strong organic bases and are, therefore, almost completely unabsorbed from the gut. Their most serious toxic effect, when given parenterally, is to the vestibular apparatus and, to a lesser extent, to the cochlea (Igarashi et al., 1966). The main damage is to the sensory epithelium of the labyrinth. Toxicity is more severe and more frequent in elderly patients and in those with a significant reduction of the glomerular filtration rate and azotaemia. There is probably some potentiation between the ototoxic effects of these antibiotics and those of ethacrynic acid or frusemide.

Streptomycin and gentamicin are more active against bacteria at a pH above 7.8, and activity is much reduced at a pH below 6.0. Since bacteria rapidly become resistant to streptomycin, the urine should be pre-alkalinized with sodium bicarbonate if this antibiotic is used in the treatment of urinary infections (Harris et al., 1947).

Gentamicin is chiefly used against *Pseudomonas* infections (Brayton and Louria, 1964; Klein et al., 1964), where it is synergistic with carbenicillin. In addition, the antibiotic has additive bactericidal effects with colistin against many strains of *Pseudomonas*, and with kanamycin or ampicillin against *Proteus*. Plasma levels of gentamicin should be kept below 10 μg/ml to avoid toxic effects on the 8th nerve.

2.2.6 *Tetracyclines and chloramphenicol*

Chloramphenicol is unsuitable for treatment of urinary infections except in

TABLE I

Weak acids showing pH-dependent excretion

Acid	Importance of pH-dependent excretion*	Species investigated	References
Salicylate	1	Man, dog and rabbit	Gutman et al., 1955; Macpherson et al., 1955
Phenylbutazone	3	Man and dog	Gutman et al., 1960
Phenobarbitone	1	Man and dog	Waddell and Butler, 1957
Probenecid	3	Dog	Weiner et al., 1960
Carinamide	3	Dog	Berglund, 1962
Nitrofurantoin	2	Dog	Woodruff et al., 1961
Nalidixic acid	2	Dog	McChesney et al., 1964
Acetazolamide	2	Man and dog	Maren, 1956
Sulphathiazole	1	Man and pig	Dalgaard-Mikkelsen and Poulsen, 1956
Sulphaethidole	1	Man	Kostenbauder et al., 1962
Sulphadimidine	1	Man	Williams et al., 1968
p-Aminosalicylate	1	Dog	Huang et al., 1960

Weak bases showing pH-dependent excretion

Base	Importance of pH-dependent excretion*	Species investigated	References
Mepacrine	3	Man	Jailer et al., 1947
Chloroquine	3	Man	Jailer et al., 1947
Quinine	3	Man and dog	Haag et al., 1943
Quinidine	2	Man	Gerhardt et al., 1969
Trimethoprim	1	Man	Sharpstone, 1969
Procaine	3	Dog and rabbit	Terp, 1951
Prilocaine	2	Man	Eriksson, 1966
Nicotine	2	Man	Haag and Larson, 1942
Mecamylamine	1	Man and dog	Baer et al., 1956; Milne et al., 1957
Pempidine	1	Man	Harington et al., 1958
Tolazoline	3	Dog	Torretti et al., 1962
Pethidine	2	Man	Asatoor et al., 1963
Levorphanol	3	Dog	Braun et al., 1963
Methadone	2	Man	Baselt and Casarett, 1972
Amphetamine	1	Man	Asatoor et al., 1965
Fenfluramine	2	Man	Riley et al., 1969
Amitriptyline	3	Man	Sjöqvist et al., 1969
Nortriptyline	3	Man	Sjöqvist et al., 1969
Imipramine	3	Man	Sjöqvist et al., 1969
Desmethylimipramine	3	Man	Sjöqvist et al., 1969

* Importance of pH-dependent excretion: 1 = important; 2 = intermediate; 3 = unimportant.

exceptional circumstances, as long-term therapy with this drug is particularly liable to cause aplastic anaemia. Therapy with tetracyclines is now less popular as many strains of organisms isolated from urine are resistant to these drugs, and in addition they may cause azotaemia and renal damage if given in high dosage.

By their bacteriostatic effect, these drugs may inhibit the bactericidal activity of more powerful antibiotics.

2.2.7 *Nitrofurantoin and nalidixic acid*

These drugs are only useful in urinary tract infections, as effective concentrations of the drugs are not attained elsewhere. Both substances are excreted more rapidly in alkaline urine (Table I, p. 202), but nitrofurantoin is considerably more therapeutically effective in acid urine where there is a higher relative content of the freely diffusible unionized fraction of the drug. The two drugs are often antagonistic and probably should never be prescribed in combination. Acidifying salts, e.g. ammonium chloride, potentiate the activity of nitrofurantoin, as the drug is sometimes as much as 800 times as effective if the urinary pH is below 5.4 as if it is above 7.8. This is a much more important factor than the increase of concentration in alkaline urine due to enhanced clearance. The urinary concentration and therapeutic efficacy of nalidixic acid is greatly reduced in patients with renal insufficiency. Nitrofurantoin is both ineffective and highly toxic in such cases, especially by production of an irreversible peripheral neuropathy (Loughridge, 1962; Roelsen, 1964).

2.2.8 *Hexamine mandelate*

This combination of hexamine and mandelic acid, although largely superseded by more active compounds, may be valuable for long term therapy as bacterial resistance does not occur, and the drugs often produce a significant antifungal activity in the urine. These drugs are only useful if the urinary pH can be kept below 5.0 by oral ammonium chloride or methionine. At this pH, the action of the two compounds is synergistic as the hexamine liberates formaldehyde, and mandelic acid is largely in the active diffusible unionized form. Toxic effects, especially gastrointestinal irritation, are, however, common at the high dosage necessary for effective antibacterial action.

2.2.9 *Polymyxins and colistin*

These drugs are cyclic basic polypeptides owing their bactericidal action against many Gram-negative bacilli to damage to the bacterial plasma membrane (Kaye and Chapman, 1963). Sensitive bacteria do not easily develop resistance to these antibiotics, and there is a synergistic effect with sulphonamides and trimethoprim. Nephrotoxicity, especially in patients with previously damaged kidneys, limits the use of these drugs.

2.3 URICOSURIC DRUGS

Urate is both secreted and reabsorbed by the proximal renal tubule (Berliner et al., 1950; Gutman et al., 1959), although in man there is net tubular reabsorption, the clearance of urate averaging 5–10% of the glomerular filtration rate. Most organic acids which are secreted by the proximal tubular epithelium are uricosuric agents at appropriate dosage, and will increase urate clearance to 2–5 times the basal value. At low dosage of these drugs, urate secretion is chiefly inhibited (Gutman and Yu, 1958), causing urate retention, whereas, at higher doses, the less sensitive reabsorptive mechanism is reduced (Sirota et al., 1952), with a consequent rise of urate clearance. At usual pharmacological doses, thiazides are in the low dosage range and therefore cause urate retention, whilst conventional uricosuric agents, e.g. probenecid, sulphinpyrazone, salicylates and phenylbutazone, are inhibitors of urate reabsorption. The effects are usually additive if an incomplete response has been produced by a single drug (Yu et al., 1963), but salicylates inhibit the uricosuric actions of probenecid and sulphinpyrazone. The effect of uricosuric drugs is significantly increased if there is simultaneous alkalinization of the urine by sodium bicarbonate. This also insures against dangerous crystalluria and obstructive uropathy, as sodium urate is much more soluble than is uric acid itself. Lactate and β-hydroxybutyrate reduce urate clearance, and may inhibit the normal uricosuric effects of probenecid and salicylates (Yu et al., 1957; Padova and Bendersky, 1962).

Acetazolamide, thiazides, chlorthalidone and pyrazinamide are all drugs which decrease urate clearance at normal dosage levels. Uricosuric blood levels of thiazides and chlorthalidone can only be attained by rapid intravenous injection of the drugs, as renal excretion prevents such concentrations being reached by high oral doses. The urate-retaining effect of thiazide diuretics is reversible by the usual pharmacological doses of potent uricosuric drugs (Smilo et al., 1962), e.g. probenecid or sulphinpyrazone.

2.4 IMMUNOSUPPRESSIVE THERAPY

Immunosuppression in relation to renal disease has been chiefly used in suppression of the rejection process in renal transplantation, and in reduction of immune damage to glomeruli in glomerulonephritis, polyarteritis nodosa, disseminated lupus erythematosus, Goodpasture's syndrome and other types of glomerular disease. The main drugs used have been corticosteroids, especially prednisone, azathioprine, cyclophosphamide, actinomycin C, and antilymphocytic sera (Levey and Medawar, 1966).

Corticosteroids owe their activity to production of involution of lymphoid tissue both by an antimitotic effect and a direct action on lymphocytes. Maximum immune suppression occurs if the steroid can be given before the antigen first exerts its effect. Azathioprine blocks purine synthesis by inhibition of the enzymatic conversion of inosinate to adenylate and guanylate, thus preventing DNA and RNA synthesis (Elion and Hitchings, 1965). New formation of immunologically competent cells is thereby considerably reduced. Cyclophosphamide is an alkylating agent which causes profound damage to dividing cells, with either complete failure of mitosis or cell death in the interphase stage (Koller, 1958; Brookes and Lawley, 1964). Cross-linkage of the DNA chain occurs either to an adjacent protein or to the corresponding DNA chain in the double helix (Lawley and Brookes, 1967). This prevents the affected DNA strand from effectively acting as a template for synthesis of DNA. The drug produces a rapid reduction in the amount of lymphoid tissue in the body, indicating that there is also probably damage to non-proliferating as well as actively dividing lymphoid cells. Actinomycin C prevents transcription of messenger RNA from DNA, and thus interferes with intracellular protein synthesis (Reich, 1963). The immunosuppressive effect of antilymphocyte sera is mainly by destruction and inhibition of the function of lymphoid cells. The single great advantage of ALS is its specificity, the effects on non-lymphoid cells being usually negligible. These diverse effects on the immune response suggest that immunosuppressive drugs would be synergistic, and in fact they are almost always used in combination rather than in isolation.

Combination of prednisone and azathioprine are the main drugs in control of allograft rejection after renal transplantation (Calne, 1961; Starzl, 1964). Azathioprine is usually started about one week before an elective transplantation or as soon as possible in an emergency grafting operation from a cadaveric donor. Prednisone acts more rapidly, and is given from about one day pre-operatively. Both drugs in as low a dosage as will control the rejection process are given indefinitely after the operation. Acute rejection episodes are usually inhibited by increasing the dosage of prednisone and use of a short course of actinomycin C (Alexandre et al., 1963). Cyclophosphamide is inferior to azathioprine in the control of the rejection process, but has been claimed to be superior in therapy of glomerular disease due to immune mechanisms.

Immunosuppressive drugs are synergistic in relation to their desired pharmacological effects, but also in many instances in their toxic effects, especially in depression of circulating polymorphonuclear leucocytes and platelets, with consequent diminished resistance to infection and severe haemorrhagic manifestations. In particular, large doses of prednisone often lead to peptic ulceration and haematemesis, whilst both cyclophosphamide and azathioprine (Einhorn and Davidsohn, 1964) may cause a severe hepatitis which may progress to liver cell failure. The results of immunosuppression in renal transplantation, although greatly improved in the last few years, are still far from ideal. Immunosuppression in the therapy of glomerular disease is even more problematical, as the undoubted benefit on the primary disease has to be balanced against increased mortality from the severe toxic effects of large doses of immunosuppressive drugs. To date, some controlled trials have failed to show unequivocal evidence of benefit when results are assessed by total life expectancy.

2.5 ANTICOAGULANT THERAPY IN GLOMERULAR DISEASE

Anticoagulants have been extensively used in many cases of renal disease to prevent platelet and fibrin thrombi in glomerular capillaries and other small renal vessels (Herdman et al., 1970). Experimental nephrotoxic serum nephritis causes renal lesions similar to those of rapidly progressive glomerulonephritis in man (Vassalli and McCluskey, 1964). Deposition at first of aggregations of platelets and later of mixed platelet and fibrin thrombi in glomerular capillaries occurs early in the course of both diseases. Fibrin deposits, proliferative lesions in glomeruli, and crescent formation are reduced in amount both by heparin and by Warfarin (Halpern et al., 1965; Vassalli and McCluskey, 1965). Anticoagulants have, therefore, been widely used in many renal diseases associated with deposition of mixed platelet and fibrin thrombi, including rapidly progressive acute glomerular nephritis, acute post-streptococcal glomerulonephritis complicated by severe oliguria, Goodpasture's syndrome, Wegener's granulomatosis, polyarteritis nodosa, disseminated lupus erythematosus, malignant hypertension, hypersensitivity angiitis, thrombotic thrombocytopenic purpura, Henoch–Schönlein purpura, and renal allograft rejection. Prednisone and heparin have a considerable synergistic effect in therapy, but unfortunately prednisone increases the risk of extra-renal haemorrhage as it reduces capillary and arteriolar integrity with increased sensitivity to mild trauma and even liability to spontaneous rupture.

As the thrombosis is initiated and maintained by platelet aggregation and deposition (Kincaid-Smith et al., 1970), dipyridamole has been widely used together with heparin and Warfarin. The drug reduces platelet aggregation and adhesiveness (Sullivan et al., 1968), with a consequent prolongation of platelet survival in the circulating blood. The benefit of combinations of prednisone, heparin and dipyridamole is most obvious in acute fulminating conditions, e.g. thrombotic thrombocytopenic purpura (Brain et al., 1968) and acute allograft rejection (Clyne et al., 1970), where massive thrombosis of small vessels is the predominant feature of the disease, but is more problematical in more chronic conditions. Controlled trials of therapy are only possible in a multi-centre co-operative enterprise, as many of the conditions in which this type of treatment has been advocated are fortunately comparatively uncommon.

3 Interactions of drugs and poisons causing renal toxic effects

Drugs and poisons may damage the kidney in many different ways, and it is probable that separate toxins given simultaneously will have an additive or even a potentiating effect.

The kidney is especially vulnerable to chemical damage because of its extremely rich blood supply per unit mass of tissue, and because noxious agents are often concentrated either in renal tubule cells or in the luminal fluid and the urine. The most common functional defect is the production of acute oliguric renal failure, and in most series of cases of this type approximately one quarter are directly due to the effects of drugs and poisons. There may be:

glomerular damage;
proximal tubular necrosis;
hypersensitivity reactions;
acute tubular necrosis;
interstitial nephritis;
papillary necrosis;
analgesic nephropathy.

All these various noxious effects will tend to reduce the glomerular filtration rate with consequent potentiation and prolongation of the actions of drugs which largely depend on excretion in the urine for termination of their pharmacological effects. This important aspect of drug interaction is discussed in a later section. As a general rule, agents causing oliguria and reduced renal blood flow will tend to intensify any potential nephrotoxic effect, and conversely compounds causing a diuresis and increased renal perfusion will often reduce kidney damage. Diuretics and antihypertensive drugs are particularly liable to lower both the glomerular filtration rate and the renal blood flow. Agents causing sodium depletion will reduce the extracellular and plasma volumes and this will usually lower renal perfusion. As the main action of diuretic drugs is to increase urinary sodium loss, the glomerular filtration rate often falls substantially during treatment by these drugs, and this will sometimes lead to a mild or moderate degree of azotaemia. Thiazides and triamterene often reduce the glomerular filtration rate to an amount disproportionate to their relatively moderate diuretic effect, possibly by a direct action on renal arterioles. Antihypertensive drugs, with the exception of hydralazine (Moyer, 1953), reduce the cardiac output and the renal blood flow, and as the filtration fraction remains constant or varies only slightly, a fall of the glomerular filtration rate is often produced.

By contrast, plasma expanders, including saline infusions and osmotic diuretics, e.g. mannitol and urea, may protect the kidney from noxious drugs and chemicals. These agents increase the glomerular filtration rate and reduce water reabsorption by the proximal tubular epithelial cells, and thus lessen the concentration of drugs and chemicals within the tubular lumen. The transport time from glomerulus to renal pelvis is reduced and there is correspondingly less time for tissue injury to occur. In addition, the high volume of tubular fluid and urine lessens crystallization of compounds within the collecting tubules, renal pelves, and ureters, with consequent less chance of obstructive uropathy. Potent diuretics, e.g. frusemide, have been used to prevent renal damage from drugs and from surgical shock or haemorrhage. This method is, however, less certain than protection by mannitol infusions, as diuresis is relatively transient and is inevitably followed by a period of oliguria and sodium depletion. Mannitol infusions, combined with intravenous saline (Barry and Malloy, 1962), can maintain a high urinary flow almost indefinitely, and thus prolong the protective effect throughout the whole period of risk.

3.1 GLOMERULAR DAMAGE

Diuretics and antihypertensive drugs reduce the glomerular filtration rate chiefly by lowering the renal blood flow, i.e. they produce a minor degree of acute renal circulatory failure, often incorrectly termed 'pre-renal azotaemia'. By contrast, some drugs, e.g. troxidone (Barnett et al., 1948), penicillamine (Adams et al., 1964; Rosenberg and Hayslett, 1967) and foreign sera by injection, may damage the glomerular basement membrane by deposition of immune complexes on the outer surface of the membrane itself. These drugs are haptens, and the antigen so formed combines with antibody to produce circulating immune complexes with subsequent localization within the glomeruli. The first effect is a heavy proteinuria, often leading to a nephrotic syndrome, which is fortunately usually reversible if the drug is withdrawn early in the course of the disease. With continued administration of the offending drug, the disease may progress to glomerular fibrosis and destruction with eventual chronic renal failure. Steroids e.g., prednisone, are indicated if glomerular damage has occurred, as they diminish antibody production and thus reduce formation of circulating immune complexes. Penicillamine has caused a nephrotic syndrome more often when used in the treatment of cystinuria than in Wilson's disease. Possibly the glomerular damage may be made worse by copper depletion from the chelating action of the drug, and this is obviously less likely to occur in conditions due to copper retention as in Wilson's disease.

3.2 PROXIMAL TUBULAR NECROSIS

Severe damage to the proximal tubular epithelium with massive cellular necrosis will cause acute oliguric renal failure, whereas less severe injury will result in an acquired Fanconi syndrome with renal glycosuria, aminoaciduria, and an increase of phosphate and urate clearances. Drugs and poisons causing such lesions include heavy metals, e.g. lead, cadmium, mercury, uranium, carbon tetrachloride, glycols, chlorates and bromates, phenols and cresols, chromates and bichromates, tartrate, and outdated and degraded tetracycline. A high concentration of the drug in the proximal tubular lumen and a prolonged tubular transit time will increase the liability to tubular damage and necrosis. An osmotic diuresis, e.g. by mannitol infusion, therefore, has a protective effect provided treatment is instituted almost immediately after ingestion of the poison. Appropriate chelating agents will reduce damage from heavy metals, e.g. EDTA for lead, penicillamine for mercury, and alkalinization of the urine with sodium bicarbonate may be protective both by causation of an osmotic diuresis and by reduction of the degree of ionization of the metal within the proximal tubular lumen.

Carbon tetrachloride is widely used as a dry cleaning agent, in some fire extinguishers, and as an industrial solvent. It usually causes poisoning by inhalation but may be swallowed either by accident or with suicidal intent (Schreiner and Maher, 1965). Acute oliguric renal failure often occurs from one to ten days after exposure. The duration of the oliguric stage can vary from one day only in mild cases to as long as ten weeks in the most serious cases. Simultaneous ingestion of alcohol always exacerbates the toxic effects of carbon tetrachloride, chiefly because the solubility of the compound in ethanol enhances its rate of absorption from the gut (Guild et al., 1958; New et al., 1962). Potentiation of the toxic effect by alcohol, however, is seen if the poison is inhaled as well as if taken by mouth. There is considerable evidence that a high concentration of alcohol in body fluids increases that of carbon tetrachloride in plasma with a correspondingly higher content in kidney tissue and in urine. Tetrachloroethylene is considerably less toxic than carbon tetrachloride but may sometimes cause similar renal damage. This compound is also used as an industrial solvent and as a vermifuge in the mass treatment of hook worm infestation. Its toxicity is also enhanced by simultaneous alcohol intake.

Ethylene glycol is the main component of many antifreeze solutions and may be drunk accidentally or with intent as a highly dangerous intoxicant. After absorption from the gut it is oxidised to oxalic acid via the intermediates glycollic aldehyde, glyoxal, and glycollic and glyoxylic acids (Kahn and Brotchner, 1950).

$$(CH_2OH)_2 \rightarrow CH_2OHCHO \rightarrow CH_2OHCOOH \rightarrow CHOCOOH \rightarrow (COOH)_2$$
$$\searrow \longrightarrow CHO.CHO \longrightarrow \nearrow$$

Acute oliguric failure is due to a combination of the direct nephrotoxic effects of the glycol and of its metabolites, and to tubular obstruction by deposition of calcium oxalate crystals (Pons and Custer, 1940). Treatment should always include haemodialysis which is the most effective method of removal of the unoxidised glycol from the body (Perlmutter, 1957). In addition, simultaneous ingestion of ethanol reduces the toxic effects by competing with alcohol dehydrogenase, which oxidises both ethanol and the glycol within liver cells, and thus delays the formation of toxic metabolites.

Production of a Fanconi syndrome by outdated and degraded tetracycline (Frimpter et al., 1963; Gross, 1963) is of especial interest in showing that drug interaction may occur even before ingestion. Tetracycline was originally dispensed with citric acid, whereas it is now known that lactose is a much safer excipient (Kunin, 1967). In hot humid conditions and at low pH produced by the citric acid, tetracycline may be oxidised to two nephrotoxic derivatives, anhydrotetracycline and epianhydrotetracycline (Benitz and Diermeier, 1964), both of which damage the proximal tubules with production of a reversible Fanconi syndrome.

3.3 HYPERSENSITIVITY REACTIONS

This type of renal damage is usually accompanied by extra-renal manifestations of hypersensitivity, e.g. pyrexia, blood dyscrasias, arthropathy, and rashes which may or may not be purpuric in nature. Drugs causing hypersensitivity reactions are usually haptens, the drug–protein complex acting as an antigen in the initiation of the immune response. The renal lesions include features of an arteritis, glomerulitis and interstitial nephritis. Medicaments especially liable to cause this type of reaction include gold injections (Grégoire et al., 1956), penicillins (Brauninger and Remington, 1968), phenytoin, phenindione, thiazides, thiouracils, sulphonamides (Brown et al., 1940), foreign sera and iodine-containing compounds, especially radiographic contrast media. Severe damage can often be avoided by prompt withdrawal of the sensitising drug and temporary suppression of the immune response by steroids.

3.4 ACUTE TUBULAR NECROSIS

This type of acute oliguric renal failure, associated with an abrupt reduction of renal cortical blood supply, is most commonly caused by surgical shock or haemorrhage, but may also often occur from an acute toxic reaction to drugs and poisons. These include many antibiotics, radiographic contrast media, mercurial diuretics, salicylates, *p*-aminosalicylate, and phenylbutazone.

Radiographic contrast media are especially toxic if present in high concentration in the renal vessels. When given as a bolus into the aorta or renal artery they may cause sudden arteriolar spasm as their osmolality in solution is considerably above that of body fluids. Of oral cholecystographic agents, bunamiodyl (orabilase) has caused many cases of renal damage (Rennie, 1964), probably because of its high iodine content and its relatively rapid rate of absorption from the gut. Factors increasing nephrotoxicity are jaundice and hepatic failure, which cause a greater proportion of the drug to be excreted in the urine. In addition, bunamiodyl is relatively insoluble in acidic urine and crystalluria can easily occur (Setter et al., 1963). This can be prevented by administration of sodium bicarbonate and copious fluids by mouth. Ipanoic acid (Telepaque) and sodium diatrizoate (Hypaque) have proved less nephrotoxic, but may damage the kidney, especially if in high concentration in the blood. All these compounds are weak organic acids and are secreted by the proximal tubular epithelial cells. They are, therefore, potent uricosuric agents, and if the urine is highly acidic and concentrated may cause uric acid crystalluria. Renal damage is, in general, more likely to occur if there is pre-existing chronic renal disease, if there is severe dehydration with a low urinary volume, if the urine is highly acidic, and if there is severe hyperuricaemia which tends to increase urate output. Toxicity is usually dose dependent and is, therefore, most likely after renal angiography (Crawford et al., 1957; McAfee, 1957). The concentration of the drug within renal tissue, renal circulating blood, and urine is much less after pyelography (Prendergrass et al., 1955), and here sensitivity reactions from iodine are more likely than a more specific damage from the drug itself.

Antibiotics which are potentially nephrotoxic include sulphonamides, polymyxin and colistin, kanamycin, streptomycin, gentamicin, neomycin, cephaloridine and amphotericin B. Although an obstructive nephropathy from crystalluria is the most frequent cause of renal damage by sulphonamides (Keitzer and Campbell, 1942; Plummer and Wheeler, 1944; Weinstein et al., 1960), the drugs have produced acute tubular necrosis, hypersensitivity reactions (French, 1946), and interstitial nephritis. Prevention of obstructive nephropathy lies in a choice of the most soluble type of sulphonamide which is therapeutically effective, and in forced alkaline diuresis. Neomycin is particularly liable to cause severe renal damage. Although absorption from the gut is proportionately very small, this may be increased in cases of inflammatory gut disease (Kunin et al., 1960; Last and Sherlock, 1960). Severe renal damage has been recorded when the drug has been given intraperitoneally at the termination of operations for peritonitis, as absorption from the peritoneal cavity is much more complete and rapid than from the gut (Craig et al., 1966). Cephaloridine toxicity to the kidney is potentiated by simultaneous administration of frusemide (Dodds and Foord, 1970). It has been postulated that the diuretic stimulates the renin–angiotensin system from sodium depletion, and that angiotensin considerably increases renal damage from the antibiotic. Amphotericin-B is invariably nephrotoxic at effective dosage (Utz et al., 1964), and should be reserved for cases of disseminated and serious fungal infections. The drug particularly damages the renal concentrating and acidifying capacity of the distal tubules, and therefore tends to cause polyuric renal failure complicated by a distal tubular type of acidosis with a urine of inappropriately high pH. Again, a forced alkaline diuresis has been claimed to reduce the severity of renal damage (McCurdy et al., 1968; Douglas and Healy, 1969).

Methoxyflurane (1,1-difluoro-2,2-dichloroethyl methyl ether) is another important drug which may cause polyuric renal failure (Elkington et al., 1968). It has been extensively used, chiefly in the U.S.A., as an anaesthetic agent since 1959. Nephrotoxic effects usually only occur after prolonged anaesthesia, as the effect is dose dependent (Pezzi et al., 1966; Austin and Villandry, 1967). In most cases the renal damage is transient but has been irreversible in a few patients. Toxicity has been attributed to metabolites of the anaesthetic, possibly inorganic fluoride, or organic acids containing fluorine, e.g. difluoroacetic or methoxyfluoroacetic acids. There seems to be clear-cut potentiation of the nephrotoxicity in patients treated with tetracyclines (Kuzucu, 1970).

The tetracycline group of antibiotics is not usually nephrotoxic when given alone, provided they are pure without any chemical degradation having occurred before ingestion. They have, however, a prominent anti-anabolic effect which increases the level of blood urea independent of any co-existent renal failure (Shils, 1963) and exacerbates the azotaemia in uraemic patients.

Hypercalcaemia is a further potent cause of polyuric renal failure. Renal damage is more related to increased transfer of calcium from the glomerular filtrate than to nephrocalcinosis or renal stone formation. The use of high doses of calciferol should always be controlled by frequent determinations of plasma calcium as toxic effects from hypercalcaemia can often be insidious in the early stages. Its action is potentiated by simultaneous administration of calcium salts or by high dietary intake of dairy products. Hypercalcaemia also occurs in secondary carcinoma of bone (Spencer and Lewin, 1963), and may be exacerbated by use of androgenic steroids, especially in the therapy of secondary deposits from malignant breast tumours. Factors reducing the intensity or the pharmacological effects of hypercalcaemia on the kidney include chelating agents, e.g. sodium ethylene diamine tetra-acetate (Spencer et al., 1956), infusions of sodium phosphate, large doses of cortisone or prednisone (Verner et al., 1958), and reduced dietary intake of calcium combined with oral sodium phosphate, sodium phytate, or sodium cellulose phosphate which reduce intestinal calcium absorption.

3.5 INTERSTITIAL NEPHRITIS, PAPILLARY NECROSIS AND ANALGESIC NEPHROPATHY

Acute interstitial nephritis has been reported after ingestion of phenylbutazone, phenindione, thiazides, and sulphonamides, but such acute lesions occur less frequently than the chronic papillary damage of analgesic nephropathy. This is an important cause of renal failure which particularly illustrates the importance of drug interaction in relation to kidney function and structural damage. Following the original description by Spühler and Zollinger (1953), examples of the condition have been described from all parts of the world. There seems little doubt, however, that the disease is most common in hot dry areas where relative oliguria is frequently found, and where analgesics are often taken in excess over long periods of time (Kincaid-Smith, 1969). Most patients suffering from analgesic nephropathy have taken large quantities of phenacetin in amounts usually of more than 4 kg over many years. No case has, however, been reported in which phenacetin was the sole analgesic drug, as this medicament is almost always taken as a mixture, usually with at least two other drugs. An aspirin, phenacetin and caffeine mixture at a dosage equivalent in mg/kg body weight to that taken by affected patients has produced a high incidence of renal papillary necrosis in the rat, and the proportion of affected animals increased when there was limitation of water supply (Kincaid-Smith et al., 1968; Saker and Kincaid-Smith, 1969). By contrast, phenacetin alone, at twice the dose of that in the mixture failed to cause similar renal lesions (Nanra and Kincaid-Smith, 1970). The importance of various separate analgesics in causation of the pathology of analgesic nephropathy is still uncertain. Other compounds frequently taken together with phenacetin include aspirin, phenazone, caffeine, and amidopyrine. Any one of these analgesics has been shown to be potentially nephrotoxic at high dosage (Gault et al., 1971). The chief metabolite of phenacetin, paracetamol (N-acetyl-*p*-aminophenol) is often prescribed alone, as well as in combination with other analgesics. Experimentally, this drug has been shown to be concentrated within the renal medulla of dogs (Bluemle, Jr. and Goldberg, 1968), and renal damage from this agent alone has been reported in man (Krikler, 1967).

Several factors may explain the variability of the incidence of analgesic nephropathy in different subjects and in various environments. These include the type and amount of analgesics ingested, individual susceptibility, the presence of bacterial pyelonephritis, factors influencing renal blood flow and especially medullary blood flow, e.g. the heterozygous state of sickle cell anaemia, and especially the incidence of dehydration which causes a high osmolality in medullary tissue and urine, and may increase the analgesic concentration in the renal pyramids.

A notable acute effect of all analgesics on the kidney is an increase of tubular cell excretion in the urine due to desquamation of the cellular lining of the nephron (Prescott, 1965). There is, however, no evidence that this effect is in any way related to the production of the medullary lesions of analgesic nephropathy. 'Analgesic nephropathy' is obviously a more satisfactory term than the more usual 'phenacetin kidney'. There is little, if any, advantage in the inclusion of phenacetin in analgesic mixtures, and the safest long-term mild analgesic is probably paracetamol followed by aspirin. Analgesic nephropathy has only very rarely followed the prolonged use of either of these drugs when taken alone.

4 Effects of renal function on the elimination and half lives of drugs

The two most important mechanisms in the curtailment of drug action are metabolic change, usually by the liver, and excretion in the urine. As a general rule, lipid-soluble drugs, which are well absorbed by the gut and which readily penetrate into the interior of body cells, are mainly metabolized usually to more water-soluble and less pharmacologically active compounds. By contrast, water-soluble drugs, which are poorly absorbed by the gut and which are mainly distributed in the extracellular water, are mostly excreted in the urine. If a drug is entirely excreted unchanged by the kidney, its concentration in plasma falls logarithmically, and its disappearance rate is best defined by the half-life, i.e. the time in which plasma concentrations fall to one half of the basal value. The following mathematical equation defines the relationship between the half-life of such a drug, its renal clearance, and its apparent volume of distribution within body water (Butler, 1958):

$$t_{\frac{1}{2}} = \ln_2 \cdot \frac{\text{volume of distribution in ml}}{C_X}$$

where $t_{\frac{1}{2}}$ is the half-life in minutes, $\ln_2$ is the natural logarithm of 2, i.e. 0.69, and C_X is the clearance in ml/min. Drugs are frequently bound to plasma protein, especially albumin, and the apparent volume of distribution and the clearance must be calculated in the same way, i.e. either the total plasma content must be used in the estimation of both values, or alternatively the active free fraction which is not protein bound. The half-life, therefore, varies: (a) directly with the apparent volume of distribution; (b) inversely with the renal clearance. Profound alterations of the pharmacological effect may occur by drug interactions which alter either of these two factors. Reduction of renal function is particularly prone to cause severe adverse drug reactions. Smith et al. (1966) reported that such untoward effects were about 2.5 times as frequent in patients with a blood urea nitrogen above 40 mg/100 ml as in those in whom it was in the normal range of below 20 mg/100 ml.

4.1 ALTERATIONS OF APPARENT VOLUME OF DISTRIBUTION

Drug interactions can influence the apparent volume of distribution of one compound by at least two mechanisms: displacement from protein binding sites, and alteration in the distribution ratio between the extra- and the intracellular compartments. Displacement from protein binding will enhance the pharmacological activity of a drug because the active free fraction increases, but will shorten the half-life as more of the drug is available for either metabolic change or for renal excretion. The pharmacological effects of alterations of distribution between the two compartments are more complex. Increase of the extracellular fraction will hasten renal excretion, but will usually reduce the rate of metabolic change. The effect on the activity of the drug will vary according to which of the two fractions is the more important pharmacologically.

Many drug interactions are due to displacement of an active compound from plasma protein binding sites (Brodie, 1965), the higher the affinity for binding the more likely is a drug to modify the binding of another compound. Salicylates, phenylbutazone and some sulphonamides have a high binding affinity, and may increase the pharmacological effects of many other compounds by displacement from protein-binding sites with a rise of the active non-protein bound fraction, e.g. increase of the toxic effects of methotrexate (Dixon et al., 1965). Displacement from protein binding sites will obviously also increase the rate of excretion of a drug by glomerular filtration, but the effect on tubular secretion is more variable. Protein binding up to 90% of the total plasma content of a drug usually has little if any effect on tubular secretion, as equilibration between bound and free fractions of a drug is extremely rapid, and the reaction time is in most cases only a fraction of that available for tubular uptake and concentration of the unbound fraction within the proximal tubule cell. At levels of binding above 90%, however, the free concentration may be sufficiently low to reduce the tubular secretion rate, and competitive displacement of the drug from binding sites may substantially increase the rate of secretion, with a consequent rise of urinary output.

Changes of distribution of a drug between extra- and intracellular compartments are often due to abrupt alterations of acid–base balance which disturb the normal hydrogen ion gradient between plasma and intracellular fluid. Thus, rapid alkalinization by large amounts of sodium bicarbonate increases the concentration of phenobarbitone in plasma but reduces central nervous system depression by the drug (Waddell and Butler, 1957). Production of an acute acidosis by breathing high concentrations of CO_2 will raise the plasma level of mecamylamine (Payne and Rowe, 1957), but this enhances the hypotensive action of the drug, as the effect is mainly due to the fraction in extracellular fluid. One particularly important interaction of this type is the differential effect of sodium bicarbonate and of acetazolamide on the distribution of salicylate. Both drugs will alkalinize the urine and thus increase the rate of salicylate excretion, but acetazolamide causes an extracellular acidosis, whereas sodium bicarbonate produces an alkalosis. Acetazolamide will, therefore, temporarily increase the proportion of drug within the cells, whereas sodium bicarbonate has the reverse effect. As the action of salicylate is more dependent on the cellular content, acetazolamide temporarily increases the pharmacological effect of the drug (Hill, 1971). At doses of salicylate near the LD_{50} level in rats, administration of acetazolamide increases the mortality rate, whereas sodium bicarbonate reduces it. Acetazolamide is, therefore, an undesirable drug in the treatment of aspirin poisoning, whilst a forced alkaline diuresis by administration of sodium bicarbonate and mannitol infusions will substantially improve the survival rate.

4.2 ALTERATIONS OF RENAL CLEARANCE OF DRUGS

The half-life of a drug which is eliminated by renal excretion is inversely proportional to its clearance. Therefore, other compounds which reduce the clearance rate will both potentiate and prolong its pharmacological effects. Drugs are excreted by glomerular filtration, followed in some cases by proximal tubular secretion and/or passive back diffusion which may or may not be pH dependent. In a previous section it has been shown that many drugs may reduce the glomerular filtration rate, and thus the rate of excretion of drugs dependent on glomerular filtration, either by temporary or permanent renal damage. Some drugs, e.g. probenecid, may greatly influence excretion of other compounds by competitive reduction of their rate of proximal tubular secretion without there being any change of glomerular filtration rate.

5 Transport of organic acids and bases

The kidney regulates the excretion of many organic acids and bases both by active and by passive transport processes. The proximal tubular epithelium actively secretes a large number of organic acids and bases from the peritubular blood to the tubular lumen with concentration of the compounds within the cytoplasm and intracellular fluid of the tubule cells. It is generally assumed that there is a single transport system for all secreted organic acids, and a separate single system for organic bases. This view is based on mutual competition between separate acids and bases for tubular concentration and subsequent delivery into tubular fluid without there being any cross competition between the acidic and basic systems (Weiner and Mudge, 1964). Proximal tubular secretion is surprisingly non-specific, a large number of differing bases and acids, with great variation in molecular size, chemical structure and in ionic strength being included in each of the two separate transport groups.

Secreted acids have varying maximal transport capacity (T_m). Acids with the highest T_m pass most rapidly from the blood to the tubular lumen (Sperber, 1954), and their cellular–plasma concentration ratio is relatively low. Their transport is easily depressed by reduction of temperature or by agents which act as metabolic inhibitors, especially those reducing the activity of high energy phosphate bonds. They are weak inhibitors of transport of other compounds and especially those acids with a low T_m. Conversely, acids with a low T_m pass more slowly into the tubular lumen, concentration within the interior of tubular cells is high, their rate of transport is more resistant to cold and to metabolic inhibitors, and they are particularly effective as competitive inhibitors of transport of organic acids with a high T_m (Josephson et al., 1953a, b; Kinter and Cline, 1961). Diodrast, *p*-aminohippurate, and the penicillins are typical examples of high T_m organic acids, and probenecid and carinamide of the low T_m values, averages in adult human subjects being as follows: *p*-aminohippurate 0.4 mmol/min, diodrast 0.2 mmol/min, phenolsulphonphthalein and benzylpenicillin 0.1 mmol/min, and probenecid 0.014 mmol/min. The difference is usually explained by a greater affinity of compounds such as probenecid for binding to intracellular constituents concerned in the transport system, their low T_m being due to slow release from binding sites (Foster and Hong, 1958; Kinter, 1959), this step being the rate limiting factor of the transport process. Acidic compounds transported by the proximal tubules include sulphonic and carboxylic acids, glycine and other conjugates of organic acids, heterocyclic carboxylic acids, e.g. penicillins, sulphonamides and thiazides, ester and phenolic glucuronides, ethereal sulphates, aliphatic organic acids, e.g. oxalic acid, and acyl glycines and enolic compounds, e.g. phenylbutazone. The structural requirements for transport are ill understood. The molecule must not be very large (Oliver and Shevky, 1930), it should not contain a basic as well as an acidic grouping, and there must be either a single negatively charged acidic group, or if more than one, they should not be at opposite ends of the molecule (Hober et al., 1942).

Of compounds with a low T_m, probenecid is a more potent inhibitor of proximal tubular secretion of organic acids than carinamide (Boger et al., 1950; Beyer et al., 1951), chiefly because of its longer half-life in vivo. It reduces the clearances of penicillins, sulphonamides, thiazides, salicylate, and phenylbutazone, and thus prolongs and intensifies their pharmacological effects. In addition, probenecid lowers the rate of glycine conjugation of salicylate and *p*-aminosalicylate and, therefore, prolongs the half-life of these drugs both by reducing their excretion rate and the rate of their metabolic inactivation (Beyer et al., 1950).

Proximal tubular transport of organic bases is of less pharmacological importance than secretion of acids and, therefore, has been less thoroughly examined. Many of the bases concerned are highly toxic compounds except at very low dosage. Tetraethylammonium (Rennick et al., 1947) and N-methyl-nicotinamide (Sperber, 1948) have been studied in most detail. Each base competitively inhibits the secretion of the other, but has no effect on secretion of organic acids. Pharmacologically active secreted bases include catecholamines (Rennick and Quebbemann, 1970), quinine, tolazoline and mecamylamine (Peters, 1960). Cyanine 863 is a competitive inhibitor of base secretion analogous to probenecid in the case of organic acids (Rennick et al., 1956). Like probenecid, it is strongly bound to intracellular proteins, particularly those of mitochondria, and is excreted slowly with a low renal clearance. It is, however, a toxic compound and has no useful pharmacological effects.

6 Reabsorption of drugs by back diffusion

Some drugs, e.g. streptomycin, are excreted at a clearance equal to the glomerular filtration rate, which means there is no appreciable back diffusion of the compound from the tubular fluid to the peri-tubular capillary blood. The excretion rate of such compounds is purely governed by the glomerular filtration rate and is little, if at all, influenced by variation of urine flow rate or by changes of urinary pH. Some neutral but more lipid-soluble drugs, e.g. glutethimide, are excreted at a clearance considerably below that of inulin and of streptomycin, indicating that extensive back diffusion across the tubular cells has occurred. The longer the transit time from glomerulus to renal pelvis, the greater will be the degree of passive back diffusion in relation to the amount filtered at the glomeruli. The clearance of such a drug is, therefore, greatly influenced by factors altering urine flow, e.g. diuretic drugs, osmotic diuresis, high fluid intake or dehydration, but is unaffected by changes in acid–base balance. By contrast, the clearance of many lipid-soluble organic acids and bases is dependent both on urine flow and on changes of urinary pH (Milne et al., 1958). The freely diffusible unionized fraction of the drug passes from the tubular lumen to peri-capillary blood much more readily than the ionized water-soluble fraction. Diffusion of the latter is reduced both by the impermeability of the lipid-containing cell membrane to water-soluble compounds, and by the ionic charge of the molecule. The clearance and rate of urinary excretion of many weak acids is, therefore, often greater in alkaline urine, and conversely that of many weak bases in highly acidic urine. The limits of pK_a of weak bases and acids at which pH-dependent excretion can occur are 3.0–7.5 for weak acids, and 5.0–11.3 for weak bases.

Administration of sodium or potassium bicarbonate or citrate, or acetazolamide and other carbonic anhydrase inhibitors, will alkalinize the urine and thus potentiate and prolong the actions of weak bases, e.g. amphetamine, mecamylamine, pempidine, and quinidine, and reduce that of weak acids, e.g. salicylate and phenobarbitone (Weiner and Mudge, 1964). By contrast, ammonium chloride, methionine, or intravenous arginine dihydrochloride render the urine maximally acidic and have the converse effects.

These interactions have been used in practice in the treatment of poisoning, e.g. by salicylate or phenobarbitone, by forced alkaline diuresis, in the diagnosis of drug addiction, by increasing the urinary content of the suspected drug, and in detailed pharmacokinetic analyses, which are incomplete and often misleading unless the effects of pH-dependent excretion are included in the investigation. As an extreme example, the half-life of salicylate in cases of severe poisoning with aspirin is from 24 to 30 hr with acidic urine but only

6 hr if the urine is maximally alkaline (Levy, 1965). The pharmacological effects and half-life of weak acids or bases are significantly affected by pH-dependent excretion if a substantial fraction of the ingested dose is excreted unchanged in the urine when the clearance of the compound is at its maximum value. Thus, there is clear evidence that the actions of phenobarbitone and salicylate are potentiated when the urine is acidic, and vice versa, those of mecamylamine, pempidine, amphetamine and quinidine if the urine is alkaline. By contrast, the action of drugs which are mainly inactivated by metabolic change may be little affected by alteration of urinary pH, even though their clearance is widely different in acidic and alkaline urines, e.g. morphine and its derivatives. Some drugs, however, are somewhat intermediate in this respect. Thus, pethidine is usually mainly inactivated by metabolic change, but if mistakenly prescribed in cases of severe cirrhosis of the liver or in patients treated by monoamine oxidase inhibitors which reduce access of the drug to microsomal enzymes within hepatic cells, urinary excretion may exert a much greater influence on the effects and duration of action of this hypnotic (Asatoor et al., 1963). In such patients the pH-dependent excretion of pethidine may become of major practical importance. Dosage of drugs can often modify the proportion excreted in the urine, especially if metabolic pathways are easily saturated by increasing amounts of available drug. For example, methadone at usual dosage levels is chiefly metabolised in the liver. At high dosage in drug addicts or in cases of attempted suicide, the proportion excreted in acidic urine becomes a major fraction of the total (Baselt and Casarett, 1972), and in such cases the pharmacological effects and duration of action of methadone are increased by urinary alkalinization. Table I gives details of the main drugs known to be excreted by the mechanism of pH-dependent excretion.

7 Conclusions

Interactions between drugs in relation to renal disease, structure and function have been shown to occur frequently, and often to be of major pharmacological or toxicological importance. Fortunately, not all interactions are adverse as many combinations of drugs in relation to the kidney show desirable synergistic effects in the treatment of renal disease. In some cases, use of a single drug has proved of little value, whereas wisely chosen combinations of drugs may make all the difference between recovery, and progression of renal disease to terminal uraemia.

References

Abraham, E. P. (1962): The cephalosporins. *Pharmacol. Rev.*, **14**, 473.

Adams, D. A., Goodman, R., Maxwell, M. H. and Latta, H. (1964): Nephrotic syndrome associated with penicillamine therapy of Wilson's disease. *Amer. J. Med.*, **36**, 330.

Alexandre, G. P. J., Murray, J. E., Dammin, G. J. and Nolan, B. (1963): Immunosuppressive drug therapy in canine, renal and skin homografts. *Transplantation*, **1**, 432.

Antcliff, A. C., Beevers, D. G., Hamilton, M. and Harpur, J. E. (1971): The use of amiloride hydrochloride in the correction of hypokalaemic alkalosis induced by diuretics. *Postgrad. med. J.*, **47**, 644.

Asatoor, A. M., Galman, B. R., Johnson, J. R. and Milne, M. D. (1965): The excretion of dexamphetamine and its derivatives. *Brit. J. Pharmacol.*, **24**, 293.

Asatoor, A. M., London, D. R., Milne, M. D. and Simenhoff, M. L. (1963): The excretion of pethidine and its derivatives. *Brit. J. Pharmacol.*, **20**, 285.

Austin, W. H. and Villandry, P. J. (1967): Methoxyflurane and renal function. *Anaesthesiology*, **28**, 637.

Baer, J. E., Paulson, S. F., Russo, H. F. and Beyer, K. H. (1956): Renal elimination of 3-methylaminoisocamphane hydrochloride (mecamylamine). *Amer. J. Physiol.*, **186**, 180.

Barnett, H. L., Simons, D. J. and Wells, Jr., R. E. (1948): Nephrotic syndrome occurring during tridione therapy. *Amer. J. Med.*, **4**, 760.

Barry, K. G. and Malloy, J. F. (1962): Oliguric renal failure: evaluation and therapy by the intravenous infusion of mannitol. *J. Amer. med. Assoc.*, **179**, 510.

Baselt, R. C. and Casarett, L. J. (1972): Urinary excretion of methadone in man. *Clin. Pharmacol. Therap.*, **13**, 64.

Benitz, K. F. and Diermeier, H. F. (1964): Renal toxicity of tetracycline degradation products. *Proc. Soc. exp. Biol., N.Y.*, **115**, 930.

Berglund, F. (1962): Comparison between effects of carinamide and probenecid on thiosulphate secretion in the renal tubules of the dog. *Acta Pharmacol. (Kbh)*, **19**, 371.

Berliner, H. W., Hilton, J. G., Yu, T. F. and Kennedy, Jr., T. J. (1950): The renal mechanism for urate excretion in man. *J. clin. Invest.*, **29**, 396.

Beyer, K. H., Russo, H. F., Tillson, E. K., Miller, A. K., Verwey, W. F. and Gass, S. R. (1951): Benemid: *p*-(di-*n*-propylsulfamyl)-benzoic acid: its renal affinity and its elimination. *Amer. J. Physiol.*, **166**, 625.

Beyer, K. H., Wiebelhaus, V. D., Tillson, E. K., Russo, H. F. and Wilhoyte, K. M. (1950): Benemid: *p*-(di-*n*-propylsulfamyl)-benzoic acid: inhibition of glycine conjugation reactions. *Proc. Soc. exp. Biol., N.Y.*, **74**, 772.

Bluemle, Jr., L. W. and Goldberg, M. (1968): Renal accumulation of salicylate and phenacetin: possible mechanisms in the nephropathy of analgesic abuse. *J. clin. Invest.* **47**, 2507.

Boger, W. P., Beatty, J. O., Pitts, F. W. and Flippin, H. F. (1950): The influence of a new benzoic acid derivative on the metabolism of para-aminosalicylic acid (PAS) and penicillin. *Ann. intern. Med.*, **33**, 18.

Brain, M. C., Baker, L. R. I., McBride, J. A., Rubenberg, M. L. and Dacie, J. V. (1968): Treatment of patients with microangiopathic haemolytic anaemia with heparin. *Brit. J. Haematol.*, **15**, 603.

Braun, P., Tillotson, J. R., Wilcox, C. and Finland, M. (1968): Cephalexin and cephaloglycin activity in vitro and absorption and urinary excretion of single oral doses in normal young adults. *Appl. Microbiol.*, **16**, 1684.

Braun, W., Hesse, I. and Malorny, G. (1963): Zur Bedeutung pH-abhängiger Diffususionsvorgänge für die Nierenfunktion. *Arch. exp. Pathol. Pharmacol.*, **245**, 457.

Brauninger, G. E. and Remington, J. S. (1968): Nephropathy associated with methicillin therapy. *J. Amer. med. Assoc.*, **203**, 103.

Brayton, R. G. and Louria, D. B. (1964): Gentamicin in Gram-negative primary and pulmonary infections. *Arch. intern. Med.*, **114**, 205.

Brodie, B. B. (1965): Displacement of one drug by another from carrier or receptor sites. *Proc. roy. Soc. Med.*, **58**, 946.

Brodie, B. B., Lief, P. A. and Poet, R. (1948): The fate of procaine in man following its intravenous administration and methods for the estimation of procaine and diethylaminoethanol. *J. Pharmacol. exp. Therap.*, **94**, 359.

Brookes, P. and Lawley, P. D. (1964): Alkylating agents. *Brit. med. Bull.*, **20**, 91.

Brown, G. M., Weisman, R. A. and Molnar, D. A. (1961): The biosynthesis of folic acid: I Substrate and cofactor requirements for enzymatic synthesis by cell-free extracts of *Escherichia coli. J. biol. Chem.*, **236**, 2534.

Brown, W. H., Thornton, W. B. and Wilson, J. S. (1940): An evaluation of the clinical toxicity of sulfanilamide and sulfapyridine. *J. Amer. med. Assoc.*, **114**, 1605.

Burch, G., Ray, T., Threefoot, S., Kelly, F. J. and Svedberg, A. (1950): The urinary excretion and biological decay periods of radiomercury labeling a mercurial diuretic in normal and diseased man. *J. clin. Invest.*, **29**, 1131.

Butler, T. C. (1958): Termination of drug action by elimination of unchanged drug. *Federation Proc.*, **17**, 1158.

Cafruny, E. J. and Farah, A. (1956): Effect of the mercurial diuretic mersalyl on the content of protein bound sulfydryl in the cytoplasm of dog kidney cells. *J. Pharmacol. exp. Therap.*, **117**, 101.

Calne, R. Y. (1961): Inhibition of the rejection of renal homografts in dogs by purine analogues. *Transplant. Bull.*, **28**, 65.

Clarkson, T. W., Rothstein, A. and Sutherland, R. (1965): The mechanisms of action of mercurial diuretics in rats: the metabolism of ^{203}Hg-labelled chlormerodrin. *Brit. J. Pharmacol.*, **24**, 1.

Clyne, D. H., Kincaid-Smith, P., Ribush, N. T., Morris, P. J. and Marshall, V. C. (1970): Improvement of blood flow of rejecting renal allografts during heparin infusion. *Med. J. Aust.*, **1**, 522.

Cohen, A. B. (1966): Hyperkalemic effects of triamterene. *Ann. intern. Med.*, **65**, 521.

Counihan, T. B., Evans, B. M. and Milne, M. D. (1954): Observations on the pharmacology of the carbonic anhydrase inhibitor 'diamox'. *Clin. Sci.*, **13**, 583.

Craig, H. V., Guillet, G. G., Walker, J. A. and Artz, C. P. (1966): Respiratory depression related to intraperitoneal neomycin. Experimental study and review of recent literature. *Amer. Surg.*, **32**, 37.

Crawford, E. S., Beall, A. C., Moyer, J. H. and de Bakey, M. E. (1957): Complications of aortography. *Sur. Gynec. Obstet*, **104**, 129.

Crawford, J. D. and Kennedy, G. C. (1959): Chlorothiazide in diabetes insipidus. *Nature*, **183**, 891.

Dalgaard-Mikkelsen, S. and Poulsen, E. (1956): Renal excretion of sulphathiazole and sulphadimidine in pigs. *Acta Pharmacol.* (*Kbh*), **12**, 233.

Darrell, J. H., Garrod, L. P. and Waterworth, P. M. (1968): Trimethoprim: laboratory and clinical studies. *J. clin. Pathol.*, **21**, 202.

Dixon, R. L., Henderson, E. S. and Rall, D. P. (1965): Plasma protein binding of methotrexate and its displacement by various drugs. *Federation Proc.*, **24**, 454.

Dodds, M. G. and Foord, R. D. (1970): Enhancement by potent diuretics of renal tubular necrosis induced by cephaloridine. *Brit. J. Pharmacol.*, **40**, 227.

Douglas, J. B. and Healy, J. K. (1969): Nephrotoxic effects of amphotericin B including renal tubular acidosis. *Amer. J. Med.*, **46**, 154.

Earley, L. E. and Orloff, J. (1964): Thiazide diuretics. *Ann. Rev. Med.*, **15**, 149.

Einhorn, M. and Davidsohn, I. (1964): Hepatotoxicity of mercaptopurine. *J. Amer. med. Assoc.*, **188**, 802.

Elion, J. B. and Hitchings, G. H. (1965): Metabolic basis for the actions of analogs of purines and pyrimidines. *Advan. Chemotherap.*, **2**, 91.

Elkington, S. G., Goffinet, J. A. and Conn, H. O. (1968): Renal and hepatic injury associated with methoxyflurane anesthesia. *Ann. intern. Med.*, **69**, 1229.

Eriksson, E. (1966): Prilocaine. An experimental study in man of a new local anaesthetic with special regards to efficacy, toxicity and excretion. *Acta Chir. Scand.*, Supplement, **358**, 1.

Farah, A. and Kruse, R. (1960): The relation of mercurial diuretics to cellular protein-bound sulfydryl changes in renal cells. *J. Pharmacol. exp. Therap.*, **130**, 13.

Farah, A., Bender, C. H., Kruse, R. and Cafruny, E. (1959): The influence of acidosis and alkalosis on mercurial-induced diuresis and sulfydryl changes in the kidney. *J. Pharmacol. exp. Therap.*, **125**, 309.

Foster, R. P. and Hong, S. K. (1958): In vitro transport of dyes by isolated renal tubules of the flounder as disclosed by direct vizualisation. Intracellular accumulation and transcellular movement. *J. cell. Comp. Physiol.*, **51**, 259.

French, A. J. (1946): Hypersensitivity in pathogenesis of histopathological changes associated with sulfonamide chemotherapy. *Amer. J. Pathol.*, **22**, 674.

Frimpter, G. W., Timpanelli, A. E., Eisenmenger, W. J., Stein, H. S. and Ehrlich, L. I. 1963): Reversible "Fanconi syndrome" caused by degraded tetracycline. *J. Amer. med. Assoc.*, **184**, 111.

Gault, M. H., Blennerhassett, J. and Muehrcke, R. C. (1971): Analgesic nephropathy. A clinico-pathological study using electron microscopy. *Amer. J. Med.*, **51**, 740.

Gerhardt, R. E., Knouss, R. F., Thyrum, P. T., Luchi, R. J. and Morris Jr., J. J. (1969): Quinidine excretion in aciduria and alkaluria. *Ann. intern. Med.*, **71**, 927.

Ginsberg, D. J., Saad, A. and Gabuzda, G. J. (1964): Metabolic studies with the diuretic triamterene in patients with cirrhosis and ascites. *New. Engl. J. Med.*, **271**, 1129.

Goldberg, M., McCurdy, D. K., Foltz, E. L. and Bluemle, Jr., L. W. (1964): Effects of ethacrynic acid (a new saluretic agent) on renal diluting and concentrating mechanisms: evidence for site of action in the loop of Henle. *J. clin. Invest.*, **43**, 201.

Grégoire, F., Malmendier, C. and Lambert, P. (1956): Syndrome néphrotique après traitement aux sels d'or. *J. d'Urol.*, **62**, 140.

Gross, J. M. (1963): Fanconi syndrome (adult type) developing secondary to the ingestion of outdated tetracycline. *Ann. intern. Med.*, **58**, 523.

Grossman, J., Weston, R. E., Lehman, R. A., Halperin, J. P., Ullman, T. D. and Leiter, L. (1951): Urinary and fecal excretion of mercury in man following administration of mercurial diuretics. *J. clin. Invest.*, **30**, 1208.

Guild, W. R., Young, J. V. and Merrill, J. P. (1958): Anuria due to carbon tetrachloride intoxication. *Ann. intern. Med.*, **48**, 1221.

Gutman, A. B. and Yu, T. F. (1958): Renal regulation of uric acid excretion in normal and gouty man: modification by uricosuric agents. *Bull. N.Y. Acad. Med.*, **34**, 287.

Gutman, A. B., Yu, T. F. and Sirota, J. H. (1955): A study by simultaneous clearance techniques of salicylate excretion in man. Effect of alkalinization of the urine by bicarbonate administration; effect of probenecid. *J. clin. Invest.*, **34**, 711.

Gutman, A. B., Yu, T. F. and Berger, L. (1959). Tubular secretion of urate in man. *J. clin. Invest.*, **38**, 1778.

Gutman, A. B., Dayton, P. G., Yu, T. F., Berger, L., Chen, W., Sicam, L. E. and Burns, J. J. (1960): A study of the inverse relationship between pK_a and rate of renal excretion of phenylbutazone analogs in man and dog. *Amer. J. Med.*, **29**, 1017.

Haag, H. B. and Larson, P. S. (1942): Studies of the fate of nicotine in the body. 1. The effect of pH on the urinary excretion of nicotine by tobacco smokers. *J. Pharmacol. exp. Therap.*, **76**, 235.

Haag, H. B., Larson, P. S. and Schwartz, J. J. (1943): The effect of urinary pH on the elimination of quinine in man. *J. Pharmacol. exp. Therap.*, **79**, 136.

Halpern, B., Lagrue, G., Fray, A., Morard, J. C. and Milliez, P. (1965): Sur le traitement des néphropathies expérimentales par l'héparine. Perspectives d'application clinique. *Presse Médicale*, **73**, 57.

Harington, M., Kincaid-Smith, P. and Milne, M. D. (1958): Pharmacology and clinical use of pempidine in the treatment of hypertension. *Lancet*, **ii**, 6.

Harris, H. W., Murray, R., Paine, T. F., Kilham, L. and Finland, M. (1947): Streptomycin treatment of urinary tract infections. With special reference to the use of alkali. *Amer. J. Med.*, **2**, 229.

Harrison, A. R. and Rose, G. A. (1968): The effect of bendrofluazide on urinary and faecal calcium and phosphorus. *Clin. Sci.*, **34**, 343.

Herdman, R. C., Edson, J. R., Pickering, R. J., Fish, A. J., Marker, S. and Good, R. A. (1970): Anticoagulants in renal disease in children. *Amer. J. Dis. Child.*, **119**, 27.

Hill, J. B. (1971): Experimental salicylate poisoning: observations on the effects of altering blood pH on tissue and plasma salicylate concentrations. *Pediatrics*, **47**, 658.

Hitchings, G. H. (1961): A biochemical approach to chemotherapy. *Trans. N.Y. Acad. Sci.*, **23**, 700.

Hober, R., Woolley, P. M. B., Green, J. W. and Zimmerman, M. (1942): Further studies on the correlation between secretory powers of the frog kidney of molecular configuration of organic compounds. *J. cell. comp. Physiol.*, **19**, 183.

Hook, J. B. and Williamson, H. E. (1965): Addition of the saluretic action of furosemide to the saluretic action of certain other agents. *J. Pharmacol. exp. Therap.*, **148**, 88.

Huang, K. C., Moore, K. B. and Campbell, Jr., P. C. (1960): Renal excretion of para-aminosalicylic acid: a two way transport system in the dog. *Amer. J. Physiol.*, **199**, 5.

Hutner, S. H., Nathan, H. A. and Baker, H. (1959): Metabolism of folic acid and other pterin-pteridine vitamins. *Vitam. Horm.*, **17**, 1.

Igarashi, M., McLeod, M. E. and Graybiel, A. (1966): Clinical pathological correlations in squirrel monkeys after suppression of semicircular canal function by streptomycin sulfate. *Acta Oto-laryngol., Supplement* **214**, 1.

Jailer, J. W., Rosenfeld, M. and Shannon, J. A. (1947): The influence of orally administered alkali and acid on the renal excretion of quinacrine, chloroquine and santoquine. *J. clin. Invest.*, **26**, 1168.

Jawetz, E. and Gunnison, J. B. (1952): Studies on antibiotic synergism and antagonism: a scheme of combined antibiotic action. *Antibiot. Chemotherap.*, **2**, 243.

Josephson, B., Ek, J., Bucht, H., Werko, L., Kallas, J. and Grieg, A. (1953a): The competition between p-aminohippuric acid (PAH) and diodrast for renal excretion and extraction in man. *J. clin. Invest.*, **32**, 1184.

Josephson, B., Grieg, A., Kakossaios, G. and Kallas, J. (1953b): Renal tubular excretion from high plasma levels of p-aminohippurate (PAH) and diodrast (D) in unanaesthetized rabbits. *Acta physiol. Scand.*, **30**, 11.

Kahn, H. S. and Brotchner, R. J. (1950): A recovery from ethylene glycol (anti-freeze) intoxication: a case of survival and two fatalities from ethylene glycol including autopsy findings. *Ann. intern. Med.*, **32**, 284.

Kahn, S. B., Fein, S. A. and Brodsky, I. (1968): Effects of trimethoprim on folate metabolism in man. *Clin. Pharmacol. Therap.*, **9**, 550.

Kaye, J. J. and Chapman, G. B. (1963): Cytological aspects of antimicrobial antibiotics. III. Cytological distinguishable stages in antibiotic action of colistin sulfate on *Escherichia coli*. *J. Bacteriol.*, **86**, 536.

Keitzer, W. A. and Campbell, J. A. (1942): Renal complications of sulfadiazine. *J. Amer. med. Assoc.*, **119**, 701.

Kessler, R. H., Lozano, R. and Pitts, R. F. (1957): Studies on structure diuretic activity relationships of organic compounds of mercury. *J. clin. Invest.*, **36**, 656.

Kincaid-Smith, P. (1969): Analgesic nephropathy. A common form of renal disease in Australia. *Med. J. Aust.*, **11**, 1131.

Kincaid-Smith, P., Laver, M. C. and Fairley, K. F. (1970): Dipyridamole and anticoagulants in renal disease due to glomerular and vascular lesions: a new approach to therapy. *Med. J. Aust.*, **1**, 145.

Kincaid-Smith, P., Saker, B. M. and McKenzie, I. F. C. (1968): Lesions in the vasa recta in experimental analgesic nephropathy. *Lancet*, **1**, 24.

Kinter, W. B. (1959): Renal tubular transport of Diodrast-I^{131} and PAH in necturus. Evidence for simultaneous reabsorption and secretion. *Amer. J. Physiol.*, **196**, 1141.

Kinter, W. B. and Cline, A. L. (1961): Exchange diffusion and runout of diodrast-I^{131}

CHAPTER 11

Narcotic analgesics and drug interaction in man

H. W. KOSTERLITZ

1 Introduction

Narcotic analgesic drugs have a highly selective action in man and in animals. Although they have many effects on the peripheral autonomic nervous system, their main clinical use is for actions that are mediated by largely unknown structures in the central nervous system. There are therefore many possibilities for a modification of the effects of narcotic analgesic drugs by psychotropic drugs and vice versa. Most of these interactions will be of a physiological rather than a pharmacological nature. This chapter will deal only with interactions between drugs, i.e. when either the effect of a narcotic analgesic is modified by another drug given simultaneously or earlier or later, or when a narcotic analgesic drug modifies the action of another drug. Thus, effects such as the stimulating action of an analeptic (e.g. bemegride or nikethamide) on respiration depressed by a narcotic analgesic will not be considered because the analeptic stimulates the respiratory centre independently, that is without interacting with the analgesic. On the other hand, the restoration of normal respiration by a specific antagonist, such as naloxone or nalorphine, is included in the discussion because such an antagonist interacts with the narcotic analgesic at the receptor.

2 Drugs interfering with the absorption of narcotic analgesics

Very little is known about drugs that affect absorption of the orally administered narcotic analgesics. Evidence has recently been adduced by Nimmo et al. (1973) that propantheline retards and metoclopramide accelerates absorption of paracetamol in man by modifying gastric emptying. It is very likely that similar effects apply to the absorption of those narcotic analgesics which are readily absorbed from the intestinal mucosa, as for instance, pethidine and methadone.

3 Interactions affecting biotransformation of narcotic analgesic drugs

Of the various possible biotransformations of morphine and its closely related congeners, conjugation with glucuronic acid is probably the most important means of inactivation in man, whereas N-demethylation has little or no importance (Way and Adler, 1961, 1962). This seems to hold also for the degradation of levorphanol. On the other hand, N-demethylation plays an important role in the degradation of pethidine, and norpethidine in the urine accounts for about one-third of the total administered dose of pethidine.

N-Demethylation is depressed or accelerated by drugs inhibiting or enhancing the activity of liver microsomal enzymes. It would appear from clinical observations that the effects of monoamine oxidase inhibitors (MAOI) are or particular importance for a modification of the action of pethidine. Doses of 100 mg of pethidine given to patients treated with iproniazid, phenelzine of pargyline have been shown to have serious and sometimes fatal effects. Central excitation with depression of respiration are the most commonly observed symptoms. These interactions have been observed by many authors, e.g. Papp and Benaim (1958), Palmer (1960), Shee (1960), Taylor (1962) and Vigran (1964). This effect of the MAOI may last for perhaps 2 or 3 weeks after withdrawal of the drug.

It is generally assumed that morphine may be similarly affected by MAOI but reliable information is not available. It has already been pointed out that in man, N-demethylation is of less importance for the degradation of morphine than is conjugation with glucuronic acid. Since Sanchez et al. (1969) have shown that in rats chloroquine increases the lethal dose of morphine, apparently by causing an increase in conjugation, it would be of interest to know whether chloroquine shortens the action of morphine in man. No information is available for man as to possible interactions between the enzyme inducers of the barbiturate group and narcotic analgesics.

It is not known whether anticholinesterases affect the duration of the action of pethidine in man. Pethidine is partly catabolised by hydrolysis of the ethoxy-group in position 4 of the molecule; Bernheim and Bernheim (1945) showed that this hydrolysis is inhibited by physostigmine in rat liver in vitro.

During chronic administration of morphine-like drugs, the activity of the microsomal enzymes of the male rat is reduced and the metabolism of non-narcotic drugs is depressed (see Scrafani and Clouet, 1971) but it is not known whether this phenomenon applies to man.

Morphine and its congeners are not themselves enzyme inducers (Scrafani and Clouet, 1971).

4 Possible interactions with depressants of the central nervous system

The most important problem is the possible potentiation of the action of narcotic analgesics by central depressants of the tranquilliser group, i.e. the combined action is greater than can be accounted for by the added effects of the individual drugs. There are a number of very well-controlled observations which show that the effects of narcotic analgesics and phenothiazines are additive; there are only very few observations which indicate that potentiation may occur. Thus, Keats et al. (1961) showed that in post-operative pain the effects of pethidine and promethazine are only additive. Similar findings were obtained by Lasagna (1965) for pethidine and triflupromazine in post-operative pain (Fig. 1).

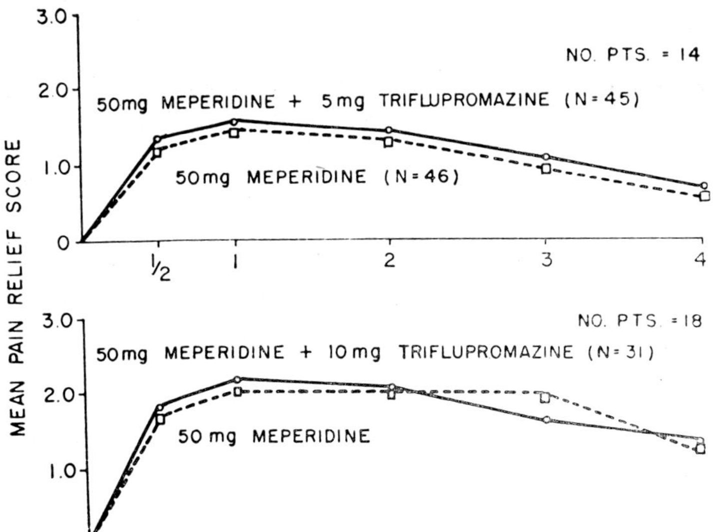

Fig. 1. Analgesic effects of pethidine and of mixtures of pethidine with triflupromazine in patients with post-operative pain. Reproduced, with permission, from Lasagna (1965).

Gorodetzky and Martin (1965) showed that, in healthy adult male post-addict volunteers, fentanyl is at least as euphorogenic as morphine. A combination of fentanyl and droperidol alters some of the morphine-like effects of fentanyl in the direction of the effects of droperidol. When the fentanyl content of the mixture is increased, the pattern of the signs and symptoms becomes more similar to that of fentanyl. For equimiotic doses, the euphorogenic potency of the mixture is at least not greater than that of the fentanyl contained in it. None of the effects is greater than can be accounted for by the additive effects of the drugs given alone and no potentiation has been observed.

Similarly, Dundee et al. (1963) found that, in patients whose response to graded pressure applied to the anterior surface of the tibia is tested prior to induction of anaesthesia, there is no potentiation of the analgesic effects of 100 mg of pethidine by promazine (25 mg), propiomazine (20 mg) and triflupromazine (10 mg); perphenazine (5 mg) or promethazine (12–50 mg) reduces the analgesic effect but a larger dose of promazine (50 mg) has possibly a potentiating effect (Table I). Promazine (50 mg) given alone increases sensitivity to pain (Moore and Dundee, 1961a). In another paper, Moore and Dundee (1961b) suggest that chlorpromazine may potentiate the analgesic action of pethidine.

TABLE I

Effect of phenothiazine derivatives on the analgesia index, 60–90 min after injection of pethidine[a]

Drug	Dose (mg)	Phenothiazine +pethidine analgesia index	No. of observations	Significance of phenothiazine effect (P)
Pethidine	100	+0.58	166	–
Promazine	50	+0.73	60	<0.05
Promazine	25	+0.62	72	N.S.[b]
Propiomazine	20	+0.59	51	N.S.[b]
Triflupromazine	10	+0.44	60	N.S.[b]
Perphenazine	5	+0.30	58	<0.001
Promethazine	12	+0.15	60	<0.001
Promethazine	25	+0.23	51	<0.001
Promethazine	50	+0.03	80	<0.001

[a] Modified from Dundee et al. (1963).
[b] N.S. – not significant.

The phenothiazine derivative, methotrimeprazine, has analgesic effects in post-operative and labour pain (Lasagna and DeKornfeld, 1961; DeKornfeld et al., 1964). When a mixture of methotrimeprazine and morphine is given, the depression of respiration is the same as that caused by the morphine present in the mixture (Pearson and DeKornfeld, 1963). On the other hand,

Lambertsen et al. (1961) showed that a combination of chlorpromazine and pethidine given to normal men depressed pulmonary minute volume and respiratory rate more than the individual drugs; tidal volume was not affected.

5 Possible interactions with drugs affecting the endocrine system

5.1 GENERAL

In patients hospitalized for various reasons, the response of plasma hydrocortisone to 2 U. vasopressin, but not to 1 U. ACTH, was reduced 60 min after injection of 16 mg of morphine sulphate (MacDonald et al., 1959).

During a cycle of addiction to morphine in post-addict volunteers the excretion of 17-ketosteroids was depressed. During addiction the absolute increase in daily urinary 17-ketosteroid excretion in response to administration of ACTH was reduced but the percentage increases were not different in the period of addiction and the pre- and post-addiction periods. The enhancing effect of chorionic gonadotrophins on 17-ketosteroid excretion was increased during the addiction period, the percentage increases being greater than the absolute increases.

6 Agonist-antagonist interactions

Narcotic analgesic drugs have a wide spectrum of agonist and antagonist actions. Compounds with mainly agonist effects comprise of morphine, heroin, levorphanol, fentanyl, pethidine, methadone, codeine and many other drugs used clinically for their analgesic and euphorogenic effects. At the other end of the spectrum are compounds which are antagonists with little or no agonist components. At present, the principal example of this kind of compound is naloxone (N-allylnoroxymorphone). In the middle of the spectrum there are compounds of dual agonist and antagonist actions which are sometimes called 'antagonist analgesics'; to this group belong nalorphine and levallorphan which were used as antagonists in morphine overdosage before the purer antagonist, naloxone, had become available. Pentazocine, which has relatively weak agonist and antagonist actions, also belongs to this group. Other compounds of similar actions have been investigated in animals but have not yet been introduced into clinical use. Compounds with dual agonist and antagonist actions were the subject of a recent symposium (Kosterlitz et al., 1972).

Many attempts have been made to separate analgesic, euphorogenic and respiratory depressant effects by the simultaneous use of a compound with mainly agonist actions, e.g. morphine or pethidine, and a compound with dual agonist and antagonist actions. Telford and Keats (1961) stated then that there was no pharmacological basis for the use of 'narcotic–narcotic antagonist' mixtures. They arrived at the conclusion that analgesia produced by such mixtures is accompanied by side-effects similar to those observed in analgesia of a similar degree when obtained by narcotic analgesics without addition of antagonists. It would appear that there is no advantage of using such mixtures for pre-anaesthetic medication or for the treatment of post-operative or labour pain.

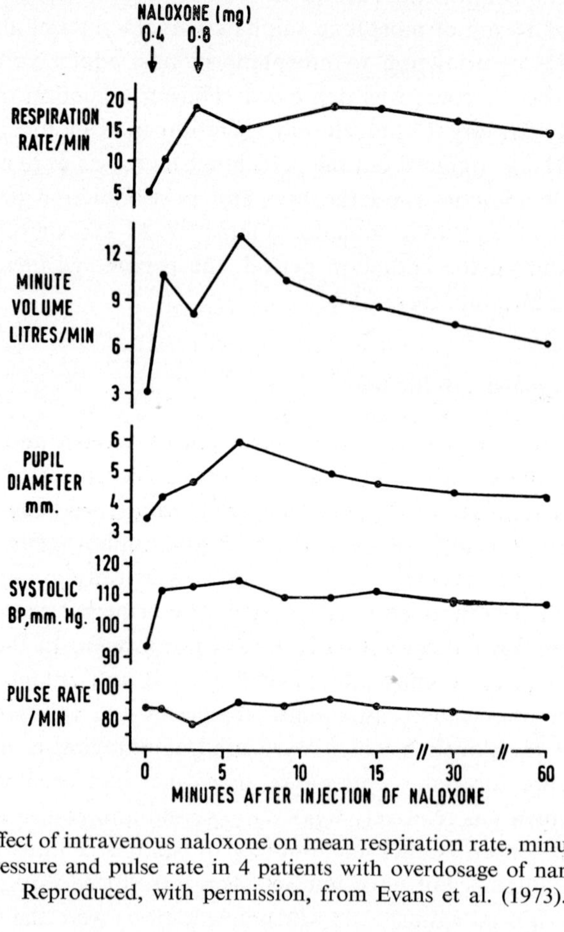

Fig. 2. The effect of intravenous naloxone on mean respiration rate, minute volume, pupil size, blood pressure and pulse rate in 4 patients with overdosage of narcotic analgesics. Reproduced, with permission, from Evans et al. (1973).

Nalorphine and levallorphan have been used for many years as antagonists in poisoning by overdosage of morphine-like drugs. When drugs with dual agonist and antagonist action, such as pentazocine, were introduced into clinical use for their analgesic effects it was found that their effects are not antagonized by nalorphine or levallorphan. For instance, the respiratory depressant effect caused by pentazocine is not antagonized by nalorphine. For satisfactory antagonism, an antagonist devoid of agonist action has to be used. Kallos and Smith (1968) showed that in human volunteers who had been given 0.7–0.8 mg/kg of pentazocine intravenously, the depressant effect on respiration was antagonized by naloxone; its median effective dose (ED_{50}) was 2–10 μg/kg. Evans et al. (1973) recently investigated the effects of naloxone in patients suffering from overdosage of various narcotic analgesic drugs. They confirmed that the effect of naloxone is highly specific. The effects on various parameters in 4 patients with narcotic analgesic overdosage is shown in Fig. 2. The authors also state that naloxone immediately reversed the effects of pentazocine in an apnoeic comatose patient.

Narcotic antagonists, e.g. cyclazocine and naloxone, have been used in the treatment of addicts dependent on heroin or other morphine-like drugs. Fink et al. (1972) have recently discussed the problems associated with this therapeutic approach. Cyclazocine, the N-cyclopropylmethyl analogue of pentazocine, is a potent analgesic with strong agonist and antagonist actions; the agonist effects are responsible for the dysphoria, vivid imagery and anxiety produced in some people. Since the 'pure' antagonist naloxone antagonizes the dysphoric effects of cyclazocine, a combination of the two drugs can be helpful in the treatment of addicts. The principal shortcomings of both cyclazocine and naloxone are their short duration of action and efforts at developing a long-acting antagonist are imperative.

References

Bernheim, F. and Bernheim, M. L. C. (1945): The hydrolysis of demerol by liver in vitro. *Anesthesiology*, **22**, 34.

DeKornfeld, T. J., Pearson, J. W. and Lasagna, L. (1964): Methotrimeprazine in the treatment of labor pain. *New Engl. J. Med.*, **270**, 391.

Dundee, J. W., Love, W. J. and Moore, J. (1963): Alterations in response to somatic pain associated with anaesthesia. XV. Further studies with phenothiazine derivatives and similar drugs. *Brit. J. Anaesthes.*, **35**, 597.

Evans, L. E. J., Roscoe, P., Swainson, C. P. and Prescott, L. F. (1973): Treatment of drug overdosage with naloxone, a specific narcotic antagonist. *Lancet*, **1**, 452.

Fink, M., Freedman, A. M., Resnick, R. and Zaks, A. (1972): Clinical status of the narcotic antagonists in opiate dependence. In: *Agonist and Antagonist Actions of Narcotic Analgesic Drugs*, p. 266. Editors: H. W. Kosterlitz, H. O. J. Collier and J. E. Villarreal. Macmillan, London and Basingstoke.

Gorodetzky, C. W. and Martin, W. R. (1965): A comparison of fentanyl, droperidol and morphine. *Clin. Pharmacol. Therap.*, **6**, 731.

Kallos, T. and Smith, T. C. (1968): Naloxone reversal of pentazocine-induced respiratory depression. *J. Amer. med. Assoc.*, **204**, 932.

Keats, A. S., Telford, J. and Kurosu, Y. (1961): 'Potentiation' of meperidine by promethazine. *Anesthesiology*, **22**, 34.

Kosterlitz, H. W., Collier, H. O. J. and Villarreal, J. E. (eds.) (1972): *Agonist and Antagonist Actions of Narcotic Analgesic Drugs*. Macmillan, London and Basingstoke.

Lambertsen, C. J., Wendel, H. and Longenhagen, J. B. (1961): The separate and combined respiratory effects of chlorpromazine and meperidine in normal men controlled at 46 mm Hg alveolar pCO_2. *J. Pharmacol. exp. Therap.*, **131**, 381.

Lasagna, L. (1965): Drug interaction in the field of analgesic drugs. *Proc. roy. Soc. Med.*, **58**, 978.

Lasagna, L. and DeKornfeld, T. J. (1961): Methotrimeprazine. A new phenothiazine derivative with analgesic properties. *J. Amer. med. Assoc.*, **178**, 887.

Macdonald, R. K., Evans, F. T., Weise, V. K. and Patrick, R. W. (1959): Effect of morphine and nalorphine on plasma hydrocortisone levels in man. *J. Pharmacol. exp. Therap.*, **125**, 241.

Moore, J. and Dundee, J. W. (1961a): Alterations in response to somatic pain associated with anaesthesia. V. The effect of promethazine. *Brit. J. Anaesthes.*, **33**, 3.

Moore, J. and Dundee, J. W. (1961b): Alterations in response to somatic pain associated with anaesthesia. VII. The effects of nine phenothiazine derivatives. *Brit. J. Anaesthes.*, **33**, 422.

Nimmo. J., Heading, R. C., Tothill, P. and Prescott, L. F. (1973): Pharmacological modification of gastric emptying: effects of propantheline and metoclopramide on paracetamol absorption. *Brit. med. J.*, **1**, 587.

Palmer, H. (1960): Potentiation of pethidine. *Brit. med. J.*, **2**, 944.

Papp, C. and Benaim, S. (1958): Toxic effects of iproniazid in a patient with angina. *Brit. med. J.*, **2**, 1070.

Pearson, J. W. and DeKornfeld, T. J. (1963): Effect of methotrimeprazine on respiration. *Anesthesiology*, **24**, 38.

Sanchez, E., Tampier, L. and Mardones, J. (1969): Effects of chloroquine pretreatment on lethal dose of morphine and on morphine metabolism in rats. *Eur. J. Pharmacol.*, **7**, 106.

Scrafani, J. T. and Clouet, D. H. (1971): Biotransformations. In: *Narcotic Drugs. Biochemical Pharmacology*, p. 137. Editor: D. H. Clouet. Plenum Press. New York and London.

Shee, J. C. (1960): Dangerous potentiation of pethidine by iproniazid, and its treatment. *Brit. med. J.*, **2**, 507.

Taylor, D. C. (1962): Alarming reaction of pethidine in patients on phenelzine. *Lancet*, **2**, 401.

Telford, J. and Keats, A. S. (1961): Narcotic–narcotic antagonist mixtures. *Anesthesiology*, **22**, 465.

Vigran, I. M. (1964): Dangerous potentiation of meperidine hydrochloride by pargyline hydrochloride. *J. Amer. med. Assoc.*, **187**, 953.

Way, E. L. and Adler, T. K. (1961): The biological disposition of morphine and its surrogates. I. *Bull. World Health Organization*, **25**, 227.

Way, E. L. and Adler, T. K. (1962): The biological disposition of morphine and its surrogates. 4. *Bull. World Health Organization*, **27**, 359.

CHAPTER 12

Drug interaction in general practice

J. C. PETRIE, D. DURNO AND J. G. R. HOWIE

1 Introduction

Although the general practitioner is required to have a wide range of knowledge in many different spheres he cannot realistically be expected to have a detailed knowledge of all the rapidly expanding technology of hospital and laboratory medicine.

Pharmacologically active substances are prescribed at 70% of general practice consultations (Cartwright, 1967) and there is no doubt that practitioners wish relevant and practical advice about the rational use of medicines. However, a 'credibility' gap has developed between laboratory and hospital medicine and the practitioner, who sees little clinical relevance in the extremely detailed and often lavishly produced information which he receives from many different sources of widely varying quality.

It is not surprising that practitioners have adopted a somewhat resigned and cynical attitude and direct much of the circulating information straight into a waste-paper basket without reading it, whether it is bad or brilliant! Many respected practitioners claim that they interpret the latest advice with extreme caution and change their own prescribing patterns only when they themselves have recognised that the information is relevant to their own practice, experience and patients.

Drug interactions are the newest factor which practitioners have to consider when they issue a prescription. However, the relative contribution of drug interactions to morbidity and mortality against other factors which affect the response of a patient to medicines is at present almost totally unquantified outside hospital.

The un-informed use of a wide number of medicines is hazardous as, perhaps unfortunately, the days of placebos and coloured waters are gone and most products now satisfy criteria of efficacy. There is a clear need to assess the extent to which the theoretical risks of multiple therapy are matched by clinically significant interactions relevant to general practice, particularly as over 90% of all medicines are prescribed outside hospital (Editorial, 1971a).

2 The extent of drug interaction in general practice

Illness in general practice is superficially less dramatic than in hospital where patients are exposed to, on average, 6 different substances during an average 16-day admission (Dollery, 1972). However, the time spent by any one patient in hospital is usually short compared to his lifetime in the community.

The potential for interactions is staggeringly large (Dollery, 1972). Fortunately clinically significant adverse interactions appear to be less frequent than might be expected from the prescriptions issued annually – 266.5 million in 1971 for England and Wales (Department of Health and Social Security, 1972), the annual tonnage of medicines produced and the increasing number of substances, often of different formulations, listed in the Pharmacopoeias or available as proprietary preparations. In the United States as many as 22,000 preparations are available (Task Force on Prescription Drugs, 1968).

There is wide concern about the so-called 'drug explosion'. In the U.S.A. 1 person in 3 between the ages of 18 and 74 was issued with a prescription for a minor tranquilliser in one year (Editorial, 1971b). One night's sleep in every 10 is induced by hypnotics (Dunlop, 1970). An assessment of the extent of prescription of some of the most widely prescribed medicines in the U.K. is shown in Table I. In this table no attempt has been made to quantitate the extent of sales of medicines available 'over-the-counter' for self-medication. There are national variations in pharmaceutical and medical practice and these have been discussed for Europe by Dunlop and Inch (1972).

In addition studies on patients outside hospital have been carried out. The average number of drugs obtained by prescription being taken by patients referred from general practice to medical units was 3.2 for females and 2.3 for males. Only 11% of the patients were not taking medicines (Starr and Petrie, 1972). In a study from Cincinnati on 821 outpatients the average number of medicines taken was 2 although a few patients were receiving as many as 8 medicines at one time. Fifteen per cent of these patients were not taking medicines (Sigell and Flessa, 1970). In a study of ambulant patients from Florida the average number of different medicines taken was 3.5 (including 'over-the-counter' medicines) during the two months prior to the outpatient clinic visit. Only 9% of these patients denied taking any medicines (Meleney and Fraser, 1968).

TABLE I

A selection of the major groups of drugs associated with clinically significant drug interactions supplied by prescription for 1970 in the United Kingdom (Department of Health and Social Security, 1972)

Drug group	Annual prescriptions (Millions)	Table
Barbiturate[a]	22	III VI VII VIII IX
Antihistamine	20	VI VII VIII IX
Penicillin	18	V
Tetracycline	16	III V
Benzodiazepine	15	VII VIII IX
Cold and cough cures[b]	14	II IV VII
Antidepressant (tricyclic)	6.4	II VI VII VIII IX
Phenothiazine	6	II IV VI VIII IX
Sulphonamide	3.5	III IV V
Steroid (oral)	3	IV VI VIII
Antihypertensive adrenergic neurone-blocking agent	1.3	II IV VII
Sulphonylurea	1.0	III IV V VI IX
Antidepressant (MAOI)	0.4	II IV VII VIII IX
Warfarin	0.15	III IV V VIII
Phenindione	0.15	III
Total	126.9	

[a] Excludes totals from combined preparations.
[b] Containing phenylpropanolamine, phenylephrine, ephedrine, pseudoephedrine.

This widespread use and consumption of medicines arises because of many factors. Most practitioners attempt to initiate treatment only with medicines with which they are familiar. Nevertheless, much prescribing is initiated by partners, other practices and specialists, and in each year many general practitioners prescribe more than 150 different drugs (Wilson, 1971; Durno, personal communication). As the number of different medicines prescribed increases, so inevitably does the knowledge about the individual characteristics of each diminish. In addition to these factors, there are many persuasive influences to prescribe outside the usually small range of 30–40 medicines which each practitioner prescribes regularly. These influences, which will not be discussed in detail, include:

(a) the convenience of combined preparations;
(b) the expectation for medicines by the public;
(c) the desire to evaluate new products;
(d) a 'spirit of adventure';
(e) skilled advertising, including visits by representatives, samples in the post, buffet suppers, dinners and film shows, etc.

3 Communication about medicines

3.1 GENERAL

One of the main difficulties associated with the evaluation of the extent and clinical importance of drug interactions in general practice is that measurement depends on the detection of the interaction by both the patient and by his practitioner. At present, spontaneous detection rates of drug interaction in general practice are extremely low because the facilities for communication about medicines are not satisfactory and there is a lack of awareness and recognition of drug interactions. In addition there is a natural reluctance to report interactions which, in retrospect were preventable.

The 'medicines history' obtained at the initial medical consultation is notoriously unreliable. Patients often fail to mention major prescribed medicines that they are taking, such as hypnotics, analgesics, and the 'pill'. Indeed, patients are extremely confused about the nature and names of current medicines and usually are unable to indicate the dose or the time or the frequency of administration of the medicines that they are taking or their own allergic status to the medicines.

This is regrettable and remarkable, but not surprising because medicines may be supplied or issued from many different sources and the patient may not understand the instructions that he is given at the time the medicine is obtained.

Within each general practice a patient tends to consult a specific practitioner but because of the advent of larger group practices, health centres and off-duty rosters, a patient may be seen by several different doctors or by a locum tenens, who may be unaware of the precise details of current therapy. The consultation may take place at a surgery or in the patient's home. In either situation, because of the severe limitations of the record systems used there is considerable risk of a drug interaction being initiated unintentionally.

A further potential source of drug interaction arises because medicines are often issued without a personal patient–doctor contact. In such circumstances a formal entry is frequently not made in the patient's notes about the prescription issued. This omission may arise because the patient may not consider that a formal medical consultation is necessary, or simply, the patient may not wish to trouble his doctor. The patient arranges for the receptionist to the practice to prepare a 'repeat' prescription which is later signed by the practitioner, often among 20–30 other prescriptions which he signs at the end of a surgery session. Alternatively, the medicine may be obtained from a chemist or pharmacist who issues a preparation to a patient and at a later stage asks the practitioner to sign the completed prescription forms.

Medicines issued for previous illnesses and friends' medicines also contribute. The potential importance of this problem has been hinted at in the 'Spring-clean for Safety' campaign carried out in Scotland. Unwanted medicines in the home were handed in for destruction and in a short time a total of 4.5 million tablets and capsules were collected, almost half of which were hypnotics or tranquillisers (Wilson, 1972).

A further source of drug interaction concerns combined proprietary preparations, some of which contain hidden constituents such as barbiturates and sympathomimetic substances, available 'over-the-counter'.

Medicines initiated during a hospital admission are considered by many general practitioners to be an increasingly important source of medicines with a potential to interact. A delay in communication with the practitioner in the high-risk period immediately after the patient has been discharged is not unusual, and medicines incompatible with current treatment may be prescribed before the information is forthcoming. In addition, few hospital doctors supply advice in their letters about the newer medicines which have been issued to patients and some of these hospital-initiated medicines may be outside the previous experience of the general practitioner. It is false to offer idealistic advice to practitioners to restrict their therapy to a few medicines that they know well when many of their patients are being treated by different specialists; some of whom are introducing new medicines without guidance as to what precautions the practitioner should take. Patients may also obtain medicines from different 'specialty' outpatient departments and each department may be unaware of the exact therapy prescribed by the other and, in turn, by the practitioner.

A further source of medicines involves self-medication (Dunnell and Cartwright, 1972). In British studies, 66% of subjects interviewed had taken drugs as self-medication in the previous month (Jefferys et al., 1960) and 50% of the patients in the previous fortnight (Beveridge and Petrie, 1972).

These many sources of medicines make it essential that communication about medicines must be adequate. Unfortunately the records systems for transferring information about medicines are less than ideal.

3.2 RECORDS IN GENERAL PRACTICE

There has been little improvement in the transfer of information about medicines between doctors, and between doctors and patients over the last 10 years. In most practices in the United Kingdom the patient's notes are kept in a standard envelope (EC6) which although not ideal has still to be superceded by an acceptable alternative. The notes within the envelope tend not to have a standard arrangement or sequence. Contributions are in many handwritings, not all of which are legible. Rapid review and retrieval of information about 'events' (Finney, 1965) and 'problems' (Weed, 1969) and medicines history is difficult.

In a survey of records from eight general practices who allowed their records to be examined Dawes (1972) found that the recording of the therapeutic agent used was the most frequently recorded item, occurring in 70% of episodes but the amount prescribed was recorded in only one quarter of the episodes and the dosage in less than one fifth. In the study no attempt was made to check the actual medicines' history of the patients.

In a Scottish study of 559 patients referred to medical units, 89% of the patients were taking medicines but in only 56% was any information supplied by the practitioner, and only 36% of the total number of medicines (1557) being taken were mentioned. The largest group of medicines not mentioned by the practitioner were those supplied by prescription (61%). These medicines included sedatives, hypnotics, analgesics, antacids and even anticoagulants, and other substances with the potential to cause an adverse interaction. Information about medicines given in emergency situations was excellent but there was no information at all about drugs taken as self-medication. The information about the allergic status of patients was minimal (Beveridge and Petrie, 1972).

Two further studies are of interest. Barnes and Hoile (1969), in a survey of letters accompanying emergency admissions, found that there was no mention of drug therapy in half the available letters. De Alarcon and Hodson (1964) in a random sample of 500 letters from case notes found that in only 23% of the letters obtained was some form of treatment mentioned, and no reference to allergic status was made. The subject of letters from general practitioners has been developed by Forsyth and Logan (1968).

In some areas systems which use computer facilities are being developed for outpatients, such as the Kaiser Permanente programme in San Francisco (Friedman et al., 1971) and for general practice (Farmer and Cross, 1972; Durno, 1973). However on a wider scale the situation and difficulties are best summarised by quoting that 20% of doctors in general practice do not keep notes (Robb, 1970). It is only recently that doctors in the United Kingdom have agreed that pharmacists should label the containers of medicines with the name of the medicine that has been supplied.

Patients continue to be extremely reluctant to carry cards on which details of current medicines are recorded even when they are on 'high-risk' preparations such as steroids or anticoagulants. It is possible that their motivation could be increased by improving their understanding of the hazards of some of the forms of therapy. However, it must be emphasised that patients must not be frightened away from low-risk therapy and the undesirability of therapeutic nihilism must be stressed.

3.3 AWARENESS OF DRUG INTERACTIONS

In addition to a readily accessible medicines history measurement of the extent of clinically significant adverse interactions depends on the awareness by the patient and doctor that some symptoms may be due to adverse effects or drug interactions.

The lack of awareness of patients on long-term anticoagulant therapy of the hazards of taking additional medicines has been documented (Starr and Petrie, 1972). Fifty-five per cent of patients were not adequately aware of the nature and possibility of haemorrhagic complications. Slightly fewer (52%) had inadequate knowledge of the hazards of taking additional medicines, or of altering their pattern of taking medicines.

The reliability of patients has also been examined. Patients forget, or discontinue therapy spontaneously. For example, in patients on long-term treatment failure rates of 50% or more have regularly been observed (Oakes et al., 1973). The information about short courses of therapy with antibiotic treatment shows that 56% of patients had stopped taking penicillin by the third day (Bergman and Werner, 1963). Porter (1969) has estimated that 69% of patients were 'compliant', 35% intermediate, and 6% 'non-compliant'. Further studies on drug defaulting have been carried out by Blackwell (1972) and on medication errors by Stewart and Cluff (1972).

The detection of adverse interactions also requires awareness of the drug interaction by the doctors. In a survey of 253 general practitioners in the North East of Scotland (population 400,000) of the 185 doctors (74%) who replied anonymously to a 50-item questionnaire about drug interactions, the average number which the doctors claimed to have 'heard of' was 17.2 out of 50 (Petrie et al., 1974). The distribution of doctors around the mean value was of a basically normal pattern. The questions concerned 5 groups of medicines involved in drug interactions – Warfarin, adrenergic neurone-blocking antihypertensive agents, monoamine oxidase inhibitors (MAOI), hypoglycaemic and sedative agents.

The most common interactions that these practitioners claimed to be aware of were those involving MAOI. Indeed, 5 of the top 6 interactions involved these drugs (with antidepressants, 78%; with beers and wine, 71%; with phenothiazines, 64%; with hypotensive agents, 63%). This high degree of awareness presumably reflects the wide publicity that these interactions have attracted. It would thus appear that the risk of un-intentional drug interactions being initiated with this group of medicines is low, although the interactions may themselves be those with the most clinical importance. In the United Kingdom practitioners prescribed these drugs relatively infrequently and in 1970 only 400,000 prescriptions were issued compared to 6.4 million prescriptions for the tricyclic antidepressant group (Department of Health and Social Security, 1972).

Some interactions involving the oral anticoagulant, Warfarin, were claimed to have been heard of by about half the doctors who replied to the above questionnaire (with salicylates, 53%; with pentobarbitone, 48%; with butobarbitone, 48%; with Sonalgin*, 46%). Other theoretical interactions involving Warfarin sodium which have had less publicity (nalidixic acid, ethacrynic acid, dichloralphenazone, mefenamic acid) had been heard of by 10% of the doctors. This suggests that there is a need to improve the communication of information to doctors about these interactions. Nevertheless, it is possible that the less well-publicised interactions involving Warfarin are not of clinical importance, and therefore should not be over-stressed.

Interactions involving the adrenergic neurone-blocking antihypertensive agents (guanethidine, bethanidine, debrisoquine) and the tricyclic antidepressant group had been heard of by 45% of the practitioners in the above survey. However, interactions of these agents with sympathomimetic amines in cold cures – such as phenylpropanolamine and phenylephrine – had been heard of by fewer than 20% of the practitioners. Since the antihypertensive agents may cause symptoms of depression and nasal congestion in up to a third of patients, these interactions require wider publicity as antidepressants and decongestants may be given to alleviate the symptoms caused by the drug.

The awareness of practitioners of interactions involving other groups of medicines has not, to our knowledge, been measured, although such information is of interest if an indication of the effectiveness of communications about drug interaction is to be obtained.

3.4 RECOGNITION OF INTERACTIONS

In the above study, the 185 practitioners who replied were invited to report their 'experience' of the 50 specific interactions which were listed. The 6 most common interactions which they claimed to have experienced involved Warfarin. These included: interactions with salicylates (15 doctors);

* Sonalgin – butobarbitone, codeine, phenacetin.

butobarbitone (9 doctors); phenylbutazone (7 doctors); clofibrate (7 doctors); tetracycline (7 doctors); pentobarbitone (6 doctors). Eleven doctors had experienced interactions involving the adrenergic neurone-blockers with amitryptiline and 9 doctors with imipramine. Surprisingly, 6 doctors claimed to have experienced interactions involving insulin and propranolol. These reports have clear limitations, some of which have been discussed above. Nevertheless, the information is of some interest in attempting to assess the experience of practitioners of drug interactions and the relative clinical importance that they attach to the problem. An example of the limitations of the value of the information and by extrapolation the limitations of any system which invites reporting of interactions from doctors, is seen from an examination of the interactions which the doctors claimed to have experienced. For example, the most common interaction experienced involved the salicylates, but this interaction occurs only when high doses of salicylates (greater than 2 g) are given, and these adverse interactions may have had other causes. Similarly, the evidence of an effect of tetracycline on the control of Warfarin therapy is contradictory (see Chapter 7, p. 129).

An alternative method of evaluating the extent and clinical importance of drug interactions is by intensive surveillance. However, large-scale drug monitoring in general practice is not a realistic exercise at present because the quality of information about medicines cannot be guaranteed over any period of time. Furthermore, diagnoses in general practice do not correspond to those in hospital medicine and the recognition of 'events' (Finney, 1965) is difficult in a non-captive population of patients. The scale of any study would need to be extremely large, as 4000 patients have to be under very close supervision to give a 95% chance of the detection of an 'event' which occurs once in every 1000 cases.

Another method of evaluating the extent of interactions in general practice is to study groups of patients on 'high-risk' medicines. For example, in 64 patients on long-term antihypertensive adrenergic neurone-blocking agents, theoretical interactions were detected in over one third of patients, although in less than 5% was a significant loss of blood pressure control recorded at the time of the interview (Starr and Petrie, 1972). In 254 patients on long-term anticoagulant therapy with Warfarin, over a third of the patients were at theoretical risk to a drug interaction, but in only 9% was there any suggestion that a probable adverse reaction had occurred in the 6 months prior to the time of the interview (Starr and Petrie, 1972).

An alternative method of evaluation has been attempted by Durno (1973). The extent of drug interactions in a 3000-patient, two-partner practice in the year 1971 was measured using a method of data collection which involved the computer facilities made available by the University of Aberdeen. Studies of this nature are not representative of ordinary general practice, but examination of the print-out material on patients on anti-hypertensive, anticoagulant, hypoglycaemic and monoamine oxidase inhibitor agents, revealed only four cases of theoretical drug interaction and the clinical importance of these was slight.

4 Prevention of drug interactions in general practice

4.1 GENERAL

If the occurrence of interactions is to be significantly reduced, two main approaches are necessary. Firstly, systems are required to improve communications about medicines. Secondly, information must be provided for practitioners which will be favourably received because it is relevant to general practice and is not an extensive catalogue of theoretical interactions involving medicines which they never use. 'Wolf crying' reduces the effectiveness of communication of important information. This appears to be under-recognised in academic circles.

4.2 MEDICINES RECORD IN GENERAL PRACTICE

Systems for handling information about current therapy have been designed for use in hospitals (Crooks et al., 1967) and they are being developed on a national scale (Scottish Health Services Council, 1972).

In general practice, most practitioners record the diagnosis and new therapy side by side at the time of each consultation and they are reluctant to abandon this traditional method of note keeping. However, because of the demonstration of the breakdown of communication about medicines (nature, dose, frequency of administration, duration of therapy, allergic status) some practitioners may wish to consider the use of a 'medicines record' for general practice. The writing of a prescription should be the time to reappraise all aspects of current therapy and to give the patient careful instructions, both oral and written, about his therapy.

Although computer facilities may eventually provide a solution to the problem of maintaining records, at the present time, and for the next 10–20 years, they do not offer a realistic solution for the great majority of practitioners and manual systems are required.

The manual 'medicines record' must be a compact, convenient and clearly designated area within the patient's notes. In this area of the record basic information about medicines (old, current and new) could be rapidly reviewed and updated. The permanent record should remind the practitioner about other current therapy, possible interactions of medicines and contribute towards the continuity of long-term therapy in patients with diseases such as diabetes mellitus, hypertension and sub-thyroidism, etc. The 'medicines record' would also provide an estimate of the rate of tablet consumption by default of the patient, and might reduce the tendency towards polypharmacy and the problem of unrecorded 'repeat' prescriptions.

Standardisation of the forms used with the hospital discharge medicines sheets would allow more reliable communication about medicines when the patient was transferred from general practice to hospital and vice-versa. The design, in principle, would be similar to the prescribing sheets supplied for the hospital cardex system (Scottish Health Services Council, 1972).

In addition the 'medicines record' in general practice would allow the identification of patients on specific medicines for drug monitoring studies. This must be developed as it allows expansion of numerator data which are one of the limitations of the hospital system.

A 'medicines record' is one aspect of the solution of the problem of reducing iatrogenic disease in general practice. Provision of relevant information to the general practitioner is the other major factor.

4.3 RELEVANT INFORMATION

Practitioners receive information from national agencies, the pharmaceutical industry, colleagues, medical journals, bulletins, text books, university departments and pharmacists (Wilson, 1969; Macgregor, 1970; Becker et al., 1972; Stolley et al., 1972). There is clear evidence that the practitioners desire information but they have great difficulty in selecting the important facts. This problem is shared by the agencies providing information about medicines as it has not been established which aspects of the rational use of medicines require particular emphasis. Indeed, it may be less important to offer advice about drug interactions than about the inappropriate prescription of fixed doses of medicines to patients in whom wide differences in absorption, distribution, metabolism and excretion may occur, or about the inappropriate use of tetracyclines in renal failure or infancy.

In the North East of Scotland, practitioners receive information from the sources mentioned above. In addition, Neill and Barnett (1969) have designed a drug interaction disc which is shown on p. 265 (Chapter 14). This disc is not designed particularly for general practice and three further approaches are in progress.

Firstly, following the study of awareness and experience of drug interactions, tables of selected adverse drug interactions have been prepared and

TABLE II

Antihypertensive drug interactions

Drug group	Interaction with	Result
Antihypertensives	Phenothiazines; MAOI; alcohol; anaesthetics; other antihypertensive agents	Increased hypotensive effects
Adrenergic neurone-blocking agents (guanethidine; bethanidine, debrisoquine)	Cold and cough remedies[a]; tricyclic antidepressants; chlorpromazine; MAOI; inhibitors; vasopressors; amphetamines	Occasional pressor response; loss of hypotensive effect
Clonidine	Tricyclic antidepressants	Loss of hypotensive effect

[a] Containing phenylpropanolamine, phenylephrine and ephedrine.

Table III

Oral anticoagulant drug interactions. The clinical importance of many of these interactions is not established.

Drug group	Interaction with	Result
Oral anti-coagulants Warfarin, phenindione	Enzyme inducing agents, e.g. barbiturates; dichloralphenazone and sedatives (not nitrazepam); griseofulvin; chronic alcohol intake	Reduced anticoagulant effect. *Danger* if dose of anticoagulant increased to restore desired effect and then concurrent enzyme inducer (e.g. barbiturate) is *Stopped* (→ haemorrhage)
	Displacement from protein binding, e.g. phenylbutazone[a], clofibrate, quinidine, sulphonamides, sulphonylureas[a], ethacrynic acid, nalidixic acid, mefenamic acid ? chloral hydrate ? aspirin > 2 g/day ? indomethacin, phenytoin, diazoxide	Temporary intcrease in anticoagulant effect
	Vitamin C, cholestyramine, oral contraceptives	Reduced effect
	Liver disease; alcohol or drug-induced liver disease; Vitamin K deficiency (laxatives?; broad spectrum antibiotics on gut flora); steroids; thyroxine; heparin	Increased anticoagulant effect

[a] Also enzyme inhibitor effect.

circulated to practitioners. These Tables (II–IX) do not include every known drug interaction, but concentrate on the principal medicines prescribed and on the 'high-risk' interactions that are relevant to general practice. Such tables would be of added value if they were designed not on a local, but on a national or international collaborative basis as there is no reason to suppose that the awareness of drug interactions by the practitioners of the North East of Scotland is different from practitioners in other areas. Detailed tables of drug interactions have been compiled and are also accessible to the practitioners (Garb, 1971; Martin, 1971).

TABLE IV

Hypoglycaemic drug interactions

Drug group	Interaction with	Result
Insulins, oral hypoglycaemics	Drugs which influence glucose metabolism, e.g. salicylates; β-blockers, adrenergic neurone-blockers; MAOI; diazoxide	Increased hypoglycaemic effect
	Chlorpromazine; diuretics; steroids; oestrogens; thyroxine; sympathomimetics	Reduced hypoglycaemic effect
Sulphonylureas	Enzyme inhibitor agents, e.g. coumarin anticoagulant; MAOI; chloramphenicol (2 g/day)	Increased hypoglycaemic effect
	Displacement from protein binding, e.g. clofibrate; phenylbutazone; sulphonamides; ethacrynic acid; probenecid	Increased hypoglycaemic effect

TABLE V

Principal chemotherapeutic drugs used in general practice. 15% total prescriptions in 1971 were for medicines acting systemically in treatment of infection.

Drug group	Interaction with	Result
Tetracyclines	Iron salts; antacids (calcium, magnesium, aluminium, sodium bicarbonate); food	Reduced absorption (up to 50%)
Penicillins	Food	Reduced absorption. Take on empty stomach
	Tetracycline	Reduced effect. Contraindicated
Sulphonamides	Warfarin; sulphonylurea	Table III, Table IV

TABLE VI

Oral corticosteroids. 'Hidden' constituents of combined preparations may include barbiturates, e.g. 'antiasthma' preparations.

Drug group	Interaction with	Result
Oral corticosteroids	Enzyme inducing agents, e.g. barbiturates, diphenylhydantoin	Decreased steroid effect
	Displacement from plasma protein, e.g. indomethacin; phenylbutazone	Increased steroid effect
	Vaccines (measles, smallpox, etc.)	Contraindicated
	Drugs with anticholinergic activity, e.g. tricyclic antidepressants; some antihistamines, phenothiazines, anti-parkinsonian agents	Increased risk of glaucoma in susceptible patients
	Hypoglycaemic agents	See Table IV

TABLE VII

Antidepressant drugs. Any patient on MAOI should be supplied with a list of foods and substances to avoid. All current medicines therapy must be reviewed at each consultation. MAOI are seldom initiated by general practitioners. Only 396,000 prescriptions for MAOI were written in general practice in the U.K. in 1970. (Tricyclic group 6,400,000 prescriptions.)

Drug group	Interaction with	Result
Tricyclic antidepressants, e.g. imipramine, amitriptyline, nortriptyline, protriptyline desipramine, trimipramine, etc.	Guanethidine, bethanidine, debrisoquine, clonidine	Loss of control of blood pressure
	Sympathomimetics, e.g. noradrenaline, adrenaline, phenylephrine	Pressor responsemay occur
	Drugs with anticholinergic properties, e.g. tricyclic antidepressants; some antihistamines, phenothiazines, anti-parkinsonian agents	Increase in atropine-like effect – care with glaucome, urine retention, etc.
	CNS depressants	See Table VIII
	Other antidepressants especially MAO inhibitors	Hazardous potentiation
Monoamine oxidase inhibitors in general practice	Numerous drugs and foods!	Careful supervision of all current medicines essential

TABLE VIII

Drugs acting on the central nervous system. The increased effect may result from similar sedative, anticholinergic, antihistamine, phenothiazine and other shared pharmacological properties. At least 80 million prescriptions were issued in the U.K. in 1970. In addition many combined preparations contain "hidden" barbiturates, antihistamines, etc. and other substances acting on the central nervous system.

Drug group	Interaction with	Result
Central nervous system depressants, e.g. sedative, antihistamine, tranquilliser, antidepressant, major analgesic	Other CNS depressants	Increased effect
Enzyme inducers, CNS depressants, e.g. barbiturates	Barbiturates, anticonvulsants	Tolerance
	Warfarin, steroids	Table III, Table V

TABLE IX

Alcohol

	Interaction with	Result
Alcohol	Hypnotics and sedatives; tranquillisers; antidepressants; major analgesics; antihistamines	Potentiation
	Some sulphonylureas, metronidazole (Flagyl), nitrofurantoin	Disulfiram reaction

The second approach in the North East of Scotland is for the hospital Pharmacy to issue a drug discharge sheet to the patient at the time of leaving hospital. The sheet is designed to provide information about current medicines in the interval before a detailed letter about all aspects of the hospital admission is sent to the practitioner. In addition, the hospital Pharmacy are to issue to the practitioners of patients on 'high-risk' medicines, 'stickers' to apply to the outside of patients' general practice notes. On these stickers the interactions involving the medicines are shown.

The third approach, as in many other regions, is to issue cards to the patients on the 'high-risk' medicines such as steroids, monoamine oxidase inhibitors, anticoagulants and hypoglycaemic agents.

These approaches and the development of a 'medicines record' for general practice should contribute towards a reduction in the occurrence of iatrogenic disease.

References

Barnes, P. K. and Hoile, R. W. (1969): Emergency admissions to a general medical unit: A survey of the accompanying letters, with recommendations. *Brit. med. J.*, **4**, 424.

Becker, M. H., Stolley, P. D., Lasagna, L., McEvilla, J. D. and Sloane, L. M. (1972): Differential education concerning therapeutics and resultant physician prescribing patterns. *J. med. Educ.*, **47**, 118.

Bergman, A. B. and Werner, R. J. (1963): Failure of children to receive penicillin by mouth. *New. Engl. J. Med.*, **268**, 1334.

Beveridge, T. and Petrie, J. C. (1972): Transfer of information about intake of drugs by patients referred to medical units. *Brit. med. J.*, **2**, 37.

Blackwell, B. (1972): The drug defaulter. *Clin. Pharmacol. Therap.*, **13**, 841.

Cartwright, A. (1967): *Patients and their doctors.* Routledge, London.

Crooks, J., Calder, G. and Weir, R. D. (1967): Drugs in hospital. *J. roy. Coll. Phys. London*, **1**, 233.

Dawes, K. S. (1972): Survey of general practice records. *Brit. med. J.*, **3**, 219.

De Alarcon, R. and Hodson, J. M. (1964): Value of the general practitioner's letter, a further study in medical communication. *Brit. med. J.*, **2**, 435.

Department of Health and Social Security (1972): Annual Statistics. London.

Dollery, C. T. (1972): Drug interactions. In: *Eighth Symposium on Advanced Medicine*, Vol. 9, p. 210. Editor: G. Neale. Pitman Medical, London.

Dunlop, D. (1970): Abuse of drugs by the public and doctors. *Brit. med. Bull.*, **26**, 236.

Dunlop, D. and Inch, R. S. (1972): Variations in pharmaceutical and medical practice in Europe. *Brit. med. J.*, **3**, 749.

Dunnell, K. and Cartwright, A. (1972): Medicine Takers, Prescribers and Hoarders. Routledge and Kegan Paul, London and Boston.

Durno, D. (1973): Drug interaction in a general practice. *Update*, **7**, 279.

Editorial (1971a): Drug reactions. *Lancet*, *i*, 1227.

Editorial (1971b): Drug explosion. *Lancet*, *ii*, 1381.

Farmer, R. D. T. and Cross, K. W. (1972): An automated records system for general practice. *Brit. J. Prevent. Soc. Med.*, **26**, 148.

Finney, D. J. (1965): The design and logic of a monitor of drug use. *J. chron. Dis.*, **18**, 77.

Forsyth, G. and Logan, R. F. (1968): Gateway or dividing line? *A study of hospital outpatients in the 1960's.* Oxford University Press, London, New York, Toronto.

Friedman, G. D., Collen, M. F., Harris, L. E., Van Brunt, E. E. and Davis, L. S. (1971): Experience in monitoring drug reactions in outpatients. The Kaiser-Permanente drug monitoring system. *J. Amer. med. Assoc.*, **217**, 567.

Garb, S. (1971): *Clinical Guide to Undesirable Drug Interactions and Interferences.* Springer, New York; Harvey Miller and Medcalf, London.

Jefferys, M., Brotherston, J. H. F. and Cartwright, A. (1960): Consumption of medicines on a working-class housing estate. *Brit. J. prevent. soc. Med.*, **14**, 64.

Macgregor, A. G. (1970): The communication of information about drugs to the medical profession and the general public. Royal Academies of Medicine of Belgium: In: *Proc. Intern. Symp. clin. Pharmacol.*, p. 165. St. Catherine Press, Brugge, Belgium.

Martin, E. W. (1971): *Hazards of Medication.* Lippincott, Philadelphia; Blackwell, Oxford.

Meleney, H. E. and Fraser, M. L. (1968): A retrospective study of drug usage and adverse drug reactions in hospital outpatients. *Drug Inform. Bull.*, **2**, 96.

Neil, J. M. and Barnett, J. W. (1969): Major drug interactions: A system for easy reference. *J. hosp. Pharm.*, **27**, 197.

Oakes, M., Human, R. P. and Meers, P. D. (1973): Serum-levels of four antibiotics administered orally to patients in general practice. *Lancet*, **1**, 222.

Petrie, J. C., Howie, J. G. R. and Durno, D. (1974): Awareness and experience of general practitioners of selected drug interactions. *Brit. med. J.*, **2**, 262.

Porter, A. M. W. (1969): Drug defaulting in a general practice. *Brit. med. J.*, **1**, 218.
Robb, D. F. (1970): Thoughts at random. *Practitioner*, **204**, 185.
Scottish Health Services Council (1972): Control of medicines in hospital wards and departments. Her Majesty's Stationary Office, Edinburgh.
Sigell, L. T. and Flessa, H. C. (1970): Drug interactions with anticoagulants. *J. Amer. med. Assoc.*, **214**, 2035.
Starr, K. J. and Petrie, J. C. (1972): Drug interactions in patients on long-term oral anticoagulant and antihypertensive adrenergic neurone-blocking drugs. *Brit. med. J.*, **4**, 133.
Stewart, R. B. and Cluff, L. E. (1972): A review of medication errors and compliance in ambulant patients. *Clin. Pharmacol. Therap.*, **13**, 463.
Stolley, P. D., Becker, M. H., Lasagna, L., McEvilla, J. D. and Sloane, L. M. (1972): The relationship between physician characteristics and prescribing appropriateness. *Medical Care*, **10**, 17.
Task Force on Prescription Drugs (1968): *The Drug Makers and the Drug Distributors.* U.S. Government Printing Office. Washington, D.C.
Weed, L. L. (1969): *Medical Records, Medical Education and Patient Care; the Problem-oriented Record as a Basic Tool.* Cleveland Western Reserve University Press, Cleveland.
Wilson, D. G. (1971): Domiciliary prescribing. *J. roy. Coll. Practitioners*, **21**, 558.
Wilson, G. M. (1972): Prescribing for patients leaving hospital. *Prescribers J.*, **12**, 63.

CHAPTER 13

The detection of drug interaction in a hospital environment

JAMES CROOKS AND DOROTHY C. MOIR

1 Introduction

The hospital doctor of the 1970's has a vast therapeutic armamentarium at his disposal with which to treat or at the least alter the course of disease. Patients admitted to medical wards receive on average 4 drugs during the course of a hospital admission, while one in every 5 patients receives at least ten drugs (Scottish Hospital Centre, 1967). Indeed it is not uncommon for patients to receive several drugs simultaneously. The likelihood of drugs interacting in the hospital situation is therefore considerable and the probability is increased by the fact that many new drugs are prescribed first in hospital and their potential for interacting with other drugs may not be recognized. Approximately 1000 pharmacologically active drugs in perhaps 10 times this number of formulations are now available and the potential number of pairs of drugs which might interact is therefore about 500,000. Drug interactions fall into 3 categories:

(i) unsuspected;
(ii) suspected;
(iii) established.

In the case of unsuspected interactions the problem is primarily one of detection, of suspected ones that of confirmation, and of established interactions that of incidence and clinical significance. As drug interactions are detected and investigated they will move from category (i) to (ii) and ultimately to (iii). The authors have had more experience of the last two categories and for this reason more space will be devoted to them.

2 Unsuspected drug interactions

One method whereby unsuspected drug interactions may be identified is by intensive surveillance of hospital populations and several studies have been described in the literature. While in theory it seems reasonable to assume that intensive surveillance of cohorts of patients and consequently of all the drugs administered to these patients and all events happening to them should result in the recognition of all adverse effects, this approach has in practice met with limited success. To yield useful results, intensive surveillance must be carried out in a large number of patients over a prolonged period of time and requires considerable resources including full-time medical and nursing staff. Add to this the complexities of handling the data generated by a population of sufficient size to detect what are relatively infrequent occurrences, not the least difficulty being the complications introduced by the concurrent administration of so many drugs, and the total system becomes so complex that its wide adoption as a method of detecting interactions becomes limited. However, Slone et al. (1969) with a large team of nurse monitors and considerable computer facilities reported favourably on this technique and have recently described an excess of ampicillin reactions in association with allopurinol or hyperuricaemia (Boston Collaborative Drug Surveillance Program, 1972).

An alternative method with more limited objectives is to carry out intensive surveillance of patients receiving a particular drug or combination of drugs. This approach necessitates the rapid identification of the patients immediately after the decision has been made to prescribe the drug(s) so that base-line investigations can be completed. This is not easy to achieve for large hospital populations. If, however, standardised methods of prescribing (Crooks et al., 1965) and recording the administration of drugs (Crooks et al., 1967) are in use, the operation of ward pharmacy systems (Calder, 1967) whereby ward pharmacists scan all patients' prescriptions at ward level daily and subsequently ensure adequate supplies of drugs for the ensuing 24 hr, becomes possible. Pharmacists can, therefore, readily identify patients receiving a specific drug or combination of drugs who can then be studied prospectively.

3 Suspected drug interactions

Suspicion that a drug interaction is occurring may be raised in a variety of ways including pharmacological and clinical observations, the latter being derived from individual case reports from the literature or spontaneous reporting systems. The suspected interaction can then be investigated for hospital populations by applying epidemiological techniques to retrospective data based on good drug records. The object is to increase or decrease the suspicion and to indicate the most appropriate line for detailed prospective investigation to take. A description of a number of examples of this approach follows and is based on the introduction of a standardised drug handling system (Crooks et al., 1965, Crooks et al., 1967) which as a by-product created drug records with a high degree of legibility and reliability and permitted the routine abstraction of information about the drugs prescribed for 73,000 hospital patients per annum. Subsequent data linkage with details of patient identification and other important items such as age, sex, diagnosis and length and outcome of hospital stay provides the basis of a drug information system (Coull et al., 1970) which has been computerized and which allows the identification of all patients receiving a particular drug or combination of drugs. In this way a total population at risk, i.e. the denominator can readily be identified and subsequently studied to ascertain those patients experiencing an adverse effect, i.e. the numerator. Two examples of suspected drug interactions are described in some detail below in order to illustrate the potentialities and limitations of this approach.

Antagonism of the hypotensive action of adrenergic blocking agents by the tricyclic antidepressant drugs was first reported in the experimental animal (Gokhale et al., 1966). Subsequently 7 cases were reported in the clinical situation (Mitchell et al., 1967) and the drug information system was used to investigate this suspected interaction. All patients for whom one of the adrenergic blocking agents, guanethidine, bethanidine, debrisoquine had been prescribed along with one of the tricyclic antidepressants, amitriptyline, imipramine, nortriptyline or protriptyline were identified using the data in the information system for the years 1968–1971. 23 patients were identified from a population of 930 receiving adrenergic blocking agents and 1543 receiving tricyclic antidepressants. The case records of these patients were subsequently searched for data regarding their blood pressure control. Three case records had inadequate information leaving 20 for detailed study. Poor or difficult control of hypertension defined as a mean standing diastolic level of 110 mm Hg or more was observed in 14 patients. Thus good control was achieved in only 5 out of 20 patients as compared with Leishmann's conclusion on the basis of a large series (1968) that adequate control (standing diastolic pressure less than 100 mm Hg) is likely to be achieved in 65% of patients receiving hypotensive agents. It was, therefore, of interest to note that 7 of the 15 patients who had exhibited poor control developed hypotension after withdrawal of antidepressive therapy and were subsequently well controlled on the adrenergic blocking agent.

While it was impossible to draw valid conclusions from such small numbers about the frequency with which this interaction occurs, the study was primarily concerned with methodology and an attempt was therefore made to obtain a control population 3 times the size of the test group who had received the appropriate hypotensive agent and who were also similar in respect of sex, age and diagnosis but who did not receive a tricyclic antidepressant. Fifty-seven adequately matched control patients were readily identified in the drug information system and good blood pressure control was achieved in 43 out of 57 control patients (75%) comparing favourably with Leishmann's results, whereas good control was only obtained in 5 of 20 patients receiving an adrenergic blocking agent and a tricyclic antidepressant concurrently. While the numbers are insufficient for statistical analysis the suspicion that an undesired interaction was occurring when patients were treated concurrently with an adrenergic blocking agent and a tricyclic antidepressant was strengthened and shows how good records can be used in retrospective studies to confirm or refute suspicions.

More recently Neuvonen et al. (1970) acting on a pharmacological suspicion reported significant impairment of tetracycline absorption in 5 healthy male students concurrently taking ferrous sulphate as compared with that in 5 students taking tetracycline and no ferrous sulphate. As it seemed likely that tetracycline and iron might not infrequently be prescribed simultaneously, an attempt was made to assess the importance of this reported interaction in the clinical situation. A group of 77 patients who had received tetracycline and iron simultaneously for at least 48 hr and no other drugs known to interact with tetracycline were identified in the information system and details of clinical features, including subjective improvement and changes in temperature, pulse and respiratory rates and bacteriological and radiological parameters used to investigate infective processes, were abstracted from the case records and an attempt made to assess whether or not the tetracycline had been effective. Identical information was abstracted for a control population receiving tetracycline but no iron therapy, and matched for age, sex and primary diagnosis. Adequate matching was readily achieved using data in the information system and the reasons for prescribing tetracycline in both groups were also similar. Unfortunately there was an inadequate amount of bacteriological data for statistical analysis and the clinical outcome was therefore judged on the other parameters listed above. These however were only recorded adequately before and after treatment with tetracycline in 49 of the matched pairs. The median number of days on tetracycline in the test group was 8.8 compared with 8.4 in the control group. There was, as expected, a significantly greater number of patients in the iron–tetracycline group with low haemoglobins as compared with the tetracycline control group, although it is of interest to note that some patients in the iron–tetracycline group had a normal haemoglobin at the time tetracycline was instituted while others in the tetracycline group not receiving iron therapy had abnormally low haemoglobins.

Forty-two of the 49 patients in the iron–tetracycline group improved following treatment with tetracycline as judged by the criteria listed above as compared with 33 in the control group. Similar results were obtained when the clinical outcome in both groups was analysed in respect of low and normal haemoglobins. These results, therefore, suggest that the effectiveness of tetracyclines administered in the clinical situation is not impaired by the concurrent administration of iron preparations, although further analysis will be necessary to verify this finding. The greater improvement in the iron–tetracycline group may be due to the fact that they had at least two pathological conditions initially, both of which were being treated simultaneously and it therefore does not seem unreasonable that their improvement should be greater. Using the information system it is therefore possible to investigate the effectiveness of a drug in the 'real-life' clinical situation and it seems likely that this facility may be of considerable value in the field of drug interaction in the future as many interactions may result in increased or decreased effectiveness of a particular drug.

4 Established drug interactions

The ability of barbiturates to stimulate the metabolism of coumarin anticoagulants and consequently decrease the pharmacological effect of these drugs has been well documented (Robinson and MacDonald, 1966). Nevertheless, despite a general awareness of this interaction, barbiturates continue to be prescribed simultaneously with coumarin therapy. A hospital based drug information system of the type described in the previous section can be used to determine the extent to which this unfavourable interaction occurs and 377 patients who had received phenobarbitone and Warfarin were identified by the information system for this purpose. Many other drugs are known to interact with the coumarin anticoagulants and patients who had received other barbiturates, phenothiazines, nitrazepam, diazepam, oxazepam, phenylbutazone, oxyphenbutazone, clofibrate or heparin were excluded from further study. By this criterion alone, 348 of the 377 patients identified were excluded along with 14 other patients who had been anticoagulated prophylactically or were unsuitable for some other reason. Finally, the effectiveness of anticoagulation was compared in 15 patients receiving Warfarin and phenobarbitone and 15 carefully matched controls receiving Warfarin but no phenobarbitone, prothrombin activity being used as the measure of anticoagulant control. The patients were all treated individually according to the exigencies of their condition and there was therefore little uniformity among the measurements in the records available for analysis. As expected, however, the phenobarbitone group received on average more

Warfarin than their controls. The difference in amount was not statistically significant but the number of occasions on which the patients in the phenobarbitone group were given a larger cumulative dose of Warfarin than their matched controls was significant ($p < 0.01$).

The pharmacological basis for this interaction is well documented and these results support the occurrence of this interaction in everyday clinical practice. In such situations it is desirable to assess the significance of the undesired effect and this particular example shows how retrospective study of the case notes compiled for routine clinical care can be used in this way. The results suggest that the concurrent administration of phenobarbitone and Warfarin is probably of limited importance provided clinicians are aware of the hazard and this in fact correlates well with the standard clinical practice of prescribing phenobarbitone and Warfarin sumultaneously if necessary. A therapeutically potent and less hazardous alternative would, of course, be more expedient and the effectiveness of anticoagulation in a group of patients receiving Warfarin and nitrazepam was investigated. 483 patients were identified in the system who had received Warfarin and nitrazepam and of these 462 had to be excluded for the reasons given above. Anticoagulation in 21 matched pairs was reviewed and on average the nitrazepam group were given rather less Warfarin than their respective controls and it therefore seems likely that diazepine drugs may be more appropriate than barbiturates for the concurrent administration of coumarin anticoagulants.

5 **Conclusion**

Rapid identification of populations of hospital inpatients receiving specific drugs or combinations of drugs can readily be achieved using an information system such as that described above. Subsequent problems in monitoring these populations for adverse effects however, relate to the problems of handling the information generated by a population of sufficient size to detect what are relatively infrequent occurrences. While the population at risk is easily identified subsequent identification of the patients exhibiting the suspected or previously recognized adverse effect is a function of the completeness and accuracy of the information contained in the medical record. When the adverse effect is easily measured as in the study investigating the effect of simultaneous administration of tricyclic antidepressants with adrenergic blocking agents, it is possible to determine the occurrence of the effect with a reasonable degree of accuracy, whereas failure in some instances to even record clinical features compatible with the adverse effect would provide an inaccurate estimate of the incidence of the adverse effect. It is also important to remember that active search for an adverse interaction may also distort the findings and it is therefore important to appreciate that the frequency with which an interaction occurs in association with a particular combination of drugs is only significant in the context of the frequency with which the clinical features associated with the interaction occurs in a similar population receiving only one of the drugs. The provision by the information system of control populations closely matched on parameters such as age, sex, diagnosis and length of stay in hospital greatly increases the value of the system and makes it possible to obtain meaningful results from retrospective comparison of two groups of patients only one of whom is receiving the suspected interacting drug. In view of the extent of multiple prescribing, no attempt was made to match the patients in respect of all other concurrent drug therapy and the controls were likely to be inappropriate in this respect. As the awareness of the importance of interaction between two or even more drugs increases, the development of sophisticated computer programmes to permit matching on all concurrent drug therapy may ultimately resolve this difficulty.

The limitations of retrospective studies due to the inadequacy of medical records are reduced by prospective studies which require good drug records, the use of control groups and to be economical a concentration on suspected or established drug interactions.

It is our belief that hospital based systems of studying drug interactions should be developed in a number of centres, nationally or internationally using compatible methods of data acquisition since the low frequency of many of the interactions and the widespread use of polypharmacy makes the study of large populations necessary.

References

Boston Collaborative Drug Surveillance Programme (1972): Excess of ampicillin rashes associated with allopurinol or hyperuricaemia. *New Engl. J. Med.*, **286**, 505.

Calder, G. (1967): Aspects of the integration of the pharmacist into the ward therapeutic team. *J. hosp. Pharm.*, **24**, 435.

Coull, D. C., Crooks, J., Davidson, J. F., Gallon, S. C. and Weir, R. D. (1970): A method of monitoring drugs for adverse reactions I. α-Methyldopa and haemolytic anaemia. *Europ. J. clin. Pharmacol*, **3**, 46.

Crooks, J., Clark, C. G., Caie, H. B. and Mawson, W. B. (1965): Prescribing and administration of drugs in hospital. *Lancet*, **1**, 373.

Crooks, J., Weir, R. D., Coull, D. C., McNab, J. W., Calder, G., Barnett, J. W. and Caie, H. B. (1967): Evaluation of a method of prescribing drugs in hospital and a new method of recording their administration. *Lancet*, **1**, 668.

Gokhale, S. D., Gulati, O. D. and Udwadia, B. P. (1966): Antagonism of the adrenergic neurone blocking action of guanethidine by certain antidepressant and antihistamine drugs. *Arch. int. Pharmacodynamie Therap.*, **160**, 321.

Leishman, A. W. D. (1968): The treatment of hypertension. *Hosp. Med*, **2**, 1258.

Mitchell, J. R., Arias, L. and Oates, J. A. (1967): Antagonism of the antihypertensive action of guanethidine sulfate by desipramine hydrochloride. *J. Amer. med. Assoc.*, **202**, 973.

Neuvonen, P. J., Gothoni, G., Hackman, R. and Bjorksten, K.af. (1970): Interference of iron with the absorption of tetracyclines in man. *Brit. med. J.*, **4**, 532.

Robinson, D. S. and MacDonald, M. G. (1966): The effect of phenobarbital administration on the control of coagulation achieved during warfarin therapy in man. *J. Pharmacol. exp. Therap.*, **153**, 250.

Scottish Hospital Centre (1967): Collected Conference Reports 1966. Prescribing and Administration of drugs in hospital. p. 45.

Slone, D., Gaetano, L. F., Lipworth, L., Shapiro, S., Lewis, G. P. and Jick, H. (1969): Computer analysis of epidemiologic data on effects of drugs on hospital patients. *Publ. Health Reports*, **84**, 39.

Slone, D., Gaetano, L. F., Lipworth, L., Shapiro, S., Lewis, G. P. and Jick, H. (1972): Excess of ampicillin rashes associated with allopurinol or hyperuricemia. A report from the Boston Collaborative Drug Surveillance Program. Boston University Medical Center. *New Engl. J. Med.*, **286**, 505.

CHAPTER 14

Informing the medical profession about clinically important drug interactions

ANDREW HERXHEIMER

When a drug interaction first becomes known to be clinically important, doctors must be *told*. Subsequently the information needs to be *available*, at least as a reminder, in any situation where one of the interacting drugs is liable to be prescribed. These two forms of communication differ, and are better discussed separately.

The discovery of a new drug interaction in the laboratory or in practice is usually published first in a medical journal. What happens next depends on the reactions which the publication arouses among its readers. These will probably include clinicians practising in a variety of fields, medical advisers to pharmaceutical companies, and civil servants concerned with drug safety. The three groups may differ in what interactions they consider to be clinically important, for their interests differ: the clinician is concerned about his individual patients, the pharmaceutical company wishes to have its products properly and safely used on a large scale, the civil servant must use appropriate administrative methods to protect the public at large. All will be concerned to avoid direct danger to life or health, but clinicians will be bothered more than the others by interactions that interfere with the therapeutic effect of a drug, or with the performance or interpretation of laboratory tests. The methods by which doctors will be given information about a particular interaction depend largely on how serious and how frequent the interaction appears to be to the different groups of readers.

Since the seriousness and frequency of an interaction cannot be assessed at all reliably until it has been reported several times from different centres, there is nearly always a latent period of some months or longer before a sufficiently valid general warning can be issued by a pharmaceutical company or a government agency. Even when several reports of an interaction are available many of its dimensions may remain unclear. For an interaction to be properly understood one must know the doses, timing and routes of administration of the drugs which cause it, and those which do not cause it; one also needs to know what distinguishes a susceptible individual from one who is not at risk.

Doctors receive information about drugs from three different types of sources:

(a) independent professional sources;

(b) pharmaceutical manufacturers;

(c) government agencies.

Each type of source communicates with doctors in a characteristic style.

The independent professional sources essentially represent the medical profession helping itself. They include individuals, for example every doctor's personal colleagues, and individual authors of articles in journals; and a variety of organisations, such as medical societies and associations, and publishers, which publish journals, newsletters or books. Some of these publications reach a high proportion of prescribers; in Britain the *British Medical Journal* and *Prescribers' Journal* are examples. Others, especially the large reference books on drugs, are available to only a small proportion of prescribers; they are probably more widely used among pharmacists, particularly in hospitals. Even so, many users of such books do not have access to up-to-date editions.

Manufacturers of drugs communicate with doctors by means of advertisements, brochures, package inserts, and representatives who visit doctors. Information about interactions can be transmitted by any of these methods, but it has to compete for the space or time available with other information about the drug, some of which is more important to the manufacturer. And of course the fewer 'messages' are put into a communication, the better the chance that they are received and understood.

Government agencies, especially in Britain and in the United States, have been anxious to avoid trespassing into areas of clinical responsibility, since many doctors are apt to be touchy about their 'professional freedom'. In Britain communications from governmental sources have therefore been issued only when some very serious problem has arisen that could not be adequately dealt with by the manufacturers concerned. One advantage of this approach is that infrequent communications are taken more seriously than frequent ones (Belloc, 1940). However, now that drug regulatory activities in Britain are statutory rather than voluntary, this advantage is less important.

All these publications, from whatever source, can devote only a small part of their space to drug interactions. There is therefore a place for specialised collections of information on such interactions, and several are now available (Hartshorn, 1970; Garb, 1971; Martin, 1971; Hansten, 1971; Swidler, 1971).

Most of them take the form of an index listing the interactions under each of the drugs concerned, briefly describing the interaction and citing references to the original reports. Such an arrangement can function both as an immediate alerting system and as a bibliography. However, it has the major disadvantage that the prescriber rarely has much incentive to consult a special book when he is about to write a prescription: this would require a separate, time-consuming act, which will be performed only when the prescriber feels some doubt. The problem can be partly overcome by making the information more accessible, as for example in Neil and Barnett's (1969) plastic disc interaction chart. This consists of 3 discs fixed together at their centres: the disc in the middle can be rotated to indicate the interactions of a drug or group of drugs through 'windows' in the other discs (Fig. 1).

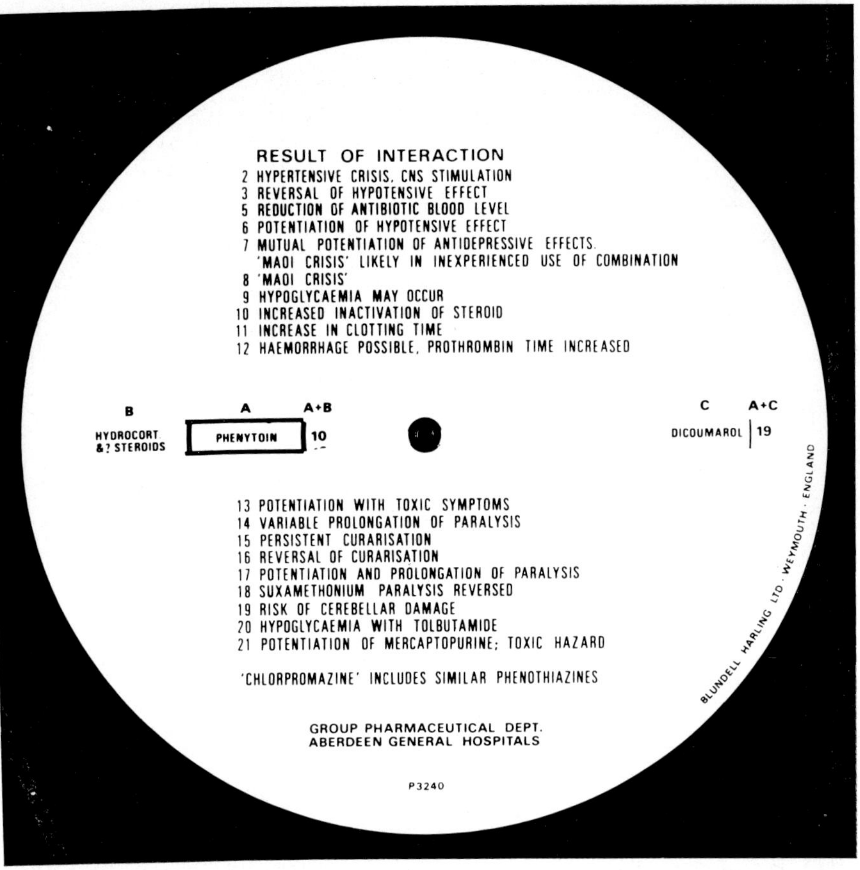
RESULT OF INTERACTION
2 HYPERTENSIVE CRISIS, CNS STIMULATION
3 REVERSAL OF HYPOTENSIVE EFFECT
5 REDUCTION OF ANTIBIOTIC BLOOD LEVEL
6 POTENTIATION OF HYPOTENSIVE EFFECT
7 MUTUAL POTENTIATION OF ANTIDEPRESSIVE EFFECTS. 'MAOI CRISIS' LIKELY IN INEXPERIENCED USE OF COMBINATION
8 'MAOI CRISIS'
9 HYPOGLYCAEMIA MAY OCCUR
10 INCREASED INACTIVATION OF STEROID
11 INCREASE IN CLOTTING TIME
12 HAEMORRHAGE POSSIBLE, PROTHROMBIN TIME INCREASED
B
HYDROCORT. &? STEROIDS
A
PHENYTOIN
A+B
10
C
DICOUMAROL
A+C
19
13 POTENTIATION WITH TOXIC SYMPTOMS
14 VARIABLE PROLONGATION OF PARALYSIS
15 PERSISTENT CURARISATION
16 REVERSAL OF CURARISATION
17 POTENTIATION AND PROLONGATION OF PARALYSIS
18 SUXAMETHONIUM PARALYSIS REVERSED
19 RISK OF CEREBELLAR DAMAGE
20 HYPOGLYCAEMIA WITH TOLBUTAMIDE
21 POTENTIATION OF MERCAPTOPURINE; TOXIC HAZARD
'CHLORPROMAZINE' INCLUDES SIMILAR PHENOTHIAZINES
GROUP PHARMACEUTICAL DEPT.
ABERDEEN GENERAL HOSPITALS
P3240
BLUNDELL HARLING LTD · WEYMOUTH · ENGLAND

Fig. 1. One side of Neil and Barnett's plastic disc interaction chart. The other side has 4 'windows' so that 4 different interactions can be shown for 1 group of drugs.

Causes of INCREASED sensitivity to oral anticoagulants

A	Vitamin K deficiency	Premature infants Starvation Malabsorption
B	Hepatic dysfunction	Decreased synthesis of clotting factors Reduced absorption of vitamin K in obstructive jaundice
C	Increased metabolic rate	Increased catabolism of Vit-K-dependent clotting factors
D	Drugs	
	1 salicylates	Several mechanisms
	2 phenylbutazone, oxyphenbutazone, mefenamic acid, nalidixic acid, ethacrynic acid, clofibrate (probably), chloral (probably)	Displacement of anticoagulant from its binding to plasma protein
	3 anabolic steroids	? hepatic dysfunction ; or as for 4
	4 phenyramidol, methylphenidate, disulfiram	Inhibition of, or competition for hepatic microsomal enzymes
	5 glucagon, quinine	? synergistic depression of clotting factors
E	Stopping a drug listed in Table II D	Reduced activity of hepatic microsomal enzymes

Causes of DECREASED sensitivity to oral anticoagulants

A	Genetic	1 Hereditary rapid metabolism of anticoagulants 2 Hereditary anomaly of the vitamin K-warfarin receptor site
B	Vitamin K	Competition for receptor site
C	Pregnancy	Elevation of clotting factors I, VII, VIII, IX, and X
	Oral contraceptives	Elevation of clotting factor X
D	Drugs barbiturates, meprobamate, glutethimide, phenazone as in dichloralphenazone, haloperidol, griseofulvin and many others	Induction of hepatic microsomal enzymes
E	Stopping a drug listed in Table I D	

These tables will fit into the British National Formulary

Reprinted from the March 31, 1972 issue of Drug & Therapeutics Bulletin published by Consumers' Association 14 Buckingham St London WC2N 6DS

A 'drug disc' of different design has recently been described by Whiting et al. (1973). It accommodates 116 different interactions, considerably more than Neil and Barnett's disc, and they are arranged more logically. The usefulness of these devices in practice will need to be assessed critically. Their greatest value may turn out to be in the education of the newly qualified doctor in hospital, but any prescriber could easily keep such a disc on his desk or even in his pocket.

However, ideally the information on interactions should appear in a compact, easily understood form together with the other prescribing information concerning the particular drug or group of drugs. The most comprehensive method of doing this is to use a computer memory store from which the prescriber can call up the required information about the drug he wishes to prescribe. In principle it is easy to compile such an information store and to keep it up to date, but in practice it will take a lot of effort, and most doctors will not have easy access to a computer in their consulting room for a long time. Such systems are now beginning to be tried out in a few hospitals.

Meanwhile there are other more practicable ways of presenting drug interaction information. One approach is illustrated in Tables I and II, taken from a brief review of the use of oral anticoagulants in *Drug and Therapeutics Bulletin* (1972). These tables refer not only to interactions between the anticoagulants and other drugs, but also to non-drug factors which can influence a patient's sensitivity to the anticoagulant. They thus give an overview of all the aspects that the prescriber should consider when he begins treatment with an anticoagulant, and subsequently when he reviews the maintenance treatment of the case. To be readily used, the tables need to be in reach wherever oral anticoagulants are prescribed, for example in medical outpatient clinics and in clinical laboratories responsible for measuring prothrombin times. They have therefore been reprinted separately (Drug and Therapeutics Bulletin, 1973) in a form suitable for use as a small wall-chart, or as a leaflet which will fit into the British National Formulary.

Although such a method of presentation could be applied to most classes of drugs, some special purposes demand a different approach. The pharmaceutical incompatibilities between certain drugs and certain infusion fluids are an example. Details of the most important of these incompatibilities must be accessible wherever a drug may be added to an infusion, i.e. in almost every ward of a general hospital. This need is met by a chart which can be displayed on the wall near the ward drug trolley, and which a doctor can also carry folded in his pocket; it is illustrated in Fig. 2. Many typographical problems had to be solved in the design of this chart. This could only be achieved with expert typographical help: without it the chart would have been difficult to use and so of less practical value (Boorman et al., 1971).

Intravenous Drugs and Infusion Fluids – some pharmaceutical incompatibilities

Explanation

1 **Inactive or toxic** products may be formed when drugs are added to intravenous infusion fluids.

2 The result of a reaction may be a colour change, formation of a cloudy solution or a precipitate, **but some reactions occur which cannot be detected visually.**

3 This guide is not comprehensive and only illustrates those incompatible combinations which have been well documented.

4 The presence of any combination of drugs in the guide is not a therapeutic recommendation of such a combination.

If you have any doubt about adding a drug to an infusion fluid, please consult the pharmacy.

May 1973

A **"drug added"** label must be completed and fixed to the bottle when a drug is added to an infusion fluid; an example of a suitable label is shown below:

Drug Added	quantity added	time	date
Return this bottle to pharmacy if unused 12 hours after addition of drugs			

Notes: checking infusion fluids

1 **All** infusion fluids should be checked for presence of particles before they are used.

2 **Sodium Bicarbonate infusions,** especially 8·4%, are particularly liable to become contaminated with particles during storage.

3 **Mannitol** infusions: crystals may be present or may form suddenly during use.

drugs incompatible with infusion fluids

Infusion fluid	**Incompatible additive**
"Aminosol" preparations	Inadvisable to add drugs.
Dextrose & laevulose (Fructose) solutions	Ampicillin, erythromycin lactobionate, novobiocin, penicillin G.
***Dextrans**	Aminocaproic acid.
"Intralipid"	Inadvisable to add drugs.
Mannitol	Inadvisable to add drugs.
Ringer-Lactate	Ampicillin, cephalothin, sodium bicarbonate, Tetracyclines.
Sodium bicarbonate	Calcium salts, cephalothin, compound vitamins, promethazine, Tetracyclines.
Whole Blood	Nothing should be added except with the express authority of the physician/surgeon in charge of the case.

incompatibilities

Occurring in the most commonly used infusion fluids i.e. 4·3% dextrose and 0·18% sodium chloride, 5% dextrose, 0·9% sodium chloride solutions.

Drug	**Incompatible with**
Aminophylline	Cephalothin, compound vitamins, promethazine, tetracyclines.
Amphotericin B	No other drug should be added (the Pharmacy has a special infusion fluid of dextrose 5% for this drug).
Ampicillin	Gentamicin, hydrocortisone sodium succinate, kanamycin, streptomycin, tetracyclines.
Carbenicillin	Erythromycin, gentamicin, kanamycin, streptomycin, tetracyclines.
Cephalothin	Aminophylline, Amylobarbitone sodium, colistin, kanamycin, tetracyclines.
Chloramphenicol sodium succinate	Compound vitamins, gentamicin, hydrocortisone sodium succinate, tetracyclines.
Cloxacillin	Gentamicin, kanamycin, streptomycin, tetracyclines.
Frusemide	Should not be administered in an infusion fluid—except the 250mg injection which is recommended for administration in compound sodium chloride injection and sodium chloride 0·9% injection.
Heparin	Erythromycin lactobionate, promethazine.
Hydrocortisone sodium succinate	Cephalothin, chloramphenicol sodium succinate, colistin, compound vitamins, methicillin, promethazine, tetracyclines.
Penicillin G	Compound vitamins, promethazine, tetracyclines.
Promethazine	Aminophylline, heparin, hydrocortisone sodium succinate, penicillin G.
Sulphadiazine sodium	Compound vitamins, tetracyclines.
Tetracyclines	Aminophylline, cephalothin, chloramphenicol sodium succinate, compound vitamins, erythromycin lactobionate, hydrocortisone sodium succinate, methicillin, penicillin G, sulphadiazine.
Compound vitamins	On theoretical grounds this preparation is likely to interact with many other drugs and therefore should not be added to an infusion fluid

* This interaction has so far been reported only between "Macrodex" and "Rheomacrodex" brands of dextran and "Epsikapron" brand of aminocaproic acid.

This chart was originally prepared for The London Hospital by G.A. Boorman, A. Campbell, C.W. Barrett, and A. Herxheimer. Details of the chart were published in the Pharmaceutical Journal issue of August 14 1971. This version has been revised by the authors for wider distribution. Further revisions are planned for the future.

Chart printed and distributed by Eli Lilly and Company Ltd, Basingstoke, Hants

Fig. 2. Drugs and intravenous infusion fluids: a chart for doctors and nurses. The chart measures 30 by 36 cm and is printed in black with green as a second colour. It is designed to be folded to 1/6 the full size, so that it fits into the British National Formulary.

We must now ask whose responsibility it is to provide the information about particular drug interactions. It seems reasonable to suggest that this responsibility rests with whoever provides the other prescribing information about the drug concerned: usually it will be an official body or a pharmaceutical manufacturer. Since an interaction usually concerns two drugs or groups of drugs, the manufacturer of each should provide the information about the interaction. This can most suitably be given on the so-called data sheet, the standard information card which manufacturers must provide for all medicines promoted to practitioners in Great Britain. In the United States the corresponding information summary is the 'drug label' (see Hollister, 1973). In fact a licensing authority should not allow manufacturers to omit it from the prescribing information for their drug, even though the other drug may be the more dangerous, or may be the newer drug. The actual wording of the section on interactions will need to be agreed or specified by the licensing authority.

So far we have considered how doctors can be given information on interactions before they write a prescription, but we must also consider what may happen when the prescription is presented to the pharmacist or when a patient wants to buy a drug which does not require a prescription. Some pharmacists believe that it would be best if they checked each prescription and each non-prescription item against the patient's drug history for pharmacological and therapeutic incompatibilities. They may be right, and such checks could certainly help to prevent some awkward interactions. But difficulties are bound to arise where the prescriber and the pharmacist communicate only through the prescription. The prescriber would often resent what he would regard as interference by the pharmacist, and any system of checking prescriptions for possible incompatibilities would need to be set up after close consultation between the prescribers and the pharmacists concerned. This may become practicable in hospitals and even in health centres, and might there be undertaken by pharmacy committees. However, for the foreseeable future the responsibility for preventing harmful interactions will remain the doctor's.

References

Belloc, H. (1940): *Cautionary Verses for Children*, Collected ed., p. 19. Duckworth, London.

Boorman, G. A., Campbell, A., Barrett, C. W. and Herxheimer, A. (1971): Drugs and intravenous infusion fluids: designing a chart for doctors and nurses. *Pharm. J.* **207**, 150.

Drug and Therapeutics Bulletin (1972): The choice of an oral anticoagulant. *Drug Therap. Bull.*, **10**, 25.

Drug and Therapeutics Bulletin (1973): Altered sensitivity to oral anticoagulants: two tables, **11**, 12.

Garb, S. (1971): *Clinical Guide to Undesirable Drug Interactions and Interferences*. Springer, New York; Harvey Miller Medcalf, London.
Hansten, P. D. (1971): *Drug Interactions: Clinical Significance of Drug–Drug Interactions and Drug Effects on Clinical Laboratory Tests*. Lea and Fabiger, Philadelphia.
Hartshorn, E. A. (1970): *Handbook of Drug Interactions*, Part I. Donald E. Francke, Cincinnati.
Hollister, L. E. (1973): New ideas about drug labels. *Clin. Pharmacol. Therap.*, **14**, 309.
Martin, E. W. (1971): *Hazards of Medication*. J. B. Lippincott, Philadelphia.
McIver, A. K. (1967): *A Guide to Drug Interactions (Chart)*. Pharmaceutical Press, London.
McIver, A. K. (1970): Table of drug interactions. In: *Pharmaceutical Handbook*, 18th ed., p. 42. Pharmaceutical Press, London.
Neil, J. M. and Barnett, J. W. (1969): Major drug interactions: a system for easy reference. *J. hosp. Pharm.*, **27**, 197.
Swidler, G. (1971): *Handbook of Drug Interactions*. Wiley – Interscience, New York.
Whiting, B., Goldberg, A. and Waldie, P. (1973): The drug disc. *Lancet*, **1**, 1037.

Subject index

* *see also* Sulphonamides